Practical Veterinary
Dental Radiography

Practical Veterinary Dental Radiography

BROOK A. NIEMIEC DVM, DipAVDC, DipEVDC, FAVD

Veterinary Dental Specialties & Oral Surgery
San Diego, California, USA

JERZY GAWOR DVM, PhD, DipAVDC, DipEVDC, FAVD

European Veterinary Specialist in Dentistry
Klinika Weterynaryjna Arka
Kraków, Poland

VLADIMÍR JEKL MVDr, PhD, DipECZM (Small Mammal Medicine and Surgery)

European Recognized Veterinary Specialist in Zoological Medicine (Small Mammal)
Avian and Exotic Animal Clinic, Faculty of Veterinary Medicine
University of Veterinary and Pharmaceutical Sciences Brno
and Exotic Companion Mammal Care Jekl & Hauptman
Brno, Czech Republic

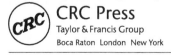

CRC Press
Taylor & Francis Group
Boca Raton   London   New York

CRC Press is an imprint of the
Taylor & Francis Group, an **informa** business

Top image on front cover kindly provided by iM3®

CRC Press
Taylor & Francis Group
6000 Broken Sound Parkway NW, Suite 300
Boca Raton, FL 33487-2742

© 2018 by Taylor & Francis Group, LLC
CRC Press is an imprint of Taylor & Francis Group, an Informa business

No claim to original U.S. Government works

Printed on acid-free paper

International Standard Book Number-13: 978-1-4822-2543-3 (Hardback)

Library of Congress Cataloging-in-Publication Data

Names: Niemiec, Brook A., author. | Gawor, Jerzy, author. | Jekl, Vladimir, author.
Title: Practical veterinary dental radiography / Brook A. Niemiec, Jerzy Gawor, and Vladimir Jekl.
Description: Boca Raton : CRC Press, [2017]
Identifiers: LCCN 2017001564| ISBN 9781482225433 (hardback : alk. paper) |
ISBN 9781315177335 (master ebook)
Subjects: LCSH: Veterinary dentistry. | Veterinary radiology. | MESH: Dentistry--veterinary |
Radiography, Dental--veterinary | Veterinary Medicine.
Classification: LCC SF867 .N538 2017 | NLM SF 867 | DDC 636.089/76--dc23
LC record available at https://lccn.loc.gov/2017001564

Visit the Taylor & Francis Web site at
http://www.taylorandfrancis.com

and the CRC Press Web site at
http://www.crcpress.com

CONTENTS

CHAPTER 9   **NASAL CAVITY PATHOLOGIES RELATED TO ORAL PROBLEMS**   **221**
Jerzy Gawor

CHAPTER 10   **RADIOGRAPHY OF THE TEMPOROMANDIBULAR JOINT AND MANDIBULAR SYMPHYSIS**   **249**
Jerzy Gawor

PREFACE

'Bene dignoscitur, bene curatur'
(Well recognized, well treated)
(Hippocrates)

Dental radiography is quickly becoming the standard of care in veterinary dentistry. This is due not only to the fact that it is crucial for proper patient care, but also because of a significant increase in client expectations. Finally, providing dental radiographs as a routine service can create significant income for a veterinary practice.

However, veterinarians and technicians (nurses) receive little to no training in veterinary dental radiology. Therefore, there is a steep learning curve involved in mastering these techniques. This text aims to bridge that knowledge gap in an easily understandable fashion. Supported by numerous images, this book will lead veterinary professionals through the various aspects of veterinary dental radiography.

The book begins with an introduction on the importance of dental radiography and increasing client acceptance of this technology. Following the introductory section we cover the various equipment options available to help practitioners choose the right equipment and then employ it properly. Next are chapters on correct exposure and development techniques for both dental and skull films. The majority of the book then covers interpretation in a stepwise and complete fashion, but one which is easily navigated. The text also covers small mammal radiography techniques and interpretation as well as future directions in imaging.

Brook Niemiec
Jerzy Gawor
Vladimír Jekl

AVDC	American Veterinary Dental College	FFD	focus film distance
CA	central ameloblastoma	MRI	magnetic resonance imaging
CBCT	cone-beam computed tomography	OT	odontogenic tumor
CCD	charge-coupled device	PD	periodontal disease
CEJ	cementoenamel junction	PDL	periodontal ligament
CMO	craniomandibular osteopathy	PID	positioning indication device
CMOS	complementary metal oxide semiconductor	PIRR	peripheral inflammatory root resorption
		PO	periostitis ossificans
CR	computed radiography	PSP	photostimulable phosphor
CT	computed tomography	PTH	parathyroid hormone
DR	digital radiography	RC	rostrocaudal
DV	dorsoventral	TMJ	temporomandibular joint
ECG	electrocardiography/electrocardiogram	TR	tooth resorption
EIRR	external inflammatory root resorption	VD	ventrodorsal

CHAPTER 1

MARKETING DENTAL RADIOGRAPHY

Brook A. Niemiec

As with any new service, incorporating dental radiography into your daily practice can be a challenge. It may be difficult to make changes, especially if it requires new techniques and training and/or may not have obvious immediate results. Therefore, many new dental radiography machines languish in the corner, significantly underused. An integral part of the process in putting this equipment and technology to good use is marketing to clients and getting these radiography services approved. Effective marketing of dental radiography truly requires a team effort, including receptionists, technicians, and veterinarians.

The critical first step in implementing dental radiography is to educate *the entire staff* on the importance of radiographs. This should start with the veterinarians and then be directed to the rest of the staff. Many national and international meetings cover this subject to a certain extent. However, this is typically best learned in a small group or one on one session. Consequently, this is covered in detail at regular educational meetings held at the San Diego Veterinary Dental Training Center.[1] For additional options to gain an understanding of the critical nature of dental radiographs, consider spending a day with a Diplomate of the American Veterinary Dental College (DipAVDC) (www.vetdentists.com). Most veterinary dentists are willing to allow visitors to come and observe at scheduled times/days.

Once all the veterinarians in the practice are in support of this service, it is essential to train the technical staff to obtain diagnostic dental radiographs. Once the staff feel comfortable with these new skills, the number of retakes and time under anesthesia will be greatly reduced. Consequently, the technician staff will be supportive as opposed to resistant to performing this vital service. Training is best achieved with hands-on instruction at either a training center or a national meeting such as the American Veterinary Dental Forum or European Congress of Veterinary Dentistry. Alternatively, a commercially available educational video is an excellent learning tool.[2] Finally, there are chairside options such as the laminated poster (**Figure 1.1**), which details the 'simplified technique' as presented in Chapter 4.[3]

In addition to properly training the technician staff to obtain dental radiographs, the entire staff (including receptionists) need to be educated on the *importance* of dental radiographs. The training should be completed by educating the reception

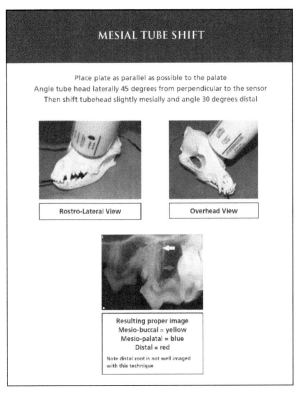

Fig. 1.1 **Sample page of the chairside laminated guide demonstrating the simplified technique of dental radiology. Available at www.vetdentalrad.com.**

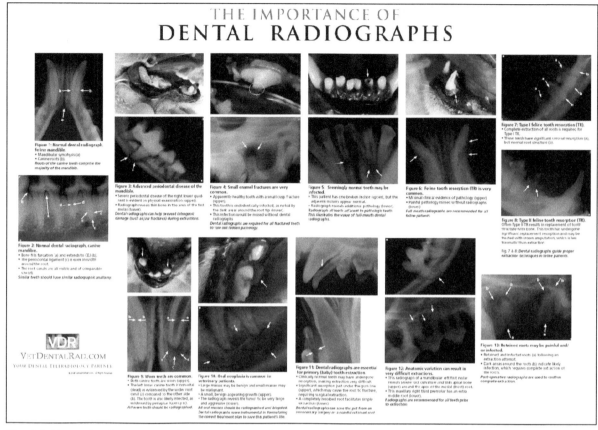

Fig. 1.2 **Example of an examination room client education poster. Available through www.vetdentalrad.com.**

staff and technicians as to the importance of dental radiographs. (See Chapter 2 for good examples of the importance of dental radiographs.) If having the staff attend a meeting or watch a video is unrealistic, consider giving a presentation yourself.

Once the entire staff understands the value of dental radiographs, it is time to start educating your clients. Clients already understand the importance of dental radiographs for themselves, as they are routinely performed by their dentist. Draw on this common experience to educate clients about utilizing dental radiography for the proper dental care of their pets. Education is by far the best way to improve client compliance of new products and procedures. Utilize the examples provided in Chapter 2 to inform and educate reluctant clients. Additionally, consider creating a personal 'smile book', which highlights cases where radiography was instrumental in the proper diagnosis and therapy of oral disease. Alternatively, an examination

room poster (**Figure 1.2**) with classic examples, which graphically demonstrates the value of dental radiography, is available to practitioners.[4]

Another way to effectively utilize dental radiographs is to simply make them mandatory with dental procedures. Clients will often try to omit 'elective' options from the estimate. Dental radiography is performed in human dentistry for almost any procedure, and humans can often direct the dentist to the problem tooth based on pain or discomfort. It can be helpful to explain to clients that because pets cannot tell us what hurts, radiographs are even *more* important for them. The information obtained from dental radiographs is crucial for the proper performance of veterinary dentistry. In fact, obtaining full-mouth radiographs on all dental patients is good practice and will greatly increase the amount of dental pathology diagnosed and improve the treatment of patients in your practice. Several studies have proven the value of full-mouth radiographs in identifying pathologic conditions in veterinary patients, which may be either painful and/or a source of infection.[5,6]

Finally, submitting radiographs for review by a board certified dentist can help to improve client acceptance of radiographs and the procedures that are being recommended based on these images. Veterinary dental telemedicine sites such as www.vetdentalrad.com are now available to help veterinarians confirm dental diagnoses and treatment planning. Including the minor cost of specialist review into the dental radiograph service is beneficial to both patients and the practice.

REFERENCES

1 San Diego Veterinary Dental Training Center: www.vdtdentaltraining.com.
2 Dental radiology simplified DVD: dogbeachvet.com
3 Dental radiology simplified chairside poster: www.dogbeachvet.com
4 Importance of dental radiographs – client educational poster: www.dogbeachvet.com
5 Verstracte FJ, Kass PH, Terpak CH (1998) Diagnostic value of full-mouth radiography in dogs. *Am J Vet Res* **59(6):**686–691.
6 Verstraete FJ, Kass PH, Terpak CH (1998) Diagnostic value of full-mouth radiography in cats. *Am J Vet Res* **59(6):**692–695.

CHAPTER 2

THE IMPORTANCE OF AND INDICATIONS FOR DENTAL RADIOGRAPHY

Brook A. Niemiec

INTRODUCTION

This chapter will cover various pathologies for which dental radiographs are indicated, demonstrating that they are often critical for proper diagnosis and treatment of oral and dental disease. The conditions that will be discussed are not unusual; they exist in many of our patients and are seen in veterinary practice on a daily basis. When they are not radiographed, often painful and/or infectious pathology is left behind.

Utilizing the knowledge gained from dental radiographs not only improves patient care, it increases acceptance of treatment recommendations. This leads to increased numbers of dental procedures performed, which is good for the patient and the practice. Finally, the information gained from radiographs facilitates the safety and efficiency of dental procedures as well as decreasing both procedure time and complications.

PERIODONTAL DISEASE

(For more information see Chapter 8, Part C.)

Periodontal disease is by far the most common problem in small animal veterinary medicine.[1,2] By the age of two, 70% of cats and 80% of dogs have some form of periodontal disease.[1,3] Small and toy breed dogs are particularly susceptible.[4] While a color change of the marginal gingiva is a reliable sign of disease, it is now known that gingival bleeding on probing is the first sign of gingivitis.[5–7] Therefore, as high as the reported incidence is, the study actually *underestimates* the level of disease.

It is widely and erroneously believed among clients and general practitioners that the amount of calculus is an accurate indicator of the level of periodontal disease. However, we now know that calculus in and of itself is relatively non-pathogenic, providing mostly an irritant effect.[3,8] Furthermore, one human study found that clinical results were not related to the amount of residual calculus following a cleaning.[9] The fact that supragingival calculus is only minimally pathogenic is a very important point, as the need for professional therapy is typically determined by clients and general practitioners by the calculus index, which may or may not be indicative of the level of disease present.[10]

Currently, the level of gingival inflammation is generally considered the best *outward* indicator of periodontal disease. However, this is not the first sign of gingivitis (as mentioned above, it is bleeding on probing, but this is not typically done on conscious oral examinations). Furthermore, it is difficult to judge the level of gingival inflammation in patients with dark pigmented gums. Therefore, further diagnostic measures (typically under general anesthesia) are required for proper diagnosis and therapy.

Periodontal probing

Periodontal probing is a critical first step in the evaluation of periodontal disease.[11,12] However, there are several reasons why dental radiographs are also required for a comprehensive evaluation of periodontal disease:[13]

1. Periodontal pockets can easily be missed due to narrow pocket width, a tight interproximal space (**Figure 2.1a**), or ledge of calculus (**Figure 2.1b**).[14] Tight interproximal spaces are typical between the molar teeth, especially in small and toy breed dogs.[15] Dental radiographs should elucidate these pathologic pockets (**Figure 2.2**).

2. Dental radiographs serve as a visual (objective) baseline to evaluate the effectiveness of

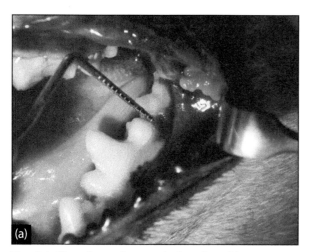
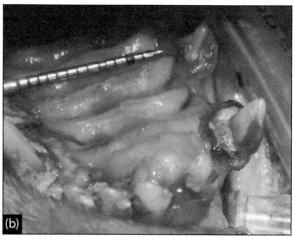

Fig. 2.1 Situations where periodontal probing may not reveal the true level of attachment loss. (a) Tight contact areas between the molars hinder the passage of the periodontal probe. In this case it is between the left mandibular first and second molars (309 and 310). Note the lack of calculus and gingival inflammation in the area. (b) Ledges of calculus, in this case on the lingual aspect of the right maxillary canine (104). Note that the periodontal probe is demonstrating a class II furcation on the second premolar (106).

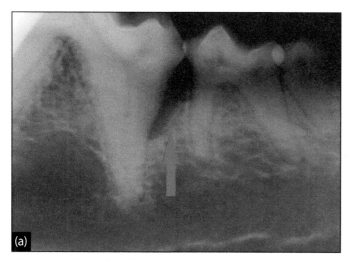
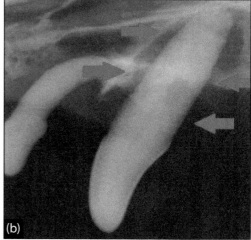

Fig. 2.2 (a) Dental radiograph of the patient in Fig. 2.1a demonstrating significant alveolar bone loss on the distal aspect of the first molar (arrow). (b) Dental radiograph of the patient in Fig. 2.1b demonstrating significant alveolar bone loss on the canine (arrows).

professional therapy and homecare.[14] This aids the practitioner to determine which teeth should be treated more aggressively or extracted, based on the trend in the level of the alveolar bone.

3 Radiographs are absolutely critical in cases of periodontal disease involving the mandible of small and toy breed dogs, as well as the mandibular canine area of cats.

In these patients, periodontal disease can cause marked weakening of the mandible[16] and significantly increase the possibility of iatrogenic fracture during extraction procedures (**Figure 2.3**).[17,18] This commonly occurs in small dogs, because the teeth roots (especially the mandibular first molar) comprise a larger percentage of the mandible

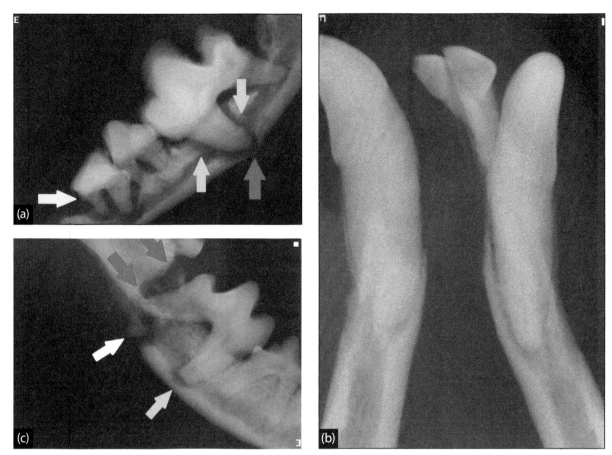

Fig. 2.3 **Dental radiographs can aid in avoiding iatrogenic pathologic mandibular fractures. (a)** In small and toy breed dogs, the mesial root of the first molar takes up virtually the entire vertical aspect of the mandible in that area (red arrow). Alveolar bone loss (blue arrows) creates a significantly weakened area in the mandible, which may result in a fracture during the extraction attempt. Note that the weak jaw could break with minor trauma regardless, and extraction is the only reliable method to allow healing. Therefore, careful extraction is required. Also note that the third premolar has lost all its periodontal attachment and is being held in the dental arch by a 'calculus bridge' to the fourth premolar. (yellow arrow). **(b)** Very wide mandibular symphyseal area and periodontal loss on the mandibular canines and incisors. This area is of significant risk of fracture when the canines are extracted. **(c)** Pathologic mandibular fracture in a small breed dog at the distal root of the right mandibular first molar (white arrow). There was significant alveolar bone loss (red arrows), which predisposed the area to fracture during the extraction attempt. Note that the practitioner did not section the tooth prior to attempting extraction. This tooth has a class II perio-endo lesion as noted by the periapical rarefaction on the mesial root (blue arrow).

compared with large breeds (**Figure 2.4**).[19] A preoperative dental radiograph can help the practitioner avoid this disastrous complication. Alternatively, if a mandibular fracture does occur during extraction, the radiograph will provide conclusive evidence as to the pre-existing periodontal disease, and will illustrate the risk of the extraction procedure.

4 While full-mouth radiographs are always recommended, in cases where several areas of the mouth are afflicted with periodontal disease, full-mouth radiographs are definitely indicated.[20,21] This will help avoid missing any pathology, which is often painful and/or infected.

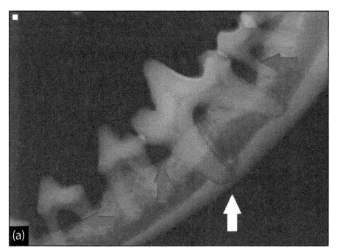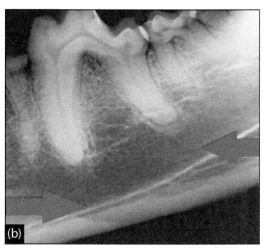

Fig. 2.4 Difference in root length between small and large breed dogs. (a) Dental radiograph of the mandible of a 4.5 kg (10 lb) dog with mild to moderate alveolar bone loss (red arrows). The mesial root of the first molar ends approximately 1 mm from the ventral cortex (white arrow). Alveolar bone loss will significantly increase the chance of a fracture in the area. (b) Dental radiograph of the mandible of a 36 kg (80 lb) dog. The mesial root of the first molar ends approximately 15 mm from the ventral cortex (arrows). Even complete loss of the bone surrounding the mesial root would generally not result in enough weakening to create a fracture.

FELINE TOOTH RESORPTION

(For more information see Chapter 8, Part E.)

Dental radiographs are absolutely critical for proper dental care in feline patients.[14,22,23] This is because resorptive lesions require intraoral dental x-rays for a definitive diagnosis and therapy.[13,24] Furthermore, these lesions are very common (up to 66% of cats presented for dental procedures in some reports).[25] Since these lesions initiate at or below the gingival margin, clinical evidence typically does not occur until fairly late in the disease course (**Figure 2.5**).[26] Therefore, severe root resorption and painful cervical crown resorption may exist undetected for significant periods of time.[14] For this reason, most veterinary dentists recommend full-mouth dental radiographs in all feline patients.[21]

Once a tooth resorption (TR) lesion is diagnosed, radiographs are critical to making appropriate therapeutic decisions.[22,23] There are two commonly recognized types of TR lesions: type 1 and type 2.[22,27] Type 3 lesions are defined as a tooth that has evidence of type 1 in one root and type 2 in the other.[28]

Type 2 lesions demonstrate replacement resorption (the lost tooth structure is replaced by bone)

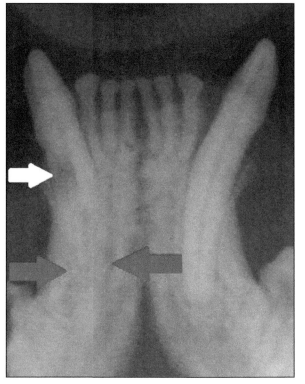

Fig. 2.5 Advanced type 2 tooth resorption with severe loss of root structure (red arrows) but only a small clinical defect (white arrow).

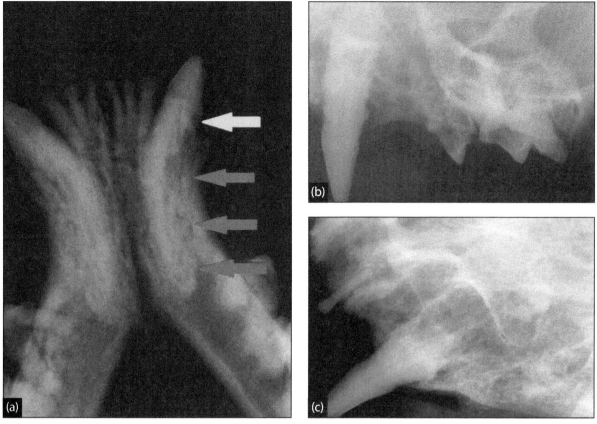

Fig. 2.6 **Type 2 tooth resorption (TR). These teeth are likely candidates for crown amputation. (a) Advanced type 2 TR of the left mandibular canine (304) with ankylosis (red arrows). There is minimal clinical involvement (blue arrow) despite the advanced root resorption. (b) Advanced type 2 TR with ankylosis of the left maxillary third premolar (207). (c) Advanced type 2 TR with ankylosis of the left maxillary canine (204). Extraction of all these affected teeth is difficult to impossible.**

of the roots, which makes extraction very difficult (**Figure 2.6**).[27] The resorption in these cases often continues until no recognizable tooth structure remains (ghost roots) (**Figure 2.7**). In cases of advanced type 2 TR lesions, endodontic infection is not known to occur.[29] This finding has resulted in the accepted therapy of crown amputation for treating these teeth.[22,24]

In stark contrast, type 1 TR lesions do not undergo replacement resorption.[22,27] These teeth typically retain sufficient normal root and pulp structure, which means that pain and possibly infection will result if inappropriately treated with crown amputation.[23] If the dental radiograph reveals intact root structure (**Figure 2.8**),

or, worse still, evidence of endodontic infection (**Figure 2.9**), complete extraction of the root is required.[13,22,24] Extraction of these teeth typically requires a *surgical* approach (mucogingival flap and buccal bone removal) due to the weakening of the tooth caused by the resorption.[14,30] Crown amputation is only acceptable for teeth with significant ankylosis and root replacement resorption (no evidence of periodontal ligaments or endodontic system), as well as no evidence of infection (endodontic or periodontal) (**Figure 2.7**).[14,22,24] Finally, patients with *caudal stomatitis* are not candidates for crown amputation. In cases of stomatitis, all the tooth roots should be removed as far as possible.[22]

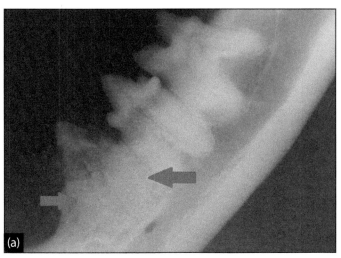
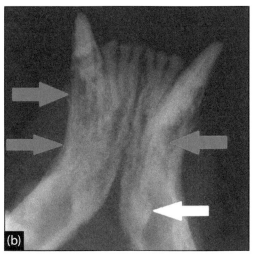

Fig. 2.7 Advanced type 2 tooth resorption (TR) with minimal to no remaining tooth structure (ghost roots). These teeth are definitely candidates for crown amputation. (a) Advanced type 2 TR with replacement resorption and ankylosis of the left mandibular third premolar (307). The roots are unidentifiable (arrows). (b) Advanced type 2 TR with replacement resorption and ankylosis of the mandibular canines (red arrows). The roots are unidentifiable other than a very small area at the apex of the left canine (white arrow). Regardless of this, these teeth can be properly treated with crown amputation.

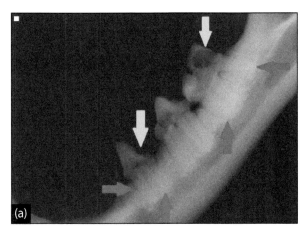
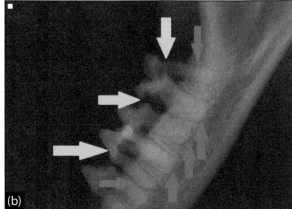

Fig. 2.8 Type 1 tooth resorption (TR). (a) Type 1 TRs on the mandibular premolars and molar of a cat. The lesions are the radiolucent areas in the crowns (blue arrows). However, there is normal appearing tooth structure with periodontal ligament and endodontic systems (red arrows). Complete extraction is required and should be fairly straightforward based on the normal periodontal ligaments. (b) Type 1 TRs on the mandibular premolars and molar of a cat. The lesions are the radiolucent areas in the crowns (blue arrows). However, there is normal appearing tooth structure with periodontal ligament and endodontic systems (red arrows). Complete extraction is required and should be fairly straightforward based on the normal periodontal ligaments. Also present is a small amount of horizontal bone loss as well as a supernumerary fourth premolar.   *(Continued)*

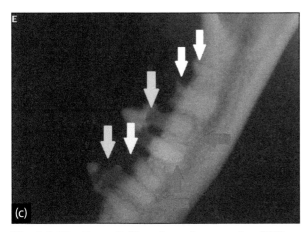

(c)

Fig. 2.8 *(Continued)* Type 1 tooth resorption (TR). (c) Type 1 TRs on the mandibular premolars and molar of a cat. The lesions are the radiolucent areas in the crowns (blue arrows). However, there is normal appearing tooth structure with periodontal ligament and endodontic systems (red arrows). Complete extraction is required and should be fairly straightforward based on the normal periodontal ligaments. These teeth also have a small amount of horizontal bone loss. The first molar was inappropriately crown amputated with identifiable tooth structure (white arrows), as was the supernumerary fourth premolar with a retained root (yellow arrow). All the teeth in this quadrant require complete extraction.

Dental radiographs will save the practitioner time and frustration by directing his/her efforts appropriately.[23] Teeth with advanced replacement resorption can be crown amputated, rather than spending time and risking complications with removing resorbed roots.[13,30] Radiographs also provide the practitioner with the ability to more accurately estimate both surgical time and cost of the procedure. In summary, radiographs are not only helpful, but absolutely required in order to diagnose and treat feline TRs in cats. In other words, crown amputation should NEVER be performed without dental radiology.[24]

CANINE TOOTH RESORPTION

(For more information see Chapter 8, Part E.)

Although much less common compared with cats, dogs do develop resorptive lesions (**Figure 2.10a**).[14,22] They are not often seen clinically (4.5% in one study), but are evident radiographically on a regular basis (56% of dogs and 11% of teeth),[31] and this occurs more often in older dogs.[24,31,32] As with feline TR, these lesions are typically first noted at the gingival margin.[22] If found radiographically, it is recommended that the cervical area of the tooth is thoroughly evaluated with a dental explorer. If there is no *clinical* evidence of resorption, no treatment is necessary.[22]

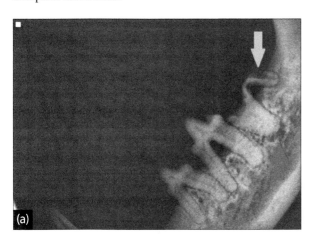

(a)

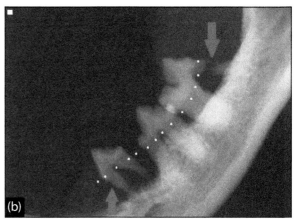

(b)

Fig. 2.9 Type 1 tooth resorption (TR) with secondary endodontic infection. (a) The left mandibular first molar (309) has a type 1 TR (blue arrow) and the crown has fractured off. However, the endodontic systems are intact and this has resulted in periapical rarefaction on the mesial root (red arrow). (b) The left mandibular third premolar and first molar (307 and 309) have a type 1 TR (arrows). However, the endodontic systems are intact. Note the advanced periodontal disease (dots).

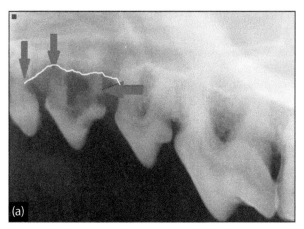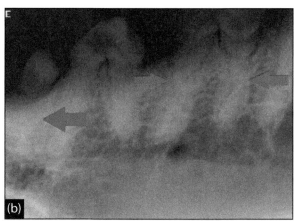

Fig. 2.10 **Canine tooth resorption (TR). (a) Advanced TR on the left maxillary first and second premolars (arrows). The involved teeth also have significant alveolar bone loss (blue line). (b) Advanced TR on the left mandibular premolar teeth of a dog (arrows). Extraction of these teeth is exceedingly difficult due to the resorption and ankylosis.**

These teeth should be evaluated clinically and radiographically under general anesthesia on a regular basis (q 6–12 months). In this author's experience, the mandibular premolar teeth are most commonly involved (**Figure 2.10b**). In addition to resorption, these teeth often have concurrent periodontal disease (**Figure 2.10a**). The resorption and secondary ankylosis (tooth and bone fusion) makes extraction by traditional means difficult to impossible, thus necessitating a surgical approach.[14,30] Imaging the condition of the roots prior to initiating surgery provides knowledge that helps in several ways.[14] First, it allows for a proper time estimate as well as a fee schedule. Furthermore, it enables the clinician to choose a surgical approach when indicated. By performing a surgical approach from the beginning, the surgeon can follow the roots during the buccal bone removal, rather than searching for fractured roots. Finally, presurgical knowledge of ankylosis allows the practitioner to use extra caution, thereby decreasing the chances of iatrogenic pathologic mandibular fracture, especially during extraction of mandibular canine or first molar teeth.

ENDODONTIC DISEASE

(For more information see Chapter 8, Part D)

Endodontic disease is very common in veterinary dentistry. It has been shown in one published report that 10% of all dogs have at least one tooth with direct pulp exposure.[33] Teeth with direct pulp exposure are exceedingly painful, and in the vast majority of cases the pulp will eventually become necrotic and likely infected as well.[22,34,35] Unfortunately, veterinary patients with endodontic disease typically suffer for a long time prior to diagnosis and definitive treatment. This is because cats and dogs very rarely show any obvious signs of oral pain or infection.[22,36,37] Therefore, the vast majority of endodontic cases go undiagnosed due to the lack of outward signs of disease (other than the broken or discolored tooth). Even in cases of obvious endodontic disease, such as a complicated crown fracture (**Figure 2.11**) or discolored (nonvital) teeth (**Figure 2.12**), radiographs may encourage clients to pursue treatment. However, dental radiographs are even more critical in cases where endodontic disease has either subtle or no clinical signs.

By far the most common situation of overlooked endodontic disease are uncomplicated crown fractures. These cases have dentinal but not direct pulp exposure (**Figures 2.13a, b**). Many of these teeth are vital, but there is a possibility that the endodontic system has been infected through the dentinal tubules.[22,38,39] This can lead to nonvitality of the tooth and subsequently infection/abscessation, just as with a tooth with direct pulp exposure. This scenario is more common in deep fractures, as

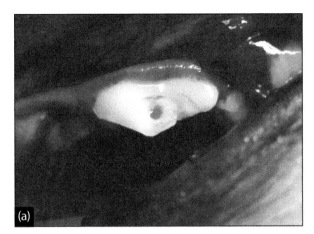

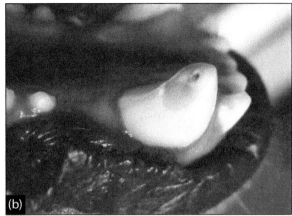

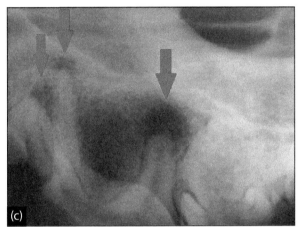

Fig. 2.11 (a) Complicated crown fracture of a left maxillary fourth premolar (208). The tooth is still vital based on the pink pulp. (b) Complicated crown fracture of a right mandibular canine (404). This tooth is nonvital based on the black pulp. (c) Intraoral dental radiograph of a left maxillary fourth premolar in a dog with a complicated crown fracture. Note the periapical rarefaction to all three roots (arrows), which indicates that the tooth is nonvital and infected. This will help convince reluctant clients of the need for therapy. Note: Even if the dental radiograph is normal, the tooth requires root canal therapy or extraction.

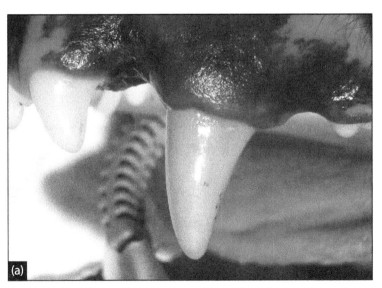

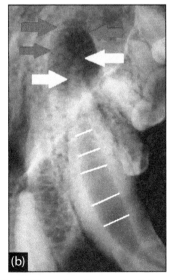

Fig. 2.12 (a) Left maxillary canine (204) with intrinsic staining (nonvital). (b) Dental radiograph of the tooth in (a), which reveals a wide endodontic system (white lines), periapical rarefaction (red arrows), and external root resorption (blue arrows), indicating chronic infection. This visual evidence will help convince clients of the need for therapy. However, discolored teeth are virtually always nonvital and often infected, therefore treatment (root canal therapy or extraction) is still indicated.

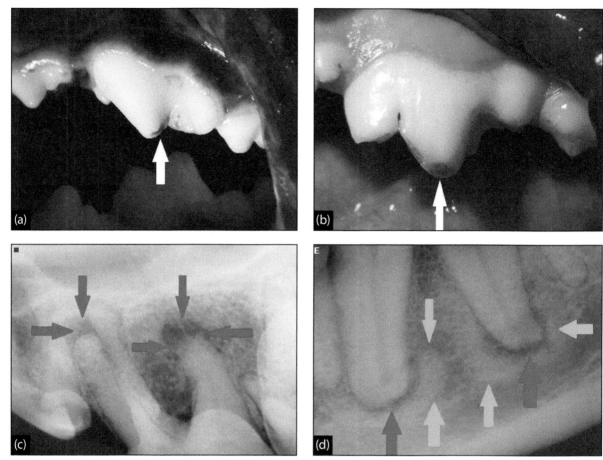

Fig. 2.13 Uncomplicated crown fractures with secondary infection. Intraoral dental pictures of a left maxillary fourth premolar (208) (a) and left mandibular first molar (309) (b) in different dogs. Both of these teeth have uncomplicated crown fractures (the crown is fractured and the dentin is exposed [arrows]). These are minor fractures but are enough to expose the dentin, which is stained dark. (c, d) Intraoral dental radiographs of the teeth in (a, b). Both of these teeth show periapical rarefaction, which is a sign of endodontic infection (red arrows). In addition, the first molar (d) also has sclerosis, which is another indication of infection (blue arrows). Both of these teeth are nonvital and in need of therapy (root canal or extraction) regardless of the very minor fractures.

the dentinal tubules are wider and more numerous nearer the pulp chamber.[38,40]

This painful inflammation (or infection) cannot be diagnosed without dental radiographs. Therefore, *every* tooth with dentin exposure should be radiographed to rule out endodontic disease.[37,39] Uncomplicated crown fractures always require some form of therapy, and proper treatment can only be determined with dental radiography. If the dental radiographs do not reveal signs of endodontic disease, a bonded sealant should be applied to

seal off the tooth from infection and decrease sensitivity.[37,39] The patient should have dental radiographs repeated in 9 months to ensure the tooth was not subclinically infected at the time of initial treatment.[22,37,39] If there is evidence of pulp nonvitality (wide root canals or periapical lucency) (**Figures 2.13c, d**), root canal therapy or extraction is mandated.[14,38,40]

Another common scenario in which teeth appear vital but may be endodontically involved, is worn teeth (attrition/abrasion).[14,22] If a tooth has

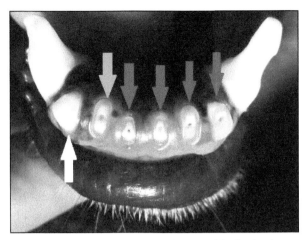

Fig. 2.14 **Severe attrition on the mandibular incisors of a dog. The right first and all three left incisors are pulp exposed and nonvital as evidenced by the dark pulps (red arrows). The right second incisor (402) is pulp exposed but still vital, as evidenced by the pink pulp (blue arrow). The pulp chamber of the right third incisor (403) is not exposed (white arrow). The five pulp exposed incisors should be extracted. The right incisor (403) should be radiographed for signs of endodontic infection and treated as directed by the radiographs.**

been worn to the point of direct pulp exposure (**Figure 2.14**), this is an obvious case of endodontic disease and requires either root canal therapy or extraction. If there is adequate reparative (tertiary) dentin in the pulp chamber (**Figure 2.15a**), the vast majority of these teeth remain vital and pain free.[41] It is critical to note, however, that there are teeth that are nonvital and infected in spite of visibly sufficient reparative dentin (**Figure 2.15b**).[41] This infection can only be determined by dental radiographs. If radiographic evidence of endodontic disease is present (i.e. wide root canals or periapical lucency), again, root canal therapy or extraction is indicated.[14,39,41] If there is no clinical or radiographic evidence of endodontic disease, a bonded sealant may be indicated and recheck radiographs in 9 months are recommended.

The final scenario of occult endodontic disease is with clinically normal teeth that are actually infected (**Figure 2.16**).[13,14] It is important to remember that infected teeth rarely present with clinical abscessation, making diagnosis without dental radiographs virtually impossible. The result is countless patients being chronically affected

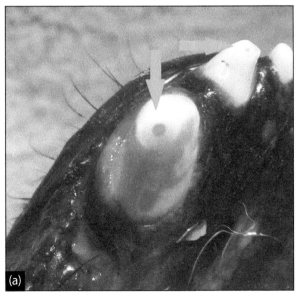
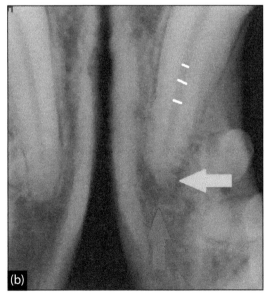

Fig. 2.15 **The importance of radiographing normal appearing teeth. (a) Abrasion of the mandibular left canine and third incisor with adequate appearing tertiary (reparative) dentin (arrows). (b) Intraoral dental radiograph of the left canine in (a). This tooth is nonvital and infected as evidenced by the periapical rarefaction (red arrow), external root resorption (blue arrow), and slightly wider endodontic system than the contralateral (white lines).**

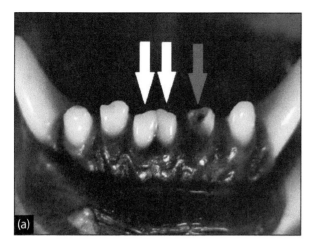

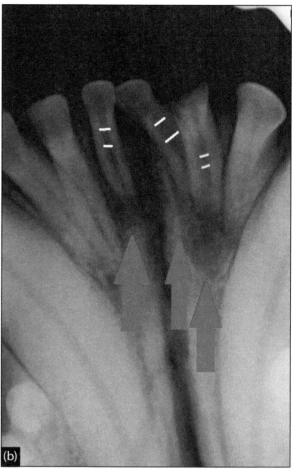

Fig. 2.16 Clinically normal appearing teeth with endodontic disease. (a) This dental picture shows a fractured left mandibular second incisor (302) (red arrow). However, the other incisors do not appear to be endodontically involved (white arrows). (b) Dental radiograph of the patient in (a). This reveals periapical rarefaction to 302, but also the first incisors (301, 401) (red arrows). In addition, the endodontic system of 302 is enlarged compared with 402 (yellow lines). Finally, the endodontic systems of 301 and 401 are even wider than 302 (white lines), indicating that they died earlier than the fractured tooth. This is a classic case of normal appearing teeth being nonvital and significantly infected.

with painful/infected teeth. Dental radiographs will elucidate the dental problem. In cases of clinical abscessation, radiographs will determine which tooth is the source of the infection. This situation is one of many that prove the value of full-mouth radiographs for all veterinary patients.[21,42]

PERSISTENT DECIDUOUS TEETH

Extraction of persistent deciduous teeth (**Figure 2.17**) is a very common procedure performed in veterinary dentistry. However, without dental radiographs this can be a very difficult and frustrating endeavor. Furthermore, many practitioners ask: 'If a deciduous tooth fractures, does it need to be

surgically extracted or will it resorb on its own?' Without the benefit of dental radiographs, this question cannot be answered.[30,43]

In some cases, the root of the deciduous tooth is normal and is held in naturally by the periodontal ligament (**Figure 2.18**). In this scenario, extraction is straightforward and root fracture should not occur if the extraction is performed correctly and carefully.[43] In most cases, however, the deciduous teeth will have undergone some to significant resorption, most often due to the pressure placed on the deciduous tooth by the erupting permanent dentition.[14] These teeth are predisposed to fracture, but an intact root canal is often still present (**Figure 2.19**). The resorption and potential

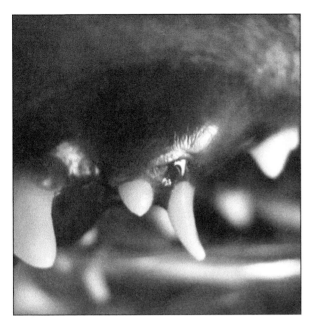

Fig. 2.17 **Persistent deciduous left maxillary canine (604). Note that the permanent tooth is just beginning to erupt; however, the deciduous tooth should still be extracted at this time.**

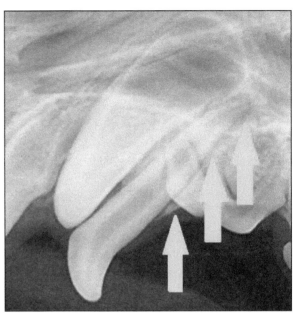

Fig. 2.18 **Persistent deciduous left maxillary canine (604), which has a radiographically appearing normal root structure (arrows). Complete extraction of this tooth is required, but should be straightforward.**

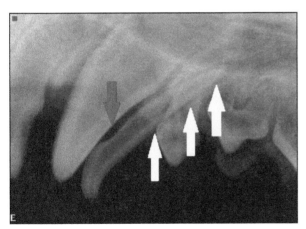

Fig. 2.19 **Persistent deciduous left maxillary canine (604), which has a radiographically appearing normal root structure for the most part (blue arrows). However, there is an area of resorption just below the gingival margin (red arrow), which was caused by the pressure of the erupting permanent tooth. This resorption will significantly weaken the tooth in the area and predispose it to fracture. Complete extraction of this tooth is required, but careful elevation is necessary and a surgical approach is likely recommended to allow the elevator to start *below* the weak area.**

ankylosis makes extraction very difficult, which commonly results in a fractured root.[43] In these cases, as with TR lesions, starting with a surgical approach from the beginning is prudent. Regardless of the surgical technique chosen, if there is an identifiable root canal, these roots require complete extraction to avoid inflammation and infection.[43,44] Contrary to popular belief, intact/normal deciduous roots do not resorb, and will affect the patient regardless of the lack of clinical signs. In one case treated by this author, a patient nearly lost his eye due to the chronic infection caused by a retained deciduous tooth root (**Figure 2.20**).

Finally, there are occasional cases where the root structure of the deciduous tooth has been almost completely resorbed and the crown is being held in place only by the gingival attachment (**Figure 2.21**).[30,43] Proper therapy for these cases requires that only the crown and the very small retaining root segment is removed. This knowledge saves the practitioner time in searching for the root, avoids undue stress or concern, and avoids unnecessary trauma to the patient.

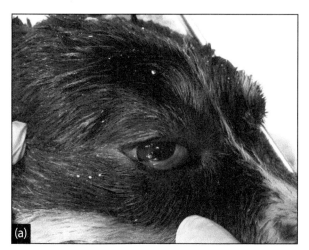
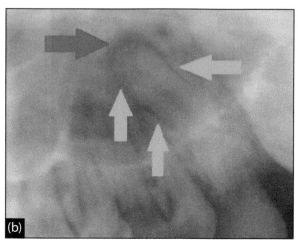

Fig. 2.20 (a) Severe chronic right ocular infection in a 12-year-old dog that responded temporarily to several different courses of antibiotics. (b) The patient was referred for dental radiographs, which revealed a retained root of the deciduous right maxillary canine (504) (blue arrows) with periapical rarefaction (red arrow). This tooth had not resorbed after 11 years and the tooth was secondarily infected, which was affecting the eye. Extraction of the root resolved the infection. This case proves the importance of complete extraction of any deciduous teeth that have not undergone significant resorption.

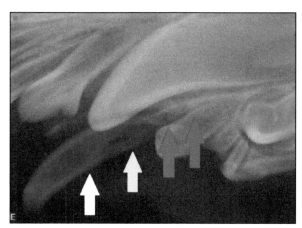

Fig. 2.21 Persistent deciduous tooth (white arrow) with significant resorption at the gingival margin (blue arrow) and complete resorption below that (red arrows). This tooth can be properly treated by removing the crown and the small area of intact root. This knowledge is important as it would avoid an unnecessary surgical search for a nonexistent root.

'MISSING' TEETH

Incomplete dental arches are quite common in veterinary patients (**Figure 2.22**). In some cases, the tooth is truly missing, but often the tooth/root is actually present and may be creating pain and/or infection. Do not assume that a tooth is truly and completely absent or was completely extracted just because it is clinically missing. Radiographs of the area are required to confirm the absence or presence of structures under the gumline.

Possible etiologies for 'missing' teeth include:[43]

1 Congenitally missing (hypo- or oligodontia) (**Figure 2.23**).[45] This is usually considered to be a genetic problem, but can occur secondary to significant infection/malnutrition during gestation or the neonatal period. There is also a genetic predisposition in Chinese Crested and Mexican Hairless breeds. This condition is also common in small, toy, and brachycephalic breeds.[46] The most common congenitally missing teeth are the premolars, maxillary second and mandibular third molars, and incisors. No specific therapy is necessary in these cases.

2 Previously extracted or exfoliated. While rare in young patients, this is quite common in mature animals. Tooth loss via exfoliation occurs most commonly due to periodontal disease, but can also be caused by trauma. However, previous extraction is a much more common scenario

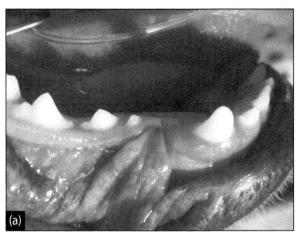
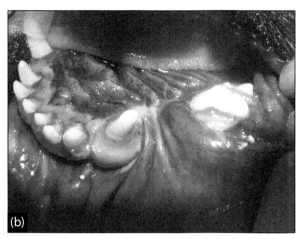

Fig. 2.22 Intraoral dental pictures of 'missing' teeth. (a) This image shows a 'missing' right mandibular first premolar (405), which is a very common condition in brachycephalic dogs. (b) An image of a patient that is 'missing' its right maxillary first three premolars (105–107).

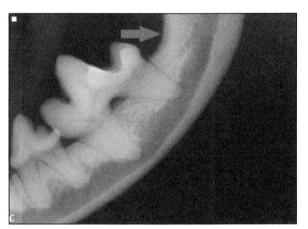
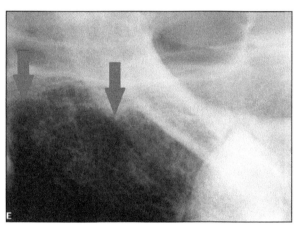

Fig. 2.23 Intraoral dental radiograph of the left mandible of a dog that is 'missing' its mandibular second and third molars (310 and 311) (arrow). There is no evidence of pathology in the area, and therefore no therapy is necessary. The fact that the bone is of the correct level in this area is evidence that this pet was likely born without the teeth.

Fig. 2.24 Intraoral dental radiograph of the left maxillary forth premolar (208) in a dog. There are no retained roots or other pathology, so no therapy is necessary. However, the dark areas (arrows) arc evidence of healing extraction sites, which indicates a fairly recent extraction.

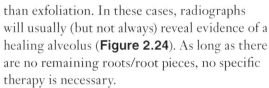

than exfoliation. In these cases, radiographs will usually (but not always) reveal evidence of a healing alveolus (**Figure 2.24**). As long as there are no remaining roots/root pieces, no specific therapy is necessary.

3 Fractured below the gingival margin (**Figure 2.25**). This may occur as a result of trauma or an incomplete extraction attempt. Retained roots following extraction attempts

are quite common. A recent study evaluating the success rates of carnassial extractions in dogs and cats revealed retained roots in almost 90% of the cases.[47] Dental radiographs will confirm the presence of a retained root, and in many cases will also reveal inflammatory bony changes, which generally demonstrates infection. If the root appears relatively normal (i.e. has not undergone significant

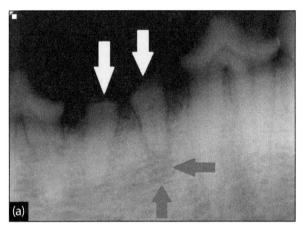

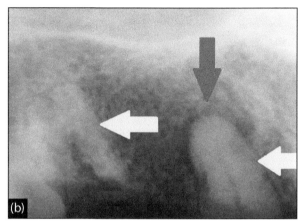

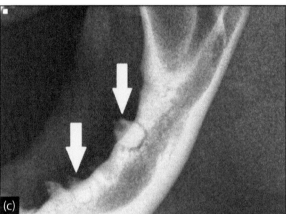

Fig. 2.25 Intraoral dental radiographs of the left mandibular premolars (a), left maxillary fourth premolar (b) in a dog, and the left mandible in a cat (c). The roots of the third premolar (307) in (a), the fourth premolar in (b) and those in (c) are retained. They are all fairly normal, with intact endodontic systems (blue arrows). In addition, the distal roots in (a) and (b) have periapical rarefaction (red arrows), which is evidence of active infection. Extraction of these roots will relieve the local infection. Dental radiographs provided critical information in these cases.

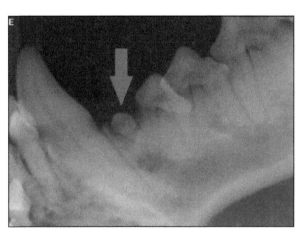

Fig. 2.26 Intraoral dental picture of the rostral left mandible of a patient with a 'missing' first premolar (305). This image reveals the embedded tooth (arrow) without evidence of cystic formation.

replacement resorption), surgical extraction is usually recommended to alleviate pain and/or infection.

4 Impacted or embedded (**Figure 2.26**). These teeth may be either malformed or normal, but do not erupt into the mouth for some reason. Often they are blocked by a structure such as bone or tooth (deciduous or permanent) or, more commonly, by an area of thick and firm gingiva called an *operculum*. However, it is also possible for *failure of passive eruption* to occur, resulting in impacted/embedded teeth. This condition is most common in the maxillary canines as well as the premolars (especially mandibular first premolars of brachiocephalic breeds) but can occur with any tooth.[48,49]

The biggest concern with leaving unerupted or impacted teeth untreated below the gumline is the development of dentigerous cysts (**Figure 2.27a**).[43,50] Dentigerous cysts arise from the enamel forming organ of the unerupted tooth.[50] The prevalence of cysts in the general population of dogs was reported to be 1.4%, with 71% of these being dentigerous.[51] The fact that many cysts are an incidental finding underscores the importance of dental radiographs for diagnosis of these lesions.[51] Despite the low numbers in the general population, dentigerous cysts are reported to occur in association with approximately 29% of impacted/embedded teeth in dogs.[52] Further, the mandibular first premolar is the most common tooth to be affected with a dentigerous cyst.[51,53] Finally, brachycephalic breeds are overrepresented, likely due to dental crowding associated with their conformation.[51,54]

As a dentigerous cyst grows, it causes bone loss by pressure. These cysts can grow quite large, resulting in weakened bone in the area of the cyst (**Figure 2.27b**). This may necessitate an extensive surgery (**Figure 2.27c**) or may even result in a pathologic fracture (**Figure 2.27d**).[55] Furthermore, dentigerous cysts can become infected and create significant swelling and pain, or they can even undergo malignant transformation.[43,51,56] For these reasons, the recommended therapy for impacted teeth is surgical extraction. If a cyst is present, extraction of the tooth and meticulous curettage of the lining should prove curative.[43,50] A biopsy of the lining is recommended and bone augmentation can be considered, especially in large lesions.[43,50]

It is critical to note that of the four causes for 'missing' teeth, two require no therapy and the other two can lead to significant pathology. Therefore, all areas of 'missing' teeth should be radiographed to ensure that the teeth are truly missing and if therapy is necessary.

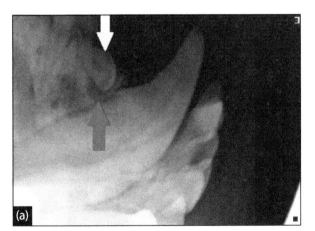
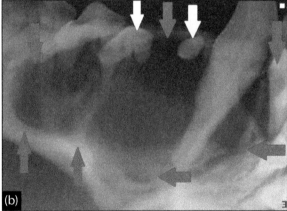

Fig. 2.27 **Dentigerous cysts. (a) Intraoral dental radiograph of the mandibular right in a dog with an impacted tooth, which reveals an embedded first premolar (405) (blue arrow), with a radiolucent area surrounding the crown (red arrow), which is indicative of an early dentigerous cyst. Extraction of the tooth and débridement of the cyst should prove curative. Since this was caught early, the surgery should be straightforward and relatively noninvasive. (b) Intraoral dental radiograph of another patient with a 'missing' mandibular first premolar. The radiograph reveals the impacted/embedded tooth (blue arrow) as well as a very large radiolucent area (red arrows), which is indicative of a large dentigerous cyst. In addition, the second and third premolars are being moved distally (white arrow). This large cyst required extraction of all teeth from the first incisor to the fourth premolar and significant débridement.** *(Continued)*

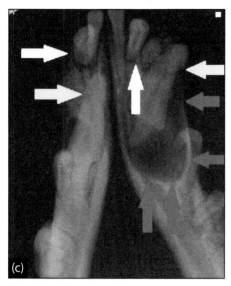

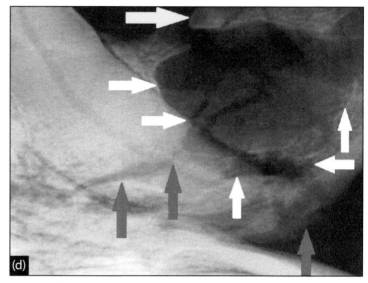

Fig. 2.27 *(Continued)* **Dentigerous cysts. (c) Intraoral dental radiograph of another patient with a 'missing' mandibular canines (304 and 404). The radiograph reveals the impacted/embedded teeth (blue arrows) as well as a very large radiolucent area (red arrows), which is indicative of a large dentigerous cyst. In addition, several incisors are malformed with short roots (white arrows). This large cyst required extraction of the canine and significant débridement. (d) Intraoral dental radiograph of another patient with a 'missing' left mandibular first premolar (305). The radiograph reveals the impacted/embedded tooth (blue arrow) as well as a very large radiolucent area (white arrows), which is indicative of a large dentigerous cyst. In addition, the mandible is fractured (red arrows). This large cyst created a pathologic fracture and required extraction of all teeth from the area, significant débridement, and jaw fracture fixation.**

MANDIBULAR FRACTURES

(For more information see Chapter 8, Parts A and F)

Mandibular fractures are a fairly common occurrence in veterinary medicine. It has been shown that the premolar/molar area makes up the majority of these fractures.[57,58] The rostral area (canines and incisors) makes up 30–45% of these fractures in dogs.[57,59] These fractures of the lower jaw are often a result of direct trauma (hit by car or dog fights), but it is becoming increasingly common for aging small breed patients to suffer from pathologic fractures.[16,17,60] In fact, 13% of mandibular fractures were considered pathologic in one study.[57]

Chronic periodontal loss causes loss of the tooth support, eventually possibly resulting in exfoliation.[11] With the majority of teeth, exfoliation will occur prior to severe bone weakening. However, in some situations, significant bone thinning will occur prior to tooth exfoliation.

Pathologic fractures are much more common in small and toy breed dogs (as opposed to large breeds) for several reasons:[11,17]

1 Small and toy-breed dogs appear to have a genetic propensity to severe periodontal disease.[4]
2 Small dogs tend to live longer, thus allowing the process of periodontal bone loss to progress further.
3 Most importantly, small dogs have proportionally larger teeth than their large breed counterparts[19] (i.e. small dogs have larger teeth in relation to smaller jaws). This places the root apex of the mandibular first molar very close to the ventral cortex of the mandible (**Figure 2.28**).[61] The next most common place for this is the mandibular canines. These teeth comprise 60–70% of the strength of the rostral mandible (**Figure 2.29**).[13,14] Therefore, when the mandibular bone/supporting structure is thinned by periodontal disease progression, this area may easily fracture before the tooth exfoliates.[16,17,60]

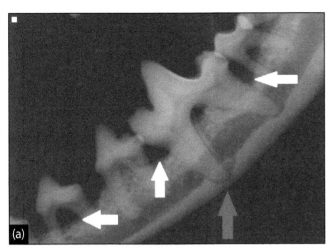
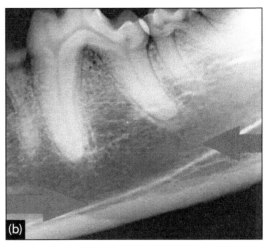

Fig. 2.28 Comparison of the mandible of a small (a) and a large (b) breed dog. In small breed dogs, the mandibular first molar is significantly larger in proportion to the mandible than it is in large breed dogs (red arrows). Advanced periodontal (or potentially endodontic) disease to the mesial root of the first molar in small and toy breed dogs can result in a pathologic fracture. The 'reserve' bone in a large breed dog makes pathologic fractures from periodontal disease highly unlikely. Figure (a) also reveals moderate horizontal alveolar bone loss (white arrows).

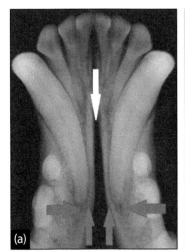
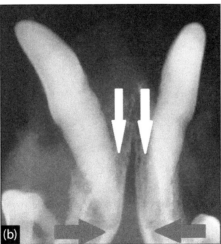
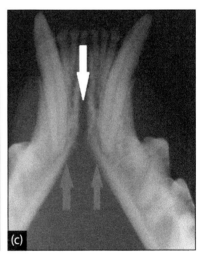

Fig. 2.29 Images of the rostral mandible in three patients demonstrating the minimal amount of bone present at the apex of the mandibular canines. (a) Intraoral dental radiograph of the mandibular canines and incisors of a normal 4.5 kg (10 lb) dog. Note that the mandible has minimal bony support even without any additional loss (red arrows). Part of the weakness results from the fibrocartilaginous mandibular symphysis (white arrow). (b) Intraoral dental radiograph of the mandibular canines and incisors of a 4.5 kg (10 lb) dog with advanced periodontal disease and secondary bone loss (white arrows). Note that the mandible has minimal bony support (red arrows). The jaw is at significant risk for fracture during extraction of these teeth. (c) Intraoral dental radiograph of the mandibular canines and incisors of a normal cat. Note that the mandible has minimal bony support even without any additional loss (red arrows). Part of the weakness results from the fibrocartilaginous mandibular symphysis (white arrow).

Note that because of the minimal remaining bone due to a combination of a low mandible/tooth volume ratio and chronic periodontally induced bone loss, pathologic fractures typically occur with a history of only mild trauma or even no trauma at all. Possible scenarios include dog fights or jumping off a bed, and some dogs have even broken their jaw while eating.[18] However, a very common situation for pathologic fractures to occur is during extraction attempts.[13,17] Elevating these roots with little or no supportive adjacent bone structure can prove disastrous. This makes dental radiology an invaluable tool for avoiding iatrogenic jaw fractures during dental procedures in small and toy breed dogs. Although this is typically thought to be a condition that would only present in older patients, this author has personally treated three cases in which the dogs have been under 3 years of age.

A pathologic fracture should be suspected in all cases of mandibular fracture, especially in the area of the mandibular first molar or canine tooth of older toy breed dogs. Additional supportive history is lack of obvious trauma, a non- or only mildly painful patient, periodontal disease elsewhere in the mouth, and/or a nonunion fracture despite apparently adequate surgical fixation.

Diagnosis of a pathologic fracture is only possible with dental radiographs, as skull films typically provide insufficient detail. The classic appearance of a pathologic fracture is bone loss around the tooth and/or periapical lucency in the area of the fracture or other root of a multirooted tooth (**Figure 2.30**).[14,17]

These fractures will NOT heal, no matter how perfect the fixation is, if the diseased tooth root is not extracted (**Figure 2.31**).[16] These teeth MUST be extracted, or they will continue to act as a nidus of infection and bone healing cannot occur.[17,61]

ORAL MASSES

(For more information see Chapter 8, Part G)

Dental radiology is very important for accurate diagnosis of oral masses.[13,23] This is because various types of growths usually have different radiographic appearances. The prudent practitioner should note

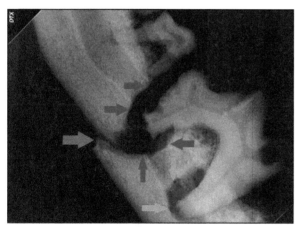

Fig. 2.30 **Intraoral dental radiograph of the right mandible of a small breed dog with advanced alveolar bone loss on the distal root (blue arrows) secondary to periodontal disease. This has resulted in a class II perio-endo abscess with periapical rarefaction on the mesial root (orange arrows). Further, the weakened bone in the area has resulted in a pathologic mandibular fracture (red arrow). The information provided by this radiograph was critical for proper therapy of this fracture and tooth.**

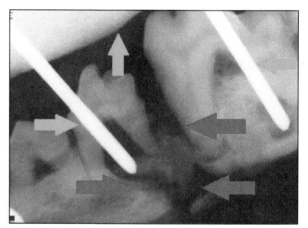

Fig. 2.31 **Intraoral dental radiograph of the left mandible of a dog that has had three external fixators applied for a mandibular fracture (blue arrows). Each fixation failed due to the infected teeth and bone in the area (red arrows). Dental radiographs provided this information and led to successful healing (bony union) of the fractured mandible.**

the type and extent of bony involvement (if any) on the histopathology request form (and ideally include copies of the radiographs and pictures) to aid the pathologist. Furthermore, it is critical to interpret the histopathology results in light of the radiographic findings. A diagnosis of a malignancy without bony involvement should be questioned prior to initiating definitive therapy such as aggressive surgery, radiation therapy, or chemotherapy (**Figure 2.32**). Conversely, a benign tumor diagnosis with significant bony reaction (**Figure 2.33**) should be further

investigated prior to assuming that the histopathologic diagnosis is correct.

Regardless of the radiographic interpretation, histopathologic testing is always necessary for accurate diagnosis of oral masses. This is for many reasons, including the fact that a variety of benign or malignant tumors can appear radiographically similar. In addition, osteomyelitis can create the same radiographic findings as malignant tumors. Finally, many aggressive tumors may show no bone involvement early in the course of disease.

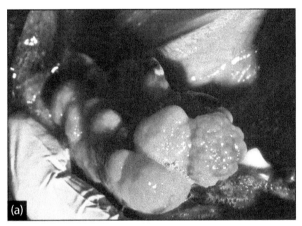
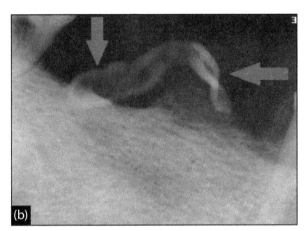

Fig. 2.32 (a) Intraoral dental picture of a large oral mass. (b) A dental radiograph of the area revealed no significant evidence of bony involvement, but demonstrated a foreign body (arrows). This led to a presumptive diagnosis of a benign lesion, which was confirmed histopathologically. Débridement of the lesion and removal of the foreign body proved curative.

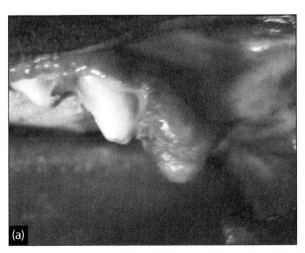
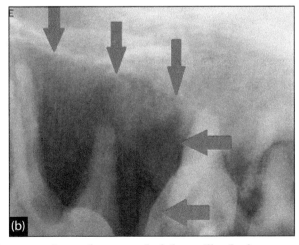

Fig. 2.33 (a) Intraoral dental picture of a small and benign appearing oral mass on the left maxilla of a dog. (b) A dental radiograph of the area revealed significant evidence of bony involvement (arrows). This led to the presumptive diagnosis of an aggressive lesion, which was confirmed histopathologically as a fibrosarcoma.

EXTRACTIONS

Pre- and postoperative dental radiographs should be obtained for all extraction procedures.[14,62,63] Pre-extraction radiographs allow the practitioner to determine the amount of disease present as well as any root abnormalities (curved [**Figure 2.34**], dilac-erated, or supernumerary [**Figure 2.35**]).[23] It has been reported that 10% of maxillary third premolars in cats actually have a third root.[64] One of the more important findings on preoperative dental radio-graphs is the presence and degree of replacement resorption and/or ankylosis (**Figure 2.36**).[13,30] In addition, the level of remaining bone will be eluci-dated (see Periodontal disease). This is particularly important when preparing for a mandibular first molar or canine extraction, as knowledge regarding the amount of remaining mandibular bone can be critical in avoiding an iatrogenic fracture (**Figure 2.37**).[13,17,30] This is especially true with the man-dibular canine teeth in cats and all breeds of dog, as there is minimal bone surrounding the apex, in addition to the mandibular first molar teeth in small and toy breed dogs, as they are proportionally larger

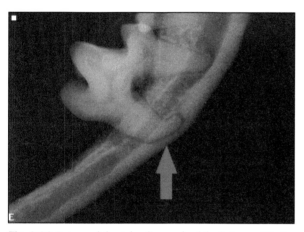

Fig. 2.34 Intraoral dental radiograph of the left mandibular first molar (309) of a small breed dog. The image reveals minimal apical bone as well as a significant 'hook' at the apex of the mesial root (arrow), which greatly predisposes the tooth and jaw to fracture during an extraction attempt.

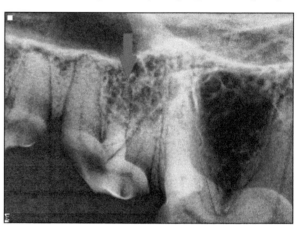

Fig. 2.35 Intraoral dental radiograph of the left maxillary third premolar (207) in a dog with a supernumerary root (arrow). This will complicate the extraction procedure.

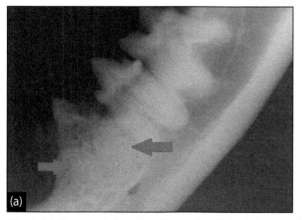

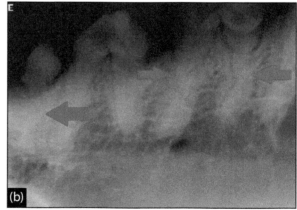

Fig. 2.36 Intraoral dental radiographs of the left mandible in a cat (a) and dog (b) with advanced tooth resorption (arrows). Extraction of the teeth in (b) is very difficult due to the advanced resorption and ankylosis. Therefore, a surgical approach is required and referral should be considered. The third premolar in (a) is a candidate for crown amputation. The knowledge provided by these images is critical for successful therapy.

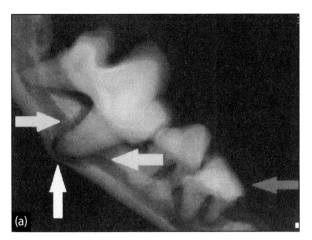

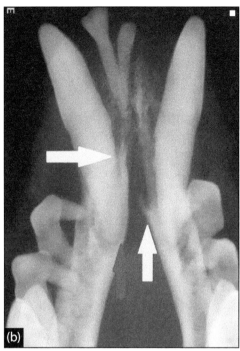

Fig. 2.37 Cases where the bone has been significantly weakened by periodontal disease and the area is highly predisposed to an iatrogenic pathologic fracture. (a) Intraoral dental radiograph of the right mandible of a 2.7 kg (6 lb) dog. The first molar has undergone significant alveolar bone loss (blue arrows) secondary to periodontal disease, which has resulted in an area of bone less than 0.5 mm thick at the apex (yellow arrow). The third premolar is being held in the dental arch by a 'calculus bridge' to the fourth premolar (red arrow). (b) Intraoral dental radiograph of the rostral mandible of a 13.6 kg (30 lb) dog with advanced alveolar bone loss secondary to periodontal disease (yellow arrows). This in combination with the normal anatomy has led to very weak bone in the area (red arrow), with a high chance of fracture.

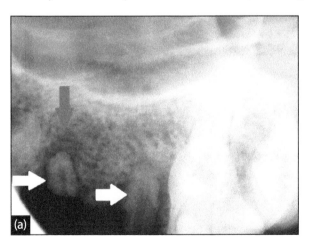

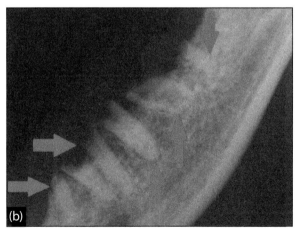

Fig. 2.38 Retained tooth roots of the left maxillary fourth premolar of a dog (a) (blue arrows) and the left mandible of a cat (b) (arrows). In (a) there is periapical rarefaction associated with the mesial root (red arrow), which indicates active infection. Extraction of these teeth is mandated.

in size compared with the jaw (**Figure 2.4**).[19] Finally, dental radiographs will serve as legal evidence of the need for extraction and as documented evidence in case of complications.[14]

Postextraction dental radiographs are equally important.[14,65,66] Regardless of the gross appearance of tooth roots following extraction, there is still a possibility of retained roots or other pathology. This makes postoperative radiographs critical in ALL extraction cases (**Figure 2.38**).[23] A recent study evaluating the success rate of extractions of carnassial teeth in dogs and cats revealed that

86.4% had retained roots, and that 66% of these roots had radiographic evidence of inflammation (i.e. likely infected).[47] There are rarely any clinical signs observed with this complication, but retained roots can be painful and/or infected.[47] Occasionally, retained roots do create a clinical abscess, and it is worth noting that there have been some lawsuits levied over these cases.

CONCLUSIONS

Considering that nearly every veterinary patient has some form of oral/dental disease, and that dental radiographs are indicated for all oral diseases, virtually every patient would benefit from the information provided by dental radiographs. In addition, dental radiographs are a critical piece of information for the veterinarian when treating oral disease, which means that dental x-ray equipment should be used on a daily basis in every general practice.

From a financial standpoint, there is not a piece of veterinary equipment that has the potential to provide the return on investment that a dental radiography machine does. If a moderately busy practice obtained radiographs whenever necessary, this equipment should be paid for in less than 3 months. This does not include the income from additional procedures that could now be performed with confidence, such as bonded sealants, scaling and root curettage, extractions, and periodontal surgery. Nor does it factor in the significant time savings during oral surgery. The information provided by radiographs regarding root and bone pathology, as well as the ability to document complete extraction, is crucial. Finally, dental radiographs will provide peace of mind to the clinician, which is priceless.

REFERENCES

1 University of Minnesota Center for Companion Animal Health (1996) *National Companion Animal Study, Uplinks*, p. 3.

2 Lund EM, Armstrong PJ, Kirkl CA *et al.* (1999) Health status and population characteristics of dogs and cats examined at private veterinary practices in the United States. *J Am Vet Med Assoc* **214:**1336–41.

3 Wiggs RB, Lobprise HB (1997) Periodontology In: *Veterinary Dentistry: Principles and Practice.* Lippincott-Raven, Philadelphia, pp. 186–231.

4 Hoffmann TH, Gaengler P (1996) Clinical and pathomorphological investigation of spontaneously occurring periodontal disease in dogs. *J Small Anim Pract* **37:**471–479.

5 Fiorellini JP, Ishikawa SO, Kim DM (2006) Clinical features of gingivitis. In: *Carranza's Clinical Periodontology.* WB Saunders, St. Louis, pp. 362–372.

6 Meitner SW, Zander H, Iker HP *et al.* (1979) Identification of inflamed gingival surfaces. *J Clin Periodontol* **6:**93.

7 Niemiec BA (2012) Gingivitis. In: *Veterinary Periodontology.* (ed. BA Niemiec) Wiley-Blackwell, Ames, pp. 41–50.

8 Niemiec BA (2008) Periodontal disease. *Top Companion Anim Med* **23(2):**72–80.

9 Sherman PR, Hutchens LH Jr, Jewson LG (1990) The effectiveness of subgingival scaling and root planing. II. Clinical responses related to residual calculus. *J Periodontol* **61(1):**9–15.

10 Niemiec BA (2012) Pathogenisis and etiology of periodontal disease. In: *Veterinary Periodontology.* (ed. BA Niemiec) Wiley-Blackwell, Ames, pp. 18–34.

11 Niemiec BA (2008) Periodontal therapy. *Top Companion Anim Med* **23(2):**81–90.

12 Huffman LJ (2010) Oral examination. In: *Small Animal Dental, Oral and Maxillofacial Disease: A Color Handbook.* (ed. BA Niemiec) Manson Publishing, London, pp. 39–61.

13 Niemiec BA (2011) The importance of dental radiology. *Eur J Comp Anim Pract* **20(3):**219–229.

14 Niemiec BA (2008) Case-based dental radiology. *Top Companion Anim Med* **24(1):**4–19.

15 Niemiec BA (2012) Advanced non-surgical therapy. In: *Veterinary Periodontology.* (ed. BA Niemiec) Wiley-Blackwell, Ames, 154–169.

16 Taney KG, Smith MM (2010) Problems with the bones, muscles and joints: In: *Small Animal Dental, Oral and Maxillofacial Disease: A Color Handbook.* (ed. BA Niemiec) Manson Publishing, London, pp. 199–224.

17 Niemiec BA (2012) Local and regional consequences of periodontal disease. In: *Veterinary Periodontology.* (BA Niemiec) Wiley-Blackwell, Ames, pp. 69–80.

18 Mulligan T Aller S, Williams C (1998) *Atlas of Canine and Feline Dental Radiography.* Veterinary Learning Systems, Trenton, pp. 176–183.

19 Gioso MA, Shofer F, Barros PS *et al.* (2001) Mandible and mandibular first molar tooth

measurements in dogs: relationship of radiographic height to body weight. *J Vet Dent* **18(2):**65–68.

20 Tsugawa AJ, Verstraete FJ (2000) How to obtain and interpret periodontal radiographs in dogs. *Clin Tech Small Anim Pract* **15(4):**204–210.

21 Verstraete FJ, Kass PH, Terpak CH (1998) Diagnostic value of full-mouth radiography in cats. *Am J Vet Res* **59(6):**692–695.

22 Dupont GA (2010) Pathologies of the dental hard tissue. In: *Small Animal Dental, Oral and Maxillofacial Disease: A Color Handbook*. (ed. BA Niemiec) Manson Publishing, London, pp. 127–157.

23 Niemiec BA (2014) Feline dental radiography and radiology: a primer. *J Feline Med Surg* **16(11):** 887–899.

24 DuPont GA (2002) Crown amputation with intentional root retention for dental resorptive lesions in cats. *J Vet Dent* **19(2):**107–110.

25 van Wessum R, Harvey CE, Hennet P (1992) Feline dental resorptive lesions. Prevalence patterns. *Vet Clin North Am Small Anim Pract* **22(6):**1405–1416.

26 Wiggs RB, Lobprise HB (1997) Domestic feline oral and dental disease. In: *Veterinary Dentistry, Principles and Practice*. Lippincott-Raven, Philadelphia, pp. 487–496.

27 DuPont GA, DeBowes LJ (2002) Comparison of periodontitis and root replacement in cat teeth with resorptive lesions. *J Vet Dent* **19(2):**71–76.

28 Bellows J (2010) Treatment of tooth resorption. In: *Feline Dentistry: Oral Assessment, Treatment, and Preventative Care*. Wiley-Blackwell, Ames, pp. 222–241.

29 Lommer MJ, Verstraete FJ (2000) Prevalence of odontoclastic resorption lesions and periapical radiographic lucencies in cats: 265 cases (1995–1998) *J Am Vet Med Assoc* **217(12):**1866–1869.

30 Niemiec BA (2012) *Dental Extractions Made Easier*. Practical Veterinary Publishing, Tustin.

31 Peralta S, Verstraete FJ, Kass PH (2001) Radiographic evaluation of the types of tooth resorption in dogs. *Am J Vet Res* **71(7):**784–793.

32 Arnbjerg J (1996) Idiopathic dental root replacement resorption in old dogs. *J Vet Dent* **13(3):**97–99.

33 Golden Al, Stoller NS, Harvey CE (1982) A survey of oral and dental diseases in dogs anesthetized at a veterinary hospital. *J Am Anim Hosp Assoc* **18:** 891–899.

34 Niemiec BA (2005) Fundamentals of endodontics. *Vet Clin North Am Small Anim Pract* **35(4):**837–868.

35 Niemiec BA (2008) Oral pathology. *Top Companion Anim Med* **23(2):**59–71.

36 Holmstrolm S, Frost P, Eisner E (1998) *Veterinary Dental Techniques*, 2nd edn. WB Saunders, Philadelphia, p. 493.

37 Woodward TM (2008) Bonded sealants for fractured teeth. *Top Companion Anim Med* **23(2):**91–96.

38 Startup S (2011) Tooth response to injury. In: *Veterinary Endodontics*. (ed. BA Niemiec) Practical Veterinary Publishing, Tustin, pp. 10–24.

39 Theuns P, Niemiec BA (2011) Bonded sealants for uncomplicated crown fractures. *J Vet Dent* **28(2):** 130–132.

40 Theuns P (2011) Endodontic anatomy. In: *Veterinary Endodontics*. (ed. BA Niemiec) Practical Veterinary Publishing, Tustin, pp. 5–9.

41 Trowbridge H, Kim S, Suda H (2002) Structure and functions of the dentin and pulp complex. In: *Pathways of the Pulp*, 8th edn. (eds S Cohen, RC Burns) Mosby, St. Louis, pp. 441–456.

42 Verstraete FJ, Kass PH, Terpak CH (1998) Diagnostic value of full-mouth radiography in dogs. *Am J Vet Res* **59(6):**686–691.

43 Niemiec BA (2010) Pathology in the pediatric patient. In: *Small Animal Dental, Oral and Maxillofacial Disease: A Color Handbook*. (ed. BA Niemiec) Manson Publishing, London, pp. 89–126.

44 Wiggs RB, Lobprise HB (1997) Pedodontics. In: *Veterinary Dentistry: Principles and Practice*. Lippincott-Raven, Philadelphia, pp. 169–174.

45 Neville BW, Damm DD, Allen CM *et al.* (2002) Abnormalities of teeth. In: *Oral and Maxillofacial Pathology*, 2nd edn. WB Saunders, Philadelphia, pp. 49–106.

46 Harvey CE, Emily PP (1993) Occlusion, occlusive abnormalities, and orthodontic treatment. In: *Small Animal Dentistry*. Mosby, St. Louis, pp. 266–296.

47 Moore JI, Niemiec BA (2014) Evaluation of extraction sites for retained roots in dogs and cats. *J Am Anim Hosp Assoc* **50(2):**77–82.

48 Shipp AD, Fahrenkrug P (1992) *Practitioner's Guide to Veterinary Dentistry*. Dr. Shipps Laboratories, Beverly Hills.

49 Harvey CE, Emily PP (1993) Occlusion, occlusive abnormalities, and orthodontic treatment. In: *Small Animal Dentistry*. Mosby, St. Louis, pp. 266–296.

50 Chamberlain TP, Verstraete FJM (2012) Clinical behavior and management of odontogenic cysts. In: *Oral and Maxillofacial Surgery in Dogs and Cats*. WB Saunders, Philadelphia, pp. 481–486.

51 Verstraete FJ, Zin BP, Kass PH *et al.* (2011) Clinical signs and histologic findings in dogs with odontogenic cysts: 41 cases (1995–2010) *J Am Vet Med Assoc* **239(11):**1470–1476.

52 Babbitt SG, Krakowski Volker M, Luskin IR (2016) Incidence of radiographic cystic lesions associated with unerupted teeth in dogs. *J Vet Dent* **33(4)**:226–233.

53 Baxter CJ (2004) Bilateral mandibular dentigerous cysts in a dog. *J Small Anim Pract* **45**:210–212.

54 Bellezza E, Angeli G, Leonardi L *et al.* (2008) A case of a mandibular dentigerous cyst in a German shepherd dog. *Vet Res Commun* **32(Suppl 1):** S235–237.

55 Ribka EP, Niemiec BA (2016) Diseases of the oral cavity and teeth. In: *Clinical Medicine of the Dog and Cat*, 3rd edn (eds. M Schaer, F Gaschen) CRC Press, Boca Raton, pp. 83–104.

56 Neville BW, Damm DD, Allen CM *et al.* (2002) *Oral and Maxillofacial Pathology*, 2nd edn. WB Saunders, Philadelphia, p. 609.

57 Lopes FM, Gioso MA, Ferro DG *et al.* (2005) Oral fractures in dogs of Brazil: a retrospective study. *J Vet Dent* **22(2)**:86–90.

58 Umphlet RC, Johnson AL (1990) Mandibular fractures in the dog. A retrospective study of 157 cases. *Vet Surg* **19(4):**272–275.

59 Matis M, Kostlin M (2012) Symphyseal separation and fractures involving the incisorve region.

60 DeBowes L (2010) Problems with the gingiva: In: *Small Animal Dental, Oral and Maxillofacial Disease: A Color Handbook*. (ed. BA Niemiec) Manson Publishing, London, pp. 159–181.

61 Verstraete FJM (1999) *Self-Assessment Color Review of Veterinary Dentistry*. Manson Publishing, London, pp. 57–58.

62 Holmstrolm SE, Frost P, Eisner ER (1998) Exodontics. In: *Veterinary Dental Techniques*, 2nd edn. WB Saunders, Philadelphia, pp. 238–242.

63 Blazejewski S, Lewis JR, Reiter AM (2006) Mucoperiosteal flap for extraction of multiple teeth in the maxillary quadrant of the cat. *J Vet Dent* **23(3):**200–205.

64 Verstraete FJ, Terpak CH (1997) Anatomical variation in the dentition of the domestic cat. *J Vet Dent* **14(4):**137–140.

65 Wiggs RB, Lobprise HB (1997) Oral surgery. In: *Veterinary Dentistry: Principles and Practice*. Lippincott–Raven, Philadelphia, pp. 312–377.

66 Holmstrom SE, Bellows J, Colmrey B *et al.* (2005) AAHA dental care guidelines for dogs and cats. *J Am Anim Hosp Assoc* **41**:42–46.

In: *Oral and Maxillofacial Surgery in Dogs and Cats*. WB Saunders, Philadelphia, pp. 265–274.

CHAPTER 3

DENTAL RADIOGRAPHY EQUIPMENT

Brook A. Niemiec

DENTAL RADIOGRAPHY UNITS

Dental radiographs are usually obtained using a wall mounted generator (**Figure 3.1a**).[1-4] Radiographic exposure is controlled by three components: kVp (kilovolt peak), mA (milliamperage), and exposure time. kVp controls the power of each particular x-ray particle, which determines the penetration of the beam through tissues. This equates to the 'quality' of the x-ray beam. The 'quantity' of the radiation is controlled by mA and the time of exposure. The higher the mA, the more x-rays produced over a given time period. The mA multiplied by exposure time determines the total number of x-rays.

There is minimal variation of tissues within the oral cavity, therefore kVP and mA are constant on most dental radiography units. Therefore, the only variable factor is time, which is typically measured in seconds (or parts thereof). Most dental radiography units have a digital control for the exposure, which is set by the operator (**Figure 3.1b**). Recently, however, veterinary-specific machines have become available with a computer setting the exposure based on the size of the patient, the speed of dental film used (or type of digital system), and the particular object tooth. This can take a lot of the guesswork out of the exposure setting. However, with a little experience and practice, it is easy to figure out which setting

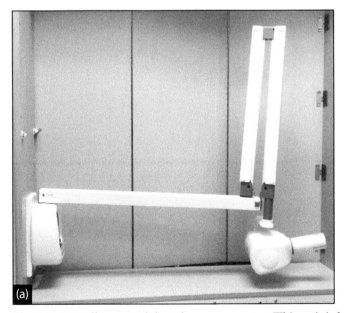

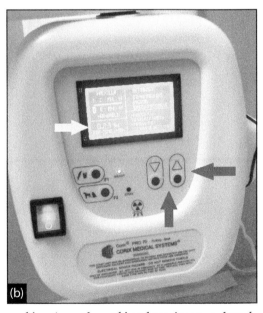

Fig. 3.1 (a) Wall mounted dental x-ray generator. This unit is housed in a 'pass through' and services two dental suites. (b) Control unit for the dental x-ray generator. The buttons on the lower right control the exposure time (red arrows). The 'up' arrow on the right increases the exposure time and darkens the image, whereas the 'down' arrow on the left decreases the exposure time and lightens the image. The LED display shows the exposure time in hundredths of a second (yellow arrow).

to use. Once it has been determined what works for a particular unit, these settings can be recorded to facilitate future radiographs.

DENTAL RADIOGRAPHIC FILM

Dental film is nonscreen, meaning it is directly exposed by the x-ray and does not require an intensifying screen. This provides much more detail than standard radiographic film. It is packaged in its own paper or plastic sleeve, protecting it from light as well as the oral environment (**Figures 3.2a, b**).[1–3,5,6]

There are three types (speeds) of dental film commonly used in dental radiography: 'D', 'E', and 'F'. The difference is the size of the silver halide crystals and subsequent to this the amount of radiation required to create an image. 'E' speed film requires approximately ½ the amount of radiation for exposure than 'D' speed film, and 'F' speed ¼–½ again (70% less than 'D').[7,8] This not only decreases exposure to the patient and

staff, but also decreases the wear and tear on the x-ray unit. There may be a slight decrease in resolution with faster films due to the larger crystal size, but according to most experts, the difference is negligible.[8,9] Therefore, it is recommended in human dentistry to use 'F' speed to decrease exposure time.[10] It is critical to note that different speed films require different safe light colors. Amber filters are used for 'D' speed films and red is correct for 'E' and 'F' speeds.[4,11]

There are several different sizes of dental film available (4, 3, 2, 1, and 0) (**Figure 3.2c**). The most common sizes used in veterinary medicine are 4, 2, and 1. Size 4 film (57 × 76 mm) is the largest available. It is used for full-mouth radiographs (especially large breed dogs) as well as major maxillofacial disease (jaw fractures and neoplasia) and extraoral images in cats. Size 4 films are fairly expensive compared with size 2 (about five times as much) so smaller films should be used when possible. Size 2 (31 × 41 mm) is the most commonly used film size for single tooth radiographs.

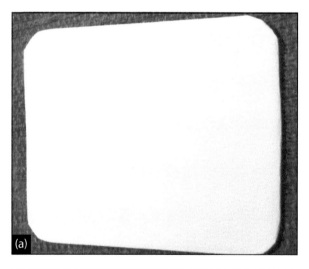

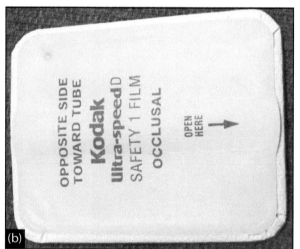

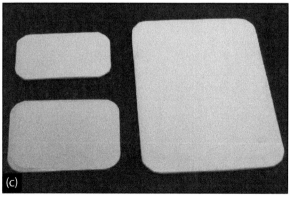

Fig. 3.2 **Dental radiographic film. (a) The front side of the film is white. This side faces the tube head. (b) The back side is colored (green in this case, but purple and other colors are possible). This side is placed away from the tube head. (c) Dental radiographic film of various sizes. Counterclockwise from top: size 1, size 2, size 4.**

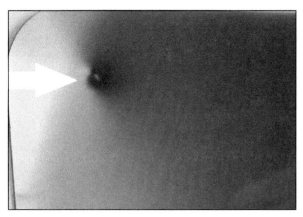

Fig. 3.3 Developed film showing the convex surface of the embossed dot (arrow). This helps to orient the film.

However, a size 4 film is required to image the canine teeth of large breed dogs as they cannot be completely imaged on a size 2 film. Size 1 (24 × 40 mm) or size 0 (22 × 35 mm) are used for small dogs and cats, especially for mandibular views.

All dental films have an embossed dot on their surface to help orient the film (**Figure 3.3**). Because of the lead backing, the convex surface of the dot *must* face the tube head. This allows the practitioner to orient the films (see Chapter 8 for a complete discussion of film orientation).

DIGITAL DENTAL RADIOGRAPHY

Digital dental radiography[12] is standard practice in human dentistry in North America and is quickly becoming so in Europe as well as in veterinary practices in both North America and Europe. Exposure techniques for digital systems are very similar to those used for standard dental radiographs, with a few minor variations. This section will cover the physics of digital radiography, the advantages (and disadvantages) of digital systems versus analog film, and the minor adjustments needed for its use. Finally, the chapter will cover the differences between the various digital radiography systems (sensor-based radiography [DR] versus photostimulable phosphor plates [CR]).

Note: There is no true definition of semidirect digital radiography. In whole-body radiography, photostimulable phosphor (PSP) plate systems (CR) are typically termed 'indirect', whereas in dental radiography semidirect generally refers to PSP. In this chapter, DR systems will be referred to as 'direct', CR as 'semidirect', and digitized analog films as 'indirect'.

The physics and technology of digital radiography
Indirect digital radiographs[13,14]
These are standard film or 'analog' radiographs that have been digitized. Ideally, this is performed by scanning with a flatbed or slide scanner. However, an easy and inexpensive way to accomplish this is to take a picture with a high-quality digital camera with a effective macro setting. This obviously requires that an analog film be exposed first, but it is an inexpensive way to experience several of the advantages of digital radiography (such as archiving and telemedicine), which are detailed below. The raw images do not match the quality of either standard digital or analog films.[15] However, if they are further digitally processed, the quality can increase significantly.[16]

Technique
This is ideally performed on a dry film, but if time is of the essence, a wet film can be used (and repeated on dry films later). Place the film on a dental radiograph viewer with the embossed dot facing out. This orients the films in the same way as other dental radiography systems (labial mounting). The light should be blocked on all sides to improve resolution. For practices that do this on a regular basis, creating a permanent mount that keeps the light out of the edges is beneficial (**Figure 3.4**). The room should be fairly dark. Place the camera in macro mode and focus just on the radiograph (**Figure 3.5**). Ideally, use a tripod for stabilization. After photographing all the radiographs desired, download and store them in a folder for the patient. Ideally, the individual images are named for each tooth/dental arch. However, if the labial mounting covenant is maintained, the teeth that are imaged can be determined just like standard digital systems (see Chapter 8). For further instructions on creating digitized radiographs, visit www.vetdentalrad.com.

True digital systems
There are two major types of true digital systems: semidirect and direct.[12,16]

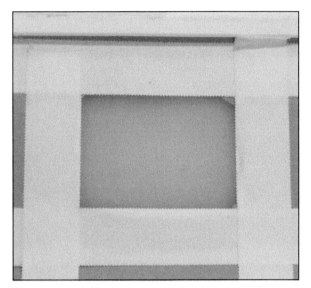

Fig. 3.4 **Dental x-ray viewer with a customized 'frame' to keep out light.**

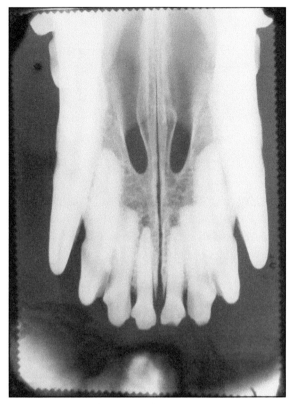

Fig. 3.5 **A properly mounted radiograph.**

Fig. 3.6 **The blank 'front' of a size 4 photostimulable phosphor plate, which faces the tube head.**

Semidirect systems

Semidirect systems utilize a PSP plate, which is covered with phosphor crystals that (temporarily) store the x-ray photon energy (**Figure 3.6**). Storage time can range from minutes to hours depending on how the plate is handled and/or stored. The plates must not be exposed to bright light prior to scanning, as this will degrade the image. Following exposure of the plate, it is removed from the patient's mouth and scanned with a near-red wavelength laser beam (**Figure 3.7**). Scanning produces an electronic 'message' of the image. This information is then sent

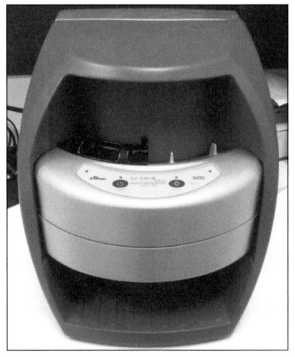

Fig. 3.7 **Photostimulable phosphor plate scanner.**

to a computer via a USB cable for processing and image creation.

When an image is scanned, some (but not all) of the energy in the plate is lost. This is valuable as an image that is overexposed can be made diagnostic by repeated scannings, depending on the system used. Once the image has been scanned, it can be 'erased' by exposure to a bright visible light. However, many current systems will automatically erase the image after scanning so that the plate is readily available for reuse.

Direct digital systems

Direct digital systems employ solid state sensors (**Figure 3.8**). The two major types of solid state sensors are CCD (charge-coupled device) and CMOS (complementary metal oxide semiconductor). These systems convert the energy from x-ray photons hitting the sensor into electronic signals. A scintillation layer is placed on top of the sensor in order to turn x-ray photons into light photons, which are subsequently absorbed by the chip. This is technologically similar to the intensifying screens used with analog films. The information is then transferred to a computer via a USB cable or Bluetooth.

Creation of the digital image

Regardless of the type of digital system, images are created in a similar fashion (**Figure 3.9**). The plates/sensors measure the intensity of the photons following passage through the oral tissues. The various energies are typically measured on a 256 unit gray scale. In this system, 0 corresponds to the maximum

measurable radiation (or black), and 255 corresponds to no exposure (or white).

These intensity measurements are performed over an array of very small regions of the sensor and are called pixels (which stands for picture element). The resolution of a digital dental image is determined by the pixels, specifically:

- Size.
- Number.
- Color depth.

Each pixel is 15–40 square micrometers (µm) in size. This means that there are thousands of pixels on a size 2 sensor. After the intensity is measured, the score of each individual pixel is transferred to the computer for image creation. The computer assigns a gray scale value to each pixel and places it in the correct location. Thus, the computer generates the diagnostic radiographic image one pixel at a time. The resultant file is termed the 'raw' image.

Software programs have the ability to manipulate this numerical information, thus changing the appearance of the image. This manipulation is performed by subjecting the information to mathematical procedures called *algorithms*. Algorithms range from quite simple to very complicated. An example of a simple algorithm is reversing the gray scale (white becomes black) to create a 'negative'. However, there are more complicated algorithms available, which improve contours or contrast and can even adjust an image that is over- or underexposed. These changes can be done manually; however, all systems have

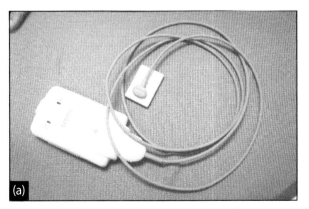
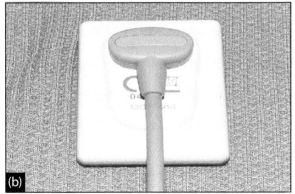

Fig. 3.8 **A digital radiography sensor. (a) The sensor and USB cable. (b) The back of the sensor where the cord enters. This faces away from the tube head.**

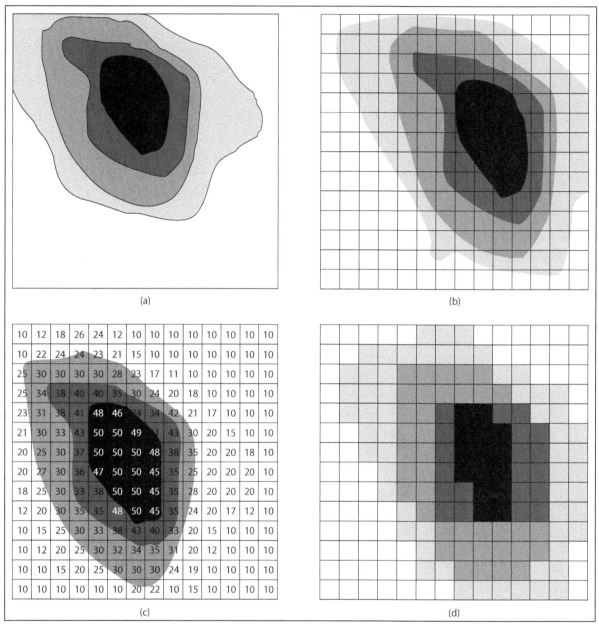

Fig. 3.9 How a digital image is created by a computer using radiology software, beginning with the x-ray shadow (a); image detected by the digital sensor where each square equals a pixel (b); numerical representation of the pixels sent to the computer (c); the digital image transferred to the computer screen (d). (Adapted from Niemiec BA (2007) Digital dental radiography. *J Vet Dent* (3):192–197.)

the ability to 'optimize' the image automatically. Algorithms are responsible for much of the differences in the appearance of the images between manufacturers. In many cases, the raw image is very similar but the algorithm gives it a different appearance. Systems are often purchased due to the perceived quality of the image, regardless of any true diagnostic difference. In fact, images may actually appear superior, even though they have a lower diagnostic quality. For a comparison of raw images produced by various sensors, visit www.vetdentalrad.com and click on 'sensor shootout'.

CR versus DR images

Numerous studies have compared DR images with CR produced images. The majority of these studies report that DR systems may have a higher resolution.[17-19] These same studies report, however, that PSP plate systems will produce quality images over a wider exposure range (see below).[17,19,20] In contrast, one study reported that PSP plates had superior image quality to solid state (DR) images.[20] The 2008 and 2010 sensor shootouts[21] showed that the PSP plate system compared favorably with the sensor systems. Finally, a good technique for determining the quality of the digital system is to compare line pairs.

Advantages of digital radiography[12,22-26]

The main advantages of *digital* radiography are reduced exposure and decreased anesthesia time. With DR technology, the image is available in seconds. Additionally, since the image is produced while the sensor and tube head are still in place, minor technique adjustments can be performed without starting over again.

Digital images are more valuable than analog films for several reasons. First, the large size of the image projected on the computer screen combined with the ability to manipulate the image allows for easier interpretation.[27] Additionally, a large computer screen allows much easier discussions with clients, and the ability to 'mark' the images further facilitates client communication. This can be used as a very effective marketing tool, gaining acceptance and approval for treatment recommendations.

Digital images are permanent (if properly stored) and therefore do not degrade over time. It is very common for analog films to fade or darken, especially if not properly fixed or rinsed. The use of toxic chemicals is avoided, as well as the trouble and expense of proper disposal. Digital images save storage space in the clinic and staff time searching for previous films. Digital images can be quickly uploaded to telemedicine sites or e-mailed to specialists for consultation. DR sensors have an additional advantage of requiring far less radiographic exposure than standard film, which, as stated by the ALARA (As Low As Reasonably Achievable) principle, is good for our patients and staff. It should be noted, however, that one study (admittedly older) actually showed an increase in exposure with a digital system using a dosimeter.[28]

The scanning of the CR phosphor plates takes about 10 seconds, and the plate must be removed from the patient's mouth. This negates some of the speed advantage, but the availability of larger plates (size 4 and even larger) can make up for this shortcoming. Experienced practitioners can actually be faster with CR systems, but for the novice, the ease of retakes with DR shortens the learning curve. This makes DR systems usually a better choice for practitioners who are initially learning to be proficient with dental radiography. That said, PSP plates have an increased latitude of exposure more than either DR or standard film, which limits retakes for experienced practitioners.

Disadvantages of digital radiography

The main argument against digital radiographs is that they provide less detail than standard radiographic film.[29-33] This is controversial at this time as other studies report similar quality, with the difference depending on several factors.[25,34-37] When general image quality is studied, digital radiographs are typically rated inferior to standard film. However, some studies report that digital images are overall superior to standard film.[38] Additionally, when particular pathology or procedural aspects are studied, digital images can be superior to plain film. Improvements in computer monitors, as well as image manipulation (enhancement), have significantly improved the quality of digital images. At this point, they are considered at least equal to and in some instances superior to standard film.[39-42] The one point of agreement in almost every study is that enhanced images are superior to the raw images.[37,42,43] Furthermore, when digital systems are compared with analog film, less exposure errors are created.[42,44]

The biggest drawback to DR systems is the lack of a size 4 sensor plate.[12] This is mostly a problem in large breed dogs, as some teeth (canines and carnassials) cannot be completely imaged on one film. In addition, exposing full-mouth radiographs in large and giant breed dogs requires significantly more exposures.

Another concern with DR sensors is the cost of replacement if they get damaged. Warrantees cover some types of damage, but drops and dog bites are typically excluded. Therefore, sensors must be handled very carefully. In fact, this author recommends that dental radiography only be performed on pets under general anesthesia with an endotracheal tube, which makes it difficult for the sensor to be damaged even if the patient is 'light' enough to bite down. Using this protocol, a sensor lasted over a decade in this author's practice.

Most DR sensors have a very narrow exposure range to create an acceptable image, which may increase the need for retakes. There is one exception (Sopix® 2 DR Intraoral Digital System), which is a DR system with a wide latitude of exposure, but it is still recommended to use the lowest possible exposure setting.

The advantages of a CR system negate many of these negative issues. First, these systems have size 4 plates (and some have even larger) and the individual plates cost less than $100 (in the USA) (smaller sizes are less). Therefore, replacement of damaged plates is not a huge expense. It is important to note that these plates do 'wear out' faster than direct digital systems and can easily be scratched, which means they will require more frequent replacement.

The major concern with CR systems is that their optimum radiographic exposure is higher than Ektaspeed film. In addition, the wide latitude of dose levels allows a diagnostic radiograph to be created with exceedingly high exposure. Practitioners must be very careful to use the lowest possible setting. Only in this way is the ALARA principle satisfied.

An additional disadvantage with all digital radiography is the initial set-up cost. Over time, however, the savings in film and development costs (not to mention staff time) will more than pay for the system. The only other disadvantage to digital systems is the need for consistent back-up of the computer information. If a computer fails, the information could be lost. Therefore, back up to a mirrored hard drive, flash drive, DVD, or, preferably, a web-based storage location is mandatory.

Differences between standard and digital radiographic techniques[12]

The most obvious difference in technique between DR and standard radiography is the decrease in radiation exposure necessary to create the image. Therefore, it is important that the x-ray generator is 'modern', as older models may not have a digital setting. This may require the purchase of a new generator. Furthermore, DR utilizes only four to five different settings between cats and the largest dog, whereas CR has a similar exposure range to that of analog films.

The lack of a true embossed dot makes determining right versus left slightly different. However, all systems still have an indicator of placement direction on the image. In addition, all digital systems utilize labial mounting, which means the image is oriented so that your vision comes from the same direction as the beam. Most systems also have a template where the image can be placed, thus permanently identifying the image.

In order to image the maxillary fourth premolar in a large breed dog with a size 2 digital sensor utilizing the distal tube shift technique, the sensor must be moved mesially on the tooth. This is because the change in projection angle will image the mesial roots over the third premolar. Therefore, the distal edge of the sensor must be set just at the distal edge of the target tooth to capture all three roots in their entirety. Finally, when using a size 2 sensor, the entire tooth (especially canines of large breed dogs) cannot be fully imaged with one exposure. Therefore, two images must be taken if an image of the crown is required.

The other major difference with DR systems is that the decreased exposure time makes a large difference with the distance between the tube head and the sensor. A few millimeters of movement away from the sensor can require an increase in the exposure time.

RECOMMENDATIONS[12]

Standard (analog) film is certainly still acceptable for intraoral dental radiography. It is of similar quality to digital images and is initially much less expensive. Therefore, it is still a great way to get started with dental radiography. However, over time, the cost of film, chemicals, and staff time will exceed the initial savings.

For most general practices considering dental radiography, a size 2 DR sensor is the best choice. It is generally faster than PSP plate or standard film systems, and this is especially true when inexperienced technicians are taking images, as retakes are much faster with a sensor because it does not need to be removed from the mouth. For more skilled technicians, size 4 (and 5) PSP plates can actually make full-mouth radiographs faster (especially in large breed dogs). Feline only practices would benefit from a size 1 or 0 sensor, as the smaller sizes better fit the feline anatomy. However, this size does not work for extraoral radiography of the temporomandibular joint.

Any practice can benefit from the variations in size offered by CR systems, but those practices performing major maxillofacial surgery (jaw fractures and oral oncologic surgery) benefit greatly from the larger images available from these systems. Furthermore, mixed practices with equine patients should consider a CR system, especially those that can take even larger films than a size 4. Finally, size 4 plates are excellent for small mammal and reptile full-body radiographs. If you are still unsure which system is best for your practice, a prepurchase consult with the dental radiographic equipment supplier can be extremely valuable (www.vetdentalrad.com).

A final thought to consider when purchasing a digital dental system is your computer monitor. The fine resolution, depth of color, and algorithms in high-end digital dental systems are likely not appreciated on inexpensive monitors. This is particularly true of laptop computer screens, which are used in many clinics. It is important to purchase a monitor that supports your investment.

CONCLUSION

Digital dental radiography is quickly becoming the standard practice of veterinary dentistry. While analog films are certainly acceptable, digital systems are more efficient and permanent, typically require less radiation exposure, utilize no toxic chemicals, allow for easy telemedicine consultations, and over time will prove less expensive than standard radiographs. In addition, numerous studies looking at many parameters have shown that digital images are at least equal to, if not superior, to standard film. Finally, the technique differences between analog and digital systems are minimal, allowing for an easy transition.

REFERENCES

1 Woodward TM (2009) Dental radiology. *Top Companion Anim Med* **24(1):**20–36.
2 Niemiec BA, Sabitino D, Gilbert T (2004) Equipment and basic geometry of dental radiography. *J Vet Dent* **21:**48–52.
3 Niemiec BA (2010) Veterinary dental radiology. In: *Small Animal Dental, Oral and Maxillofacial Disease: A Color Handbook*. (ed. BA Niemiec) Manson Publishing, London, pp. 63–87.
4 Bellows J (2008) Dental radiography. In: *Small Animal Dental Equipment, Materials, and Technique: A Primer*. Wiley-Blackwell, Ames, pp. 63–104.
5 Mulligan TW, Aller MS, Williams CA (1998) Basic equipment needs. In: *Atlas of Canine and Feline Dental Radiology*. Veterinary Learning Systems, Trenton, pp. 7–14.
6 Bellows J (2010) Radiology. In: *Feline Dentistry: Oral Assessment, Treatment, and Preventative Care*. Wiley-Blackwell, Ames, pp. 39–83.
7 Geist JR, Brand JW (2001) Sensitometric comparison of speed group E and F dental radiographic films. *Dentomaxillofac Radiol* **30(3):**147–152.
8 Farman TT, Farman AG (2000) Evaluation of a new F speed dental X-ray film. The effect of processing solutions and a comparison with D and E speed films. *Dentomaxillofac Radiol* **29(1):**41–45.
9 Ludlow JB, Platin E (1995) Densitometric comparisons of Ultra-speed, Ektaspeed, and Ektaspeed Plus intraoral films for two processing conditions. *Oral Surg Oral Med Oral Pathol Oral Radiol Endod* **79(1):**105–113.
10 Dental Radiography: Doses and Film Speed: Radiation Emiting Products: www.FDA.org accessed April 2014.
11 Niemiec BA, Sabitino D, Gilbert T (2004) Developing dental radiographs. *J Vet Dent* **21(2):**116–121.
12 Niemiec BA (2007) Digital dental radiography. *J Vet Dent* **24(3):**192–197.

13 Malleshi SN, Mahima VG, Raina A *et al*. (2013) A subjective assessment of perceived clarity of indirect digital images and processed digital images with conventional intra-oral periapical radiographs. *J Clin Diagn Res* **7(8)**:1793–1796.

14 Versteeg CH, Sanderink GC, van der Stelt PF (1997) Efficacy of digital intra-oral radiography in clinical dentistry. *J Dent* **25(3–4)**:215–224.

15 Goga R, Chandler NP, Love RM (2004) Clarity and diagnostic quality of digitized conventional intraoral radiographs. *Dentomaxillofac Radiol* **33(2)**:103–107.

16 Ajmal M, Elshinawy MI (2014) Subjective image quality comparison between two digital dental radiographic systems and conventional dental film. *Saudi Dent J* **26(4)**:145–150.

17 Borg E (1999) Some characteristics of solid-state and photo-stimulable phosphor detectors for intra-oral radiography. *Swed Dent J* **Suppl.139**:i–viii, 1–67.

18 Borg E, Attaelmanan A, Gröndahl HG (2000) Subjective image quality of solid-state and photostimulable phosphor systems for digital intra-oral radiography. *Dentomaxillofac Radiol* **29(2)**:70–75.

19 Bóscolo FN, Oliveira AE, Almeida SM *et al*. (2001) Clinical study of the sensitivity and dynamic range of three digital systems, E-speed film and digitized film. *Braz Dent J* **12(3)**:191–195.

20 Farrier SL, Drage NA, Newcombe RG *et al*. (2009) A comparative study of image quality and radiation exposure for dental radiographs produced using a charge-coupled device and a phosphor plate system. *Int Endod J* **42(10)**:900–907.

21 www.vetdentalrad.com

22 van der Stelt PF (2005) Filmless imaging: the uses of digital radiography in dental practice. *J Am Dent Assoc* **136(10)**:1379–1387.

23 van der Stelt PF (2008) Better imaging: the advantages of digital radiography. *J Am Dent Assoc* **139 Suppl**:7S–13S.

24 van der Stelt PF (1992) Improved diagnosis with digital radiography. *Curr Opin Dent* **2**:1–6.

25 Farman AG, Farman TT (1999) RVG-ui: a sensor to rival direct-exposure intra-oral x-ray film. *Int J Comput Dent* **2(3)**:183–196.

26 Hayakawa Y, Shibuya H, Ota Y *et al*. (1997) Radiation dosage reduction in general dental practice using digital intraoral radiographic systems. *Bull Tokyo Dent Coll* **38(1)**:21–25.

27 Gröndahl K (1987) Computer-assisted subtraction radiography in periodontal diagnosis. *Swed Dent J Suppl* **50**:1–44.

28 Jones GA, Schuman NJ, Woods MA (1998) Estimated skin exposure as an indicator for comparing radiovisiography (RVG) versus conventional Ektaspeed Plus dental radiography. *J Clin Pediatr Dent* **22(2)**:121–123.

29 Versteeg KH, Sanderink GC, Velders XL *et al*. (1997) In vivo study of approximal caries depth on storage phosphor plate images compared with dental x-ray film. *Oral Surg Oral Med Oral Pathol Oral Radiol Endod* **84(2)**:210–213.

30 Hintze H, Wenzel A, Frydenberg M (2002) Accuracy of caries detection with four storage phosphor systems and E-speed radiographs. *Dentomaxillofac Radiol* **31(3)**:170–175.

31 Bhaskaran V, Qualtrough AJ, Rushton VE *et al*. (2005) A laboratory comparison of three imaging systems for image quality and radiation exposure characteristics. *Int Endod J* **38(9)**:645–652.

32 Ludlow J, Mol A (2001) Image-receptor performance: a comparison of Trophy RVG UI sensor and Kodak Ektaspeed Plus film. *Oral Surg Oral Med Oral Pathol Oral Radiol Endod* **91(1)**:109–119.

33 Sanderink GC, Huiskens R, van der Stelt PF *et al*. (1994) Image quality of direct digital intraoral x-ray sensors in assessing root canal length. The RadioVisioGraphy, Visualix/VIXA, Sens-A-Ray, and Flash Dent systems compared with Ektaspeed films. *Oral Surg Oral Med Oral Pathol* **78(1)**:125–132.

34 Wenzel A (2000) Digital imaging for dental caries. *Dent Clin North Am* **44(2)**:319–338.

35 Vandre RH, Pajak JC, Abdel-Nabi H *et al*. (2000) Comparison of observer performance in determining the position of endodontic files with physical measures in the evaluation of dental X-ray imaging systems. *Dentomaxillofac Radiol* **29(4)**:216–222.

36 Eikenberg S, Vandre R (2000) Comparison of digital dental X-ray systems with self-developing film and manual processing for endodontic file length determination. *J Endod* **26(2)**:65–67.

37 Woolhiser GA, Brand JW, Hoen MM *et al*. (2005) Accuracy of film-based, digital, and enhanced digital images for endodontic length determination. *Oral Surg Oral Med Oral Pathol Oral Radiol Endod* **99(4)**:499–504.

38 Kondylidou-Sidira A, Fardi A, Giannopoulou M *et al*. (2013) Detection of experimentally induced root fractures on digital and conventional radiographs: an in vitro study. *Odontology* **101(1)**:89–95.

39 Crombie K, Parker ME, Nortje CJ *et al.* (2009) Comparing the performance of storage phosphor plate and Insight film images for the detection of proximal caries depth. *SADJ* **64(10):**452, 454–456, 458–459.

40 Shokri A, Mortazavi H, Salemi F *et al.* (2013) Diagnosis of simulated external root resorption using conventional intraoral film radiography, CCD, PSP, and CBCT: a comparison study. *Biomed J* **36(1):**18–22.

41 Shintaku WH, Venturin JS, Noujeim M *et al.* (2013) Comparison between intraoral indirect and conventional film-based imaging for the detection of dental root fractures: an ex vivo study. *Dent Traumatol* **29(6):**445–449.

42 Yoshiura K, Kawazu T, Chikui T *et al.* (1999) Assessment of image quality in dental radiography, part 2: optimum exposure conditions for detection of small mass changes in 6 intraoral radiography systems. *Oral Surg Oral Med Oral Pathol Oral Radiol Endod* **87(1):**123–129.

43 de Oliveira ML, Pinto GC, Ambrosano GM *et al.* (2012) Effect of combined digital imaging parameters on endodontic file measurements. *J Endod* **38(10):**1404–1407.

44 Zhang W, Huynh CP, Abramovitch K et al. (2012) Comparison of technique errors of intraoral radiographs taken on film v photostimulable phosphor (PSP) plates. *Tex Dent J* **129(6):**589–596.

CHAPTER 4

DENTAL RADIOGRAPHIC POSITIONING

Brook A. Niemiec

INTRODUCTION

Getting started in dental radiography can seem a daunting task, but with a little training and practice, radiography becomes fun and easy. For example, instead of measuring the bisecting angle for every radiograph, you can quickly approximate them by using the simplified technique. The following is an introduction into the exposure techniques for intraoral radiography. Further training via hands-on laboratories as well as utilization of telemedicine services can be immensely beneficial and greatly decrease the learning curve. (For a list of Hands-on Wet Laboratories, see Appendix.)

STEP 1: PATIENT POSITIONING

Position the patient so that the area of interest is convenient to the radiographic beam. In general, this is where the dental arch to be imaged is 'up'.

When imaging the mandibular canines and incisors, the patient should be in dorsal recumbency (**Figures 4.1a, b**). For mandibular cheek teeth, the patient can stay in dorsal recumbency or be placed in lateral recumbency with the side to be imaged up.

Positioning for maxillary teeth is controversial, with some veterinary dentists recommending sternal and others lateral recumbency. It is easier to visualize angles in sternal recumbency, so for the initial survey this *may* be beneficial. However, rolling patients into sternal recumbency for intra- and/or postoperative images is somewhat arduous and time-consuming. In addition, this typically displaces the monitoring (e.g. ECG) leads, adding time to the procedure. Finally, it can be traumatic to the spine of older pets as well as the hips of large breed dogs. For these reasons, in this author's practice virtually all maxillary radiographs are exposed with the patient still mostly in dorsal recumbency, with the head gently turned laterally (**Figures 4.1c, d**). This takes

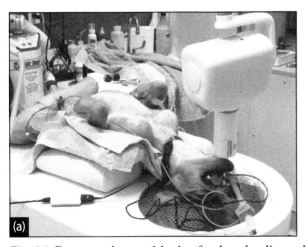
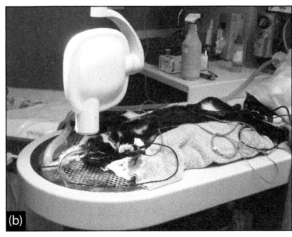

Fig. 4.1 **Proper patient positioning for dental radiographs. (a, b) A canine (a) and feline (b) patient in dorsal recumbency. This position is ideal for all rostral mandibular views (incisors, canines, mesial premolars). The remainder of the mandibular cheek teeth can also be imaged in this position.** *(Continued)*

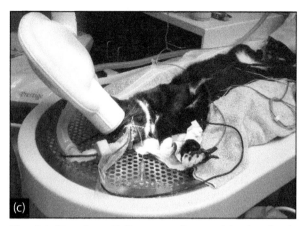

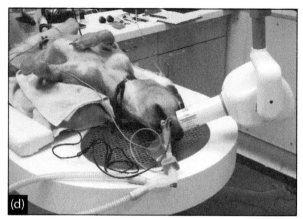

Fig. 4.1 *(Continued)* **Proper patient positioning for dental radiographs. (c, d) A feline (c) and canine (d) in dorsal recumbency with the head gently rolled laterally. All maxillary cheek teeth can easily be imaged in this position (as well as mandibular cheek teeth). Taking radiographs in this position is much more convenient and avoids rolling the patient.**

some getting used to, but decreases the number of times a patient must be rolled during surgery.

STEP 2: FILM PLACEMENT WITHIN THE PATIENT'S MOUTH[1-6]

When utilizing standard film, there is an embossed dot on the film that can be felt as a dimple on one side of the film packet (**Figure 4.2**). The side with the dimple should be placed towards the x-ray beam.

In most films, this side is pure white and the opposite or 'back' side of the film is colored. In addition, the dot should be positioned away from the structures to be imaged to avoid interference.

For digital radiography (DR) sensors, the cord will exit on the 'back' side of the sensor and this side goes away from the tube head (**Figures 4.3a, b**). For photostimulable phosphor (PSP) plates, the side with writing goes away from the tube head with the blank side towards the tube head (**Figures 4.3c, d**).

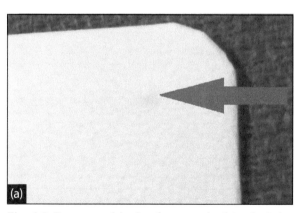

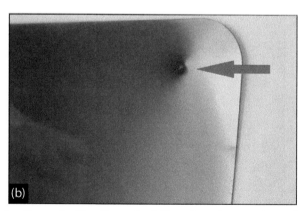

Fig. 4.2 **Proper positioning for a standard (analog) dental radiograph. On all standard film, there is an embossed dot on the film. This is shown on the packaging (a) and on a developed film (b) (arrows). The convex side of this dot *must* point out towards the x-ray beam to make a diagnostic image. This dot helps orient the film for interpretation (see Chapter 8, Part A). The white (or front) side of the film is placed towards the tube head and the colored (or back) side placed away from the tube head.**

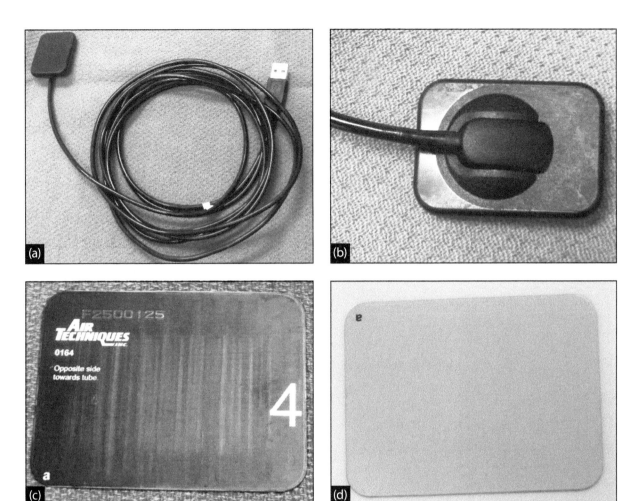

Fig. 4.3 Digital dental radiography. (a, b) A digital radiography sensor. The sensor is directly connected to the computer, which gives almost instantaneous images. Image (a) shows the USB cable as well as the flat 'front' side of the sensor. Image (b) demonstrates where the USB cable enters the 'back' side of the sensor. The back side faces away from the tube head. (c, d) Size 4 photostimulable phosphor plate from the back (c) and front (d). The side without the writing is placed towards the tube head.

Furthermore, some systems have an arrow, which simulates the dot.

The film should be placed as near as possible to (generally touching) the teeth and oral mucosa to minimize distortion (**Figure 4.4a**). Position the film/sensor/plate in the mouth so that the entire tooth (crown and entire root surface) is covered by the film/sensor (if possible). If coverage of the entire tooth is not possible with a size 2 sensor (which is common in large breed dogs), it is recommended to:

1 Position the sensor apically enough to expose the apex of the tooth and 3 mm beyond (**Figure 4.4b**). This will cut off the crown, but the crown often itself does not typically provide critical information that cannot be seen clinically.
2 Expose two images (one of root and one of crown).

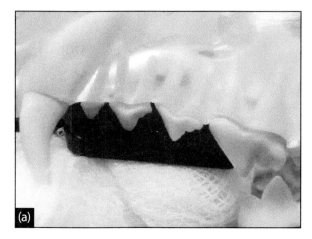

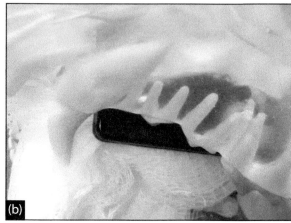

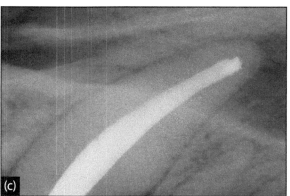

Fig. 4.4 **Placement of the film/sensor in the patient's mouth. (a) The sensor should be placed as close as possible to the objects being imaged. This is generally touching the teeth/soft tissue. The root is the most important area of the tooth to evaluate. Therefore, make sure that the sensor is placed apically enough to image the entire root and at least 3 millimeters beyond. For a maxillary canine, the sensor must be placed back at least to the mesial root of the third premolar (b) to image the apex of the root (c).**

STEP 3: POSITIONING THE TUBE HEAD[1–10]

There are two major techniques for positioning the tube head in veterinary patients, both of which are used daily.

Parallel technique
This is where the film is placed parallel to the object being radiographed and the beam placed perpendicular to both the film/sensor and the tooth/root (object) (**Figure 4.5**). This is how the majority of standard (large) films are taken and gives the most accurate image. Unfortunately, this is only useful in the mandibular cheek teeth (and not even all of them). The maxillary teeth cannot be imaged in this way due to the fact that dogs and cats do not have an arched palate. In addition, the symphysis interferes with parallel placement for the canines and incisors as well as the rostral mandibular premolars (P3 in cats and P1 and 2 in dogs). Therefore, the film/

sensor cannot be placed parallel to the tooth roots in these areas.

Bisecting angle technique
This is the most commonly used technique in veterinary dental radiography, and uses the theory of equilateral triangles to create an image that accurately represents the tooth and roots. To utilize this technique, the film is placed as parallel as possible to the tooth root. Next, the angle between the tooth root and film is measured/estimated. This angle is cut in half (bisected) and the beam placed perpendicular to the bisecting line. This gives the most accurate representation of the root.

To visualize this technique, place the sensor/film as close to parallel as possible to the tooth roots. Then place cotton tipped applicators parallel to the film and tooth roots. (**Note:** It is imperative to use the roots and not the crowns to determine the bisecting angle, as they may not be the same.

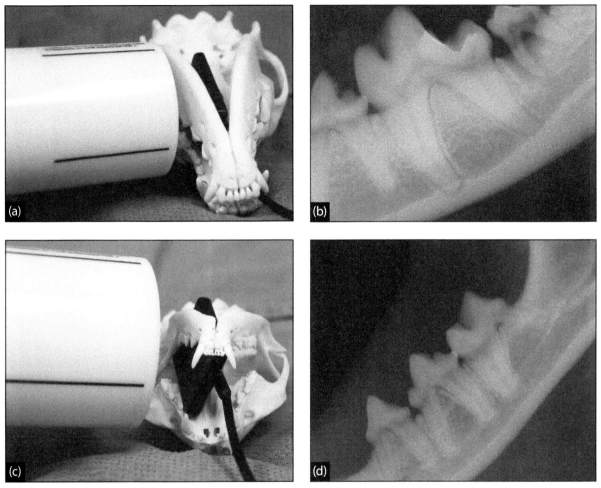

Fig. 4.5 **The parallel technique. This technique will provide the most accurate images, but is only useful for the mandibular cheek teeth. These figures demonstrate the proper placement of the sensor and tube head for the mandibular premolar and molar teeth in a canine (a, b) and a feline (c, d) patient. The patient is in dorsal recumbancy and the sensor is placed parallel to the tooth and tooth roots (a, c). The tube head is then positioned perpendicular (90 degrees) to the sensor. This will produce an excellent image of the target tooth (b, d). Note that the apex of the mesial root of the third premolar is cut off in this image. If this occurs (which is common), a bisecting angle radiograph is necessary (see Fig. 4.12).**

This is especially true of the canines and incisors [see Simplified technique, below]). Then position a third applicator halfway between these two; this is the 'bisecting' line. The tube head is positioned perpendicular to the third cotton tipped applicator (**Figure 4.6**). This is the most scientifically correct way to image veterinary patients, but is very cumbersome and time-consuming.

If the angle is incorrect, the radiographic image will be distorted. This is because the x-ray beam will create an image that is longer or shorter than the object imaged. The best way to visualize this is to think of a building and the sun. The building will create a 90-degree (right) angle to the ground. The bisecting angle in this case is 45 degrees to the ground. Early and late in the day, the sun is at an acute angle to the ground and casts a long shadow (**Figures 4.7a, b**). In radiography, this occurs when the angle of the beam to the sensor/film is too small, and is known as elongation. At some point in the late

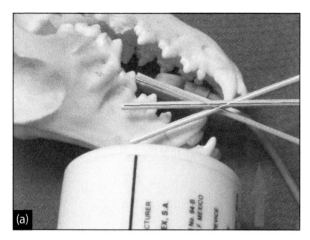

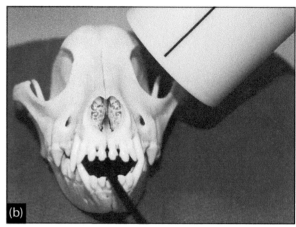

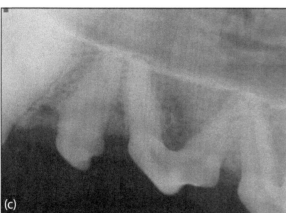

Fig. 4.6 The bisecting angle technique. This is the traditional and most scientifically correct method for imaging most teeth in dogs and cats; however, it is cumbersome. (a) Following film placement, the correct angle for the tube head is determined/measured using cotton tipped applicators. The first applicator is placed parallel to the sensor (blue line) and the second parallel to the tooth root (white line). (Note: It is important to use the root and not the crown as the angle may be different [e.g. canine and incisor teeth]). Measure the angle between these two applicators and place the third applicator at an angle half-way between the first two (red line). This is the bisecting angle and the tube head is placed perpendicular to this third applicator (arrow). (b) Proper bisecting angle for the maxillary premolars in a dog. (c) Resultant image, which correctly approximates the size of the roots.

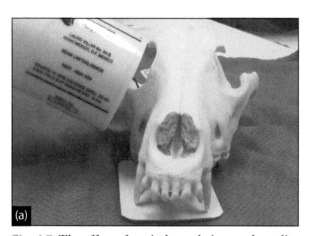

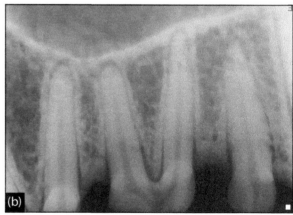

Fig. 4.7 The effect of vertical angulation on the radiographic appearance of the maxillary premolars. (a) The radiograph is exposed with the tube head too parallel to the film/sensor. This creates longer roots (b) and in radiography is called *elongation*. (Continued)

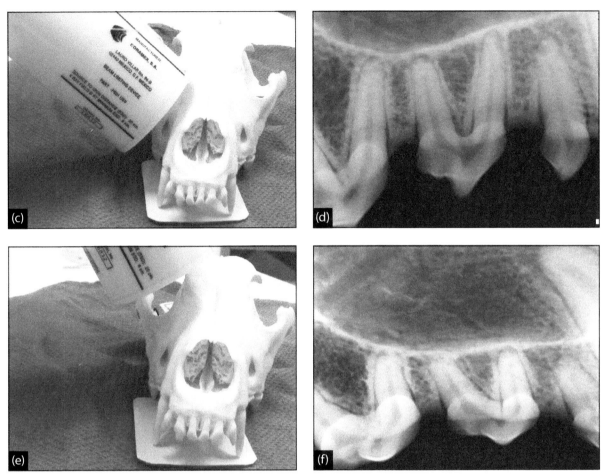

Fig. 4.7 *(Continued)* **The effect of vertical angulation on the radiographic appearance of the maxillary premolars. (c) This is the proper (45-degree) angle for imaging these teeth. The roots are the correct length and the image is of excellent diagnostic quality (d). (e) This radiograph is exposed with the tube head too perpendicular to the sensor. This creates shorter roots (f) and in radiology is called *foreshortening*.**

morning and early afternoon, the sun is at a 45-degree angle to the building, which is the bisecting angle. This produces a shadow that is an accurate representation of the building height (**Figures 4.7b, c**). As the sun continues up in the sky, the shadow shortens. This occurs in veterinary radiography when the angle of the tube head to the sensor/film is too great and the resultant distortion of the image is known as foreshortening (**Figures 4.7d, e**). Finally, at noon, the sun is straight above the building, which does not produce a shadow.

Simplified technique

The 'simplified technique' as developed by Dr. Tony Woodward,[2,11] does not utilize direct measurement of any angle, instead relying on approximate angles to create diagnostic images for almost every tooth. There are only three angles used for all radiographs in this system: 20, 45, and 90.

As above, the mandibular premolars and molars are exposed with the beam at a 90-degree angle (parallel) (**Figure 4.8**). The maxillary premolars and molars have roots that are typically straight up from

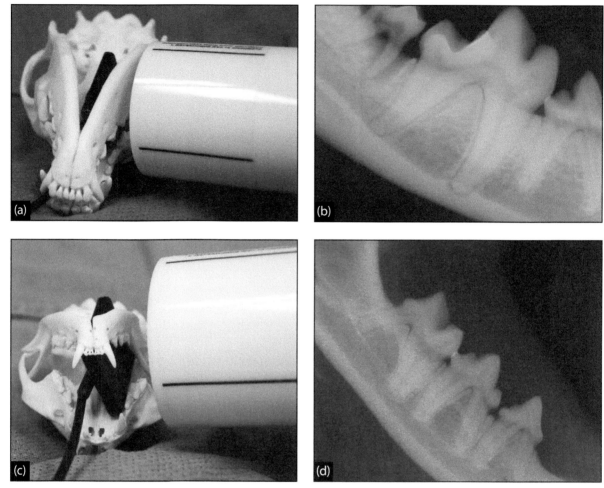

Fig. 4.8 The simplified technique for imaging the mandibular premolars and molars in a canine (a, b) and feline (c, d) patient. The patient is in dorsal recumbency and the sensor is placed parallel to the tooth and tooth roots (a, c). The tube head is then positioned 90 degrees (perpendicular) to the sensor, which produces a quality image of the target tooth (b, d).

the crowns and the sensor is essentially flat across the palate, creating an approximate 90-degree angle. Therefore, they are imaged at a 45-degree angle (**Figure 4.9**). Canines and incisors curve backward significantly (approaching a 40-degree angle to the palate) and are thus imaged with a 20 (or 70)-degree angle rostrocaudal (**Figure 4.10**).

To initiate any radiograph, place the film in the mouth and set the positioning indication device (PID) perpendicular to the film. For mandibular cheek teeth, this is the correct placement. For the maxillary premolars and molars, rotate the beam laterally to a 45-degree angle. For the incisors and mandibular

canines rotate the beam rostrally 20 degrees (to achieve the 70-degree angle to the sensor).

There are four conditions where this technique may not be sufficient.

Maxillary canines[2,12,13]

The roots of the maxillary canines are directly dorsal to the maxillary first and second premolars in dogs and the second and occasionally third premolar in cats. Therefore, an additional rotation to 20 degrees lateral is necessary to avoid superimposition with these teeth, and imaging the root over the nasal cavity, which is mostly air (**Figure 4.11**).

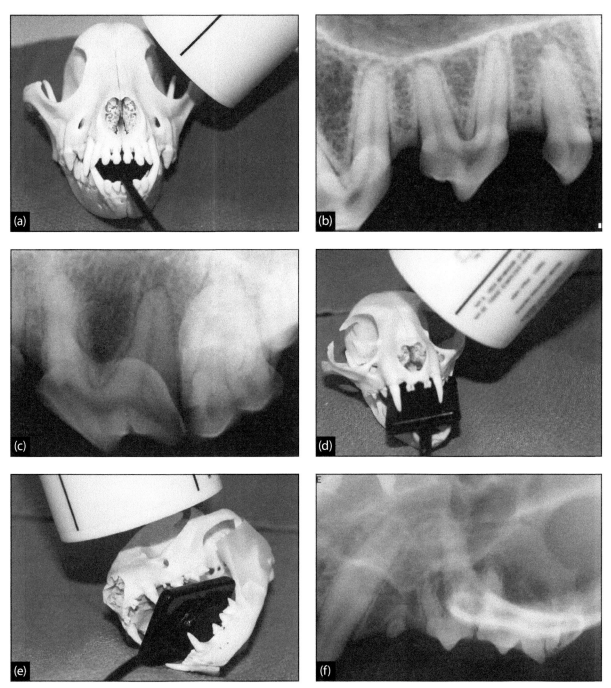

Fig. 4.9 The simplified technique for imaging the maxillary premolars and molars in a canine (a, b, c) and a feline patient (d, e, f). The patient is placed in dorsal (a, d) or lateral (e) recumbency and the sensor is placed essentially parallel to the palate. The tube head is then positioned at a 45-degree angle to the sensor, which produces quality images of the target teeth (b, c, f). Note that the mesial roots of P4 are superimposed with this image. To split these roots, the beam will need to be angled in the horizontal plane (see Figs 4.15, 4.16).

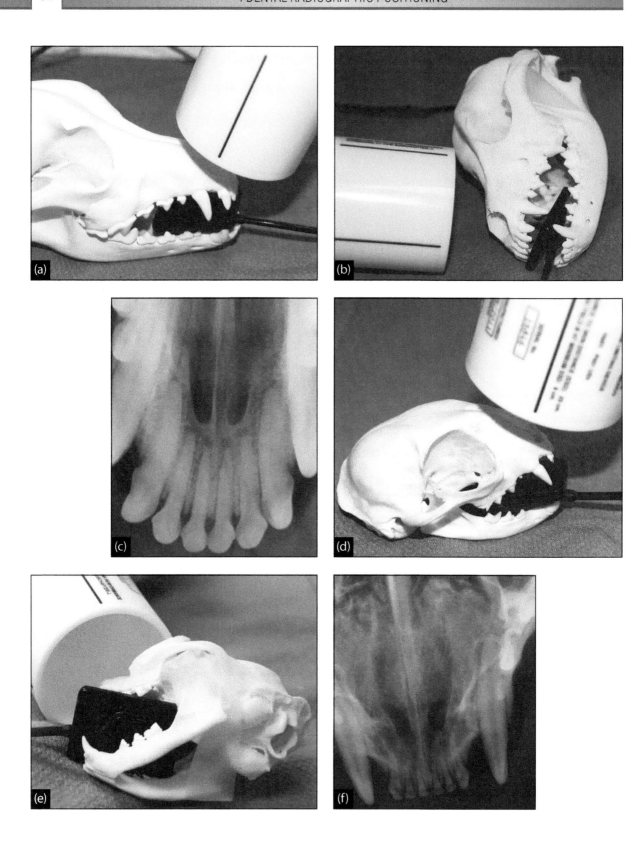

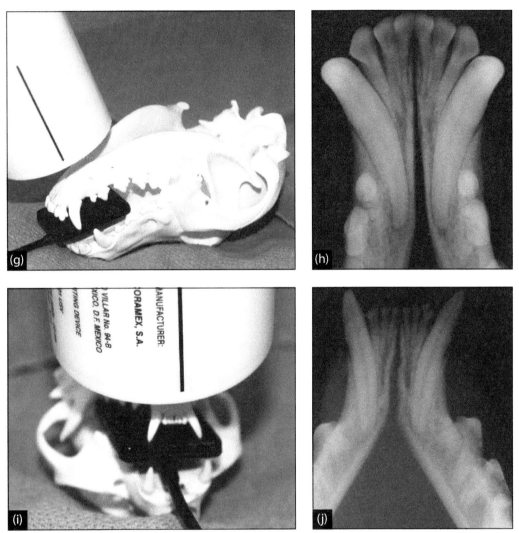

Fig. 4.10 The simplified technique for imaging the incisors and mandibular canines demonstrated using a canine and a feline skull. The patient is placed in sternal (a, d) or lateral (b, e) recumbency for the maxillary incisors and dorsal recumbency (g, i) for the mandibular dorsal incisors and canines. The sensor is placed essentially parallel to the palate or gingiva. The tube head is then positioned 70 degrees to the sensor, which produces a quality image of the target teeth (canine maxillary incisors [c], feline maxillary incisors [f], canine [h] and feline [j] mandibular canines and incisors. Note that in large breed dogs, when using size 2 sensors, separate images of the canines and incisors may be necessary.

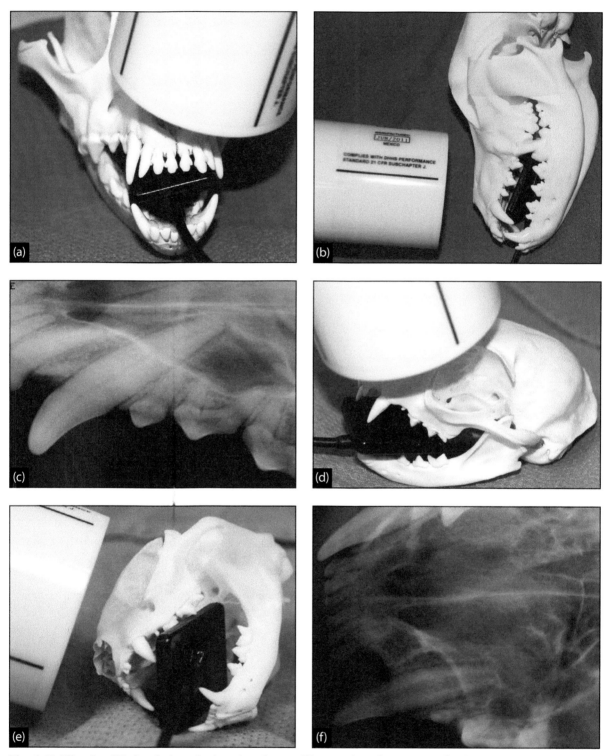

Fig. 4.11 The simplified technique for imaging the maxillary canines demonstrated using a canine (a–c) and a feline (d–f) skull. The patient is placed in sternal (a, d) or lateral (b, e) recumbency. The sensor is placed essentially parallel to the palate. The tube head is then positioned 70 degrees to the sensor in the vertical plane and 20–30 degrees lateral, which produces a quality image of the target teeth (c, f).

Rostral mandibular premolars (first and second in dogs and third in cats)[2,7,9]

The apices of these teeth are often cut off on films using the parallel technique. This is because the symphysis interferes with the placement of the film ventrally enough to image the roots. On occasion, this can be alleviated by simply rotating the tube head slightly ventrally, which will mildly foreshorten the radiograph. If this is not sufficient to image the apices, using the bisecting angle is necessary. To perform this technique, place the film/sensor in position for the canines/incisors and the tube head 45 degrees laterally (**Figure 4.12**).

Maxillary cheek teeth in cats[2,7,9]

The zygomatic arch may interfere with good visualization of the maxillary third and fourth premolars as well as the first molar with the standard intraoral bisecting angle technique (**Figure 4.9f**). This author feels that this does not significantly affect interpretation, but if the practitioner wishes to view these teeth without interference, the *extraoral technique* can be utilized. Place the film/sensor on the table and the patient's head on the sensor with the dental arch to be imaged down. Place a radiolucent mouth gag to gently hold the jaws apart. The beam is angled through the mouth to create a

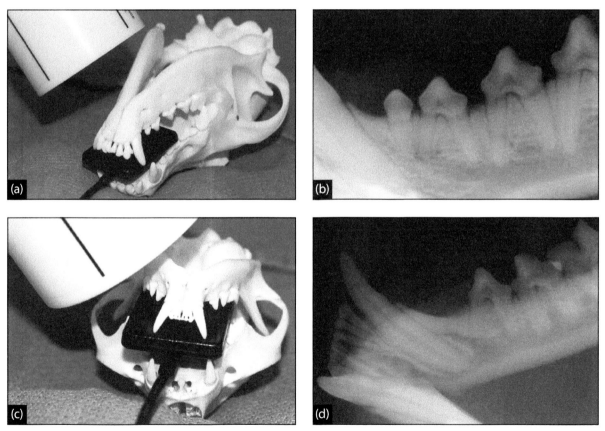

Fig. 4.12 Imaging the mesial premolars. Due to the interference of the mandibular symphysis, imaging the mesial (P1 and 2 in dogs [a, b] and P3 in cats [c, d]) premolars can be challenging. Using the bisecting angle can produce quality images of these teeth. The patient is placed in dorsal recumbency and the film/sensor is placed parallel to the gingiva, just like imaging of the mandibular canines. The beam is then placed on a 45-degree angle laterally to create the correct bisecting angle (a, c). This will create a diagnostic image of the mesial premolars (b, d).

bisecting angle, which is approximately 30 degrees (**Figure 4.13**). Remember that because this image was created extraorally, it must be labelled accordingly. This is important because it will appear to be the opposite dental arch if interpreted as an intraoral image (see Chapter 8, Part A).

The *near parallel technique* will also eliminate zygomatic arch interference. To create images with this technique, place the sensor/film across the mouth, resting it on the palatal aspect of the contralateral maxillary teeth and the lingual aspect of the ipsilateral mandibular cheek. Then place the beam almost parallel to the sensor (**Figures 4.14a, b**). This will result in an image that is less distorted than the extraoral image and also does not create confusion with regard to which side was imaged (**Figure 4.14c**).

Mesial roots of the maxillary fourth premolar[2,8]

The straight lateral 45-degree bisecting angle will give a good representation of the mesial roots but they will be superimposed (**Figure 4.9b**). If the practitioner wishes to view these roots separately, an additional angle is necessary in most cases.

This is the most difficult radiographic technique, as two precise angles are necessary to create a proper image. To split the mesial roots of a maxillary fourth premolar, the tube head (or PID) must be angled in the *horizontal* plane. This can either be in the mesial or distal direction and is called the *tube shift technique*. To perform this technique, start with the tube head in position for the straight lateral image (i.e. 45 degrees in the vertical plane). Then rotate it approximately 30 degrees in the horizontal plane. This can be done either distally or mesially. Once the roots are split, it is imperative to know which root is which. The classic way of determining the mesiobuccal root from the mesiopalatal root is to determine it via the SLOB technique (Same Lingual/Opposite Buccal).[3,10] This means that the root that is more lingual (or palatal) will be imaged in the same direction as the tube is shifted and the buccal root will be imaged in the opposite direction. Therefore, with a distal tube shift, the palatal root will move caudally in comparison to the buccal root. With a mesial tube shift, the palatal root will move rostral in relation to the buccal root.

However, there is a much simpler way to determine which root is which. If the tube head has been shifted mesially, the distal root of the fourth premolar will often be imaged over the first molar. In this case the buccal root is in the middle (**Figure 4.15**). When the tube head is shifted distally, the distal root is well

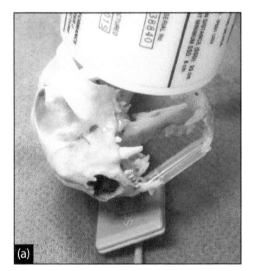

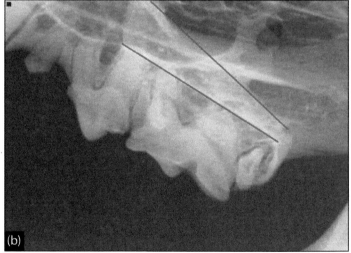

Fig. 4.13 Extraoral technique in cats for removing the zygomatic arch from the tooth roots of the maxillary cheek teeth. (a) Place the film/sensor on the table and the patient's head on the sensor with the dental arch to be imaged down. Place a radiolucent mouth gag to gently hold the jaws apart. The beam is angled through the mouth to create a bisecting angle, which is approximately 30 degrees. (b) The resultant image allows the maxillary premolars and molar to be viewed without zygomatic arch (red lines) interference.

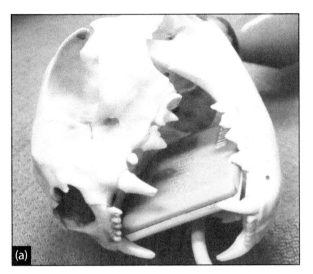

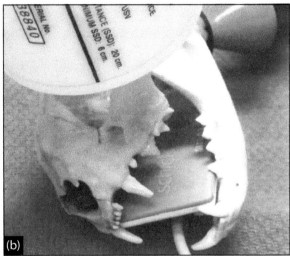

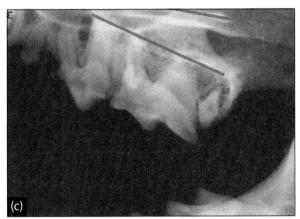

Fig. 4.14 Near parallel technique for removing the zygomatic arch from the tooth roots of the maxillary cheek teeth in cats. The patient is placed in lateral recumbency with the target teeth 'up'. The sensor/film is placed across the mouth resting on the palatal aspect of the contralateral maxillary teeth and the lingual aspect of the ipsilateral mandibular cheek. (a) The beam is positioned almost parallel to the sensor. (b) This will result in an image without zygomatic arch interference (red lines), which is less distorted than an extraoral image and does not create confusion with which side was imaged (c).

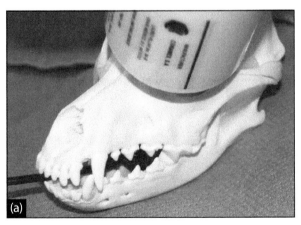

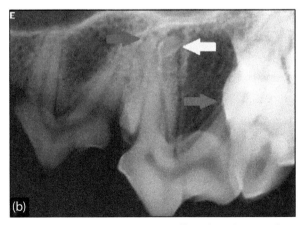

Fig. 4.15 The simplified approach to splitting and identifying the mesial roots of the maxillary fourth premolar in dogs: mesial tube shift technique. To initiate this technique, start with the sensor and tube head positioned for the standard bisecting angle technique (the tube head is 45 degrees in the vertical plane to the sensor). The tube head is then shifted mesially (a). When this is done, the distal root of the fourth premolar will often be imaged over the first molar (red arrow) (b). In this image, the buccal root is in the middle (yellow arrow) and the palatine root is in front (blue arrow).

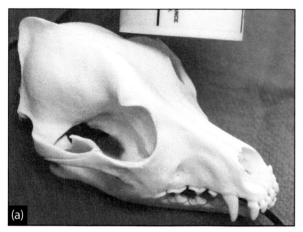
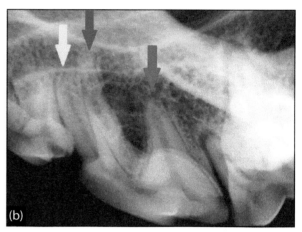

Fig. 4.16 The simplified approach to splitting and identifying the mesial roots of the maxillary fourth premolar in dogs: distal tube shift technique. To perform this technique, start with the sensor and tube head positioned for the standard bisecting angle technique (the tube head is 45 degrees in the vertical plane to the sensor). The tube head is then shifted distally (a). When the tube head is shifted distally, the distal root is well visualized away from the first molar (red arrow), and the palatal root is in the middle (blue arrow) and the buccal root in front (yellow arrow) (b).

visualized away from the first molar, and the palatal root is in the middle (**Figure 4.16**). Since the whole tooth cannot be effectively evaluated with the mesial tube shift technique, it is recommended that only the distal tube shift technique is used, thus creating a quality image of the entire tooth. **Note:** When using this technique, if the distal root is imaged well, the palatal root is in the middle.

This author has noticed that many technicians (nurses) have a particularly challenging time obtaining quality images of the maxillary P4. This is due to the zygomatic arch bulging out facially. When imaging P1–P3, the tube head is placed perpendicular to the muzzle, which is correct (**Figure 4.17a**). However, when progressing to P4, the zygomatic arch 'leads' the operator into the mesial tube shift technique, which conceals the distal root of the maxillary P4 over the first molar (**Figure 4.17b**). When correct, this accentuates the shift towards the nose of the patient (**Figure 4.16**).

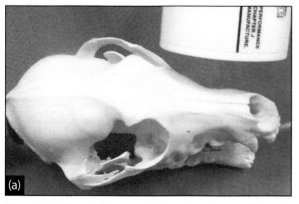
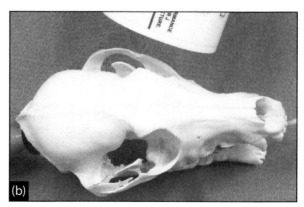

Fig. 4.17 The challenge with imaging the maxillary fourth premolar. (a) When imaging the maxillary first three premolars the tube head is placed perpendicular to the long axis of the face, which is correct. (b) However, due to the zygomatic arch bulge, the 'face' is no longer parallel to the roots. Therefore, when the beam is placed parallel to the 'face' the tube head is in position for the *mesial tubeshift technique*, which obscures the distal root over the first molar. Therefore, the zygomatic arch 'leads' the operator into the mesial tube shift technique.

STEP 4: SETTING THE EXPOSURE[1,2]

If using a machine that requires manually setting the exposure, the correct setting will need to be pre-determined. For cats there is generally one setting for the maxilla and one for the mandible, which are easily determined. For dogs, there are about five settings that are typically used. However, the vast variability in radiographic systems as well as film make creating a general technique chart impossible. The exposure time is controlled by an 'up' arrow and a 'down' arrow. This will adjust the time.

Appropriate settings can be developed after working with a few patients. If utilizing a computer controlled digital system (**Figure 4.18**), the buttons are set according to the species, film/digital system, and tooth to be imaged. Again, these settings are guidelines and minor adjustments are usually still necessary. For experienced practitioners, settings based on time are generally best.

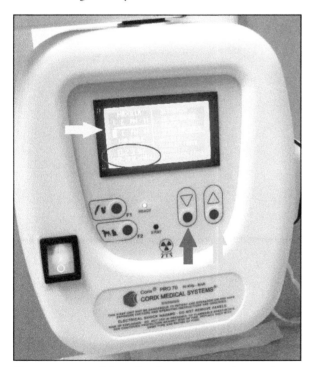

Fig. 4.18 **Typical dental radiography machine. The 'down' button (blue arrow) decreases exposure and the 'up' button (green arrow) increases exposure. The exposure time is displayed on the computer screen (red circle). The tooth that is to be imaged can also be predetermined (yellow arrow).**

STEP 5: EXPOSING THE RADIOGRAPH[1,2]

Dental radiography machines have a hand-held switch to expose the radiograph. It is best to leave the room prior to exposing the radiograph to avoid radiation exposure. Ideally, there is a 'doorbell' button placed outside the dental operatory to facilitate this. Alternatively, the operator can stand at least 2 meters (6 feet) away at a 90 to 130-degree angle to the primary beam to limit radiation exposure. It is important to remember that these switches are 'dead man's' style, which means if you let up during the exposure, it stops the production of x-ray beams. When this occurs, the unit will give an error message and the operator will have to reset the computer settings and press the switch again. Therefore, it is important to hold the button down until the machine stops beeping.

REFERENCES

1 Niemiec BA, Sabitino D, Gilbert T (2004) Equipment and basic geometry of dental radiography. *J Vet Dent* **21**:48–52.

2 Niemiec BA (2010) Veterinary dental radiology. In: *Small Animal Dental, Oral and Maxillofacial Disease: A Color Handbook.* (ed. BA Niemiec) Manson Publishing, London, pp. 63–87.

3 Mulligan TW, Aller MS, Williams CA (1998) Intraoral imaging techniques. In: *Atlas of Canine and Feline Dental Radiology.* Veterinary Learning Systems, Trenton, pp. 27–44.

4 Holmstrom SE, Frost P, Eisner ER (1998) Dental radiology. In: *Veterinary Dental Techniques*, 2nd edn. WB Saunders, Philadelphia, pp. 107–133.

5 Wiggs RB, Lobprise HB (1997) Dental and oral radiology. In: *Veterinary Dentistry: Principles and Practice.* Lippincott-Raven, Philadelphia, pp. 140–166.

6 Oakes A (2000) Introduction: radiology techniques. In: *An Atlas of Veterinary Dental Radiology.* (eds. DH DeForge, BH Colmery) Iowa State University Press, Ames, pp. xxi–xxiv.

7 Niemiec BA, Furman R (2004) Feline dental radiography. *J Vet Dent* **21(4)**:252–257.

8 Niemiec BA, Furman R (2004) Canine dental radiography. *J Vet Dent* **21(3)**:186–190.

9 Bellows J (2010) Radiology. In: *Feline Dentistry: Oral Assesment, Treatment, and Preventative Care.* Wiley-Blackwell, Ames, pp. 39–83.

10 Bellows J (2008) Dental radiography. In: *Small Animal Dental Equipment, Materials, and Technique: A Primer*. Wiley-Blackwell, Ames, pp. 63–104.

11 Woodward TM (2009) Dental radiology. *Top Companion Anim Med* **24(1):**20–36.

12 Gracis M (1999) Radiographic study of the maxillary canine tooth of four mesaticephalic cats. *J Vet Dent* **16:**115–128.

13 Gracis M, Harvey CE (1998) Radiographic study of the maxillary canine tooth in mesaticephalic dogs. *J Vet Dent* **15(2):**73–78.

CHAPTER 5

SKULL AND DENTAL RADIOGRAPHY USING MEDICAL X-RAY TECHNIQUES

Jerzy Gawor

INTRODUCTION

The term 'dental radiography' does not refer to the generator of the x-ray beam (dental or medical) or to the equipment/technology used to capture the image (digital or analog film). It is focused on oral and maxillofacial structures and utilizes intraoral and extraoral techniques. Because dental and maxillofacial structures are small, proper diagnosis and therapy depends on the resolution and quality of the radiographs. Numerous oral anatomic structures overlap, therefore dental radiography is also very technique sensitive. Slight differences in radiographic quality or positioning can significantly affect the diagnostic quality of the image. Therefore, it is important to have access to high resolution technology and create high-quality radiographs using both proper positioning and exposure (**Figures 5.1, 5.2**).

The aim of this chapter is to discuss the importance of obtaining proper skull radiographs and the possibility of producing diagnostic images of oral and maxillofacial structures with the use of nondental equipment.

Despite the fact that dental radiography is very important, most veterinary practices do not have this technology. The x-ray generator generally used is a medical machine. For dental purposes, it is always better to use a dental x-ray machine; however, diagnostic images can be produced with the use of medical x-ray machines and film/plates. When radiographing small objects (e.g. toes) or patients (e.g. small rodents), a dental x-ray machine may be utilized (**Figures 5.3, 5.4**). The major differences

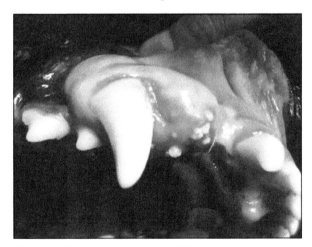

Fig. 5.1 **Clinical appearance of a hamartoma (compound odontoma) in a dog.**

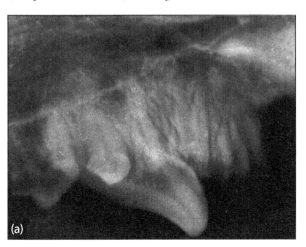

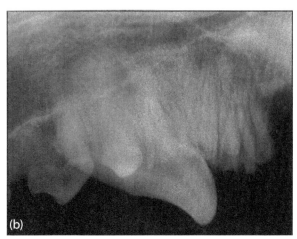

(a)

(b)

Fig. 5.2 **Intraoral radiograph of the hamartoma in Fig. 5.1. (a) Standard film in cassette; (b) dental film.**

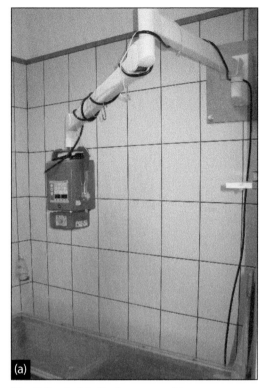

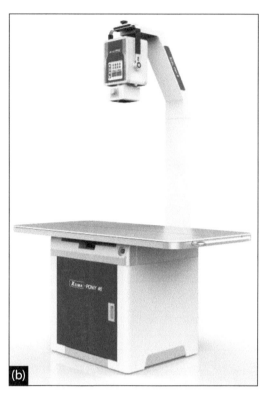

Fig. 5.3a, b Medical x-ray machines.

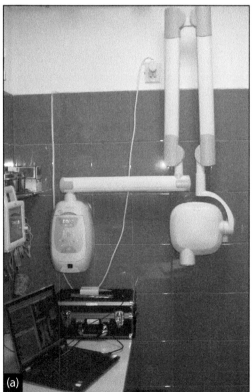

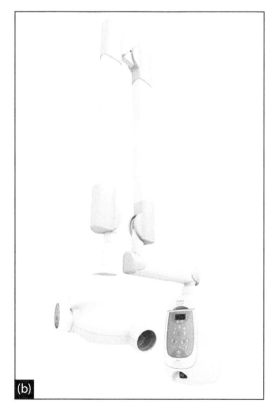

Fig. 5.4a, b Dental x-ray machines.

between dental and medical x-ray machines are listed in *Table 5.1*.

To obtain high-quality skull radiographs, positioning of the head and the rest of the body must be ideal. Therefore, patient positioning devices are necessary for appropriate placement of the body and head. Cassettes used for medical images limit their intraoral use to certain parts of the mandibles and maxillae. However, with precise extraoral positioning it is possible to obtain an image of the entire area of interest. The differences between cassettes, films, photostimulable phosphor plates, and sensors are shown in *Table 5.2*.

As the number of clinics offering CT scans increases and the value of such technology is proven, many specialists will begin offering 3D imaging. If CT/MRI is not available within the practice, standard radiographs should be performed rather that referring the patient immediately. It is important to begin the diagnostic plan with skull radiographs in the following clinical situations:

- Emergency: after head trauma when an overview is necessary to create the final diagnostic and treatment plan. It is particularly important in unconscious patients with visible head injuries to estimate the severity of the trauma (**Figure 5.5**).

Table 5.1 **Major differences between dental and medical x-ray machines**

FEATURE	DENTAL X-RAY MACHINE	MEDICAL X-RAY MACHINE
Possible applications	Limited to small areas to be radiographed intraorally and extraorally. Also for small exotic animals	More universal
Settings	Limited. Most of the parameters are fixed so that the machine can be utilized specifically for dental purposes. Not possible to set conditions other than time of exposure	Wide range of settings, which require adjusting each time for radiographed area
Head mobility	Adjustable	Fixed in most cases
Focus film distance	Limits how close the tube head can be but not how far away	Adjustable
Safety	Reduced scatter, collimation, 2 meters (6 feet) distance required	More scatter. Structural barriers often required
Positioning	Easy due to mobile parts of the machine	Often requires positioning devices

Table 5.2 **Differences between cassettes, films, photostimulable phosphor (PSP) plates, and sensors**

FEATURE	CASSETTES	DENTAL FILM	SENSORS	PSP PLATES
Screen	Yes	No	No	No
Resolution	Low, except mammography film	Highest, depending on the speed of the film (A to F)	High	High
Interpreting	Easier when image is digital	Requires magnification and negatoscope	Easy, depending on software and screen	Easy, depending on software and screen
Format	To large to apply intraorally	Sizes 0, 1, 2, and 4	Sizes 1 and 2	Sizes 1, 2, 3, 4, 4C, and 5, plus a specific rabbit format
Flexibility	None, except mammography films in flexible cassettes	Yes	None	Yes
Care	Cleaning	Disposal	Disposal sleeves required	Disposable sleeves required
Storage and care	Out of x-ray room	Temperature sensitive	Straight cables, shock sensitive	Delicate surface, sleeves required
Development time and conditions	Dark room or scanners: 1–5 minutes	Chairside darkroom, numerous conditions affecting quality: 2–5 minutes	Quick transmission: 2–4 seconds	Scanner: 0.2–1 minute time

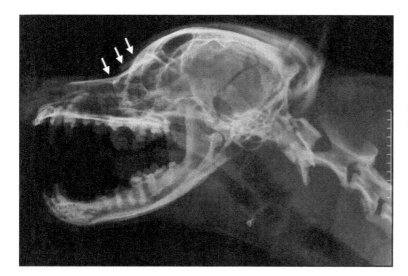

Fig. 5.5 Lateral extraoral projection in an unconscious dog after a car accident, revealing severe head injuries including fractures of the cranium (palatine bone). Additional fractures are visible at the frontal/nasal/maxillary bone (arrows). (Courtesy Dr Katarzyna Jodkowska.)

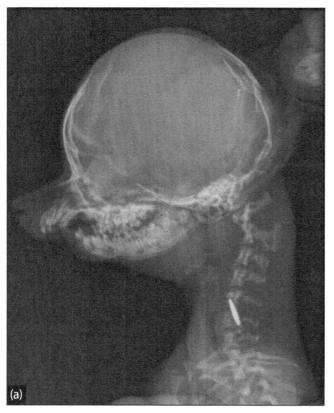

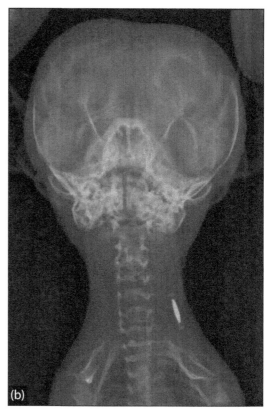

Fig. 5.6a, b Radiographs of a puppy affected by hydrocephalus. Note the ratio of cranium to the face and the presence of large and wide 'molera' (unfused fontanelle) occurring on the top of the head where the parietal and frontal bones should come together. In this puppy, the mandible had been shifted caudally, causing severe distocclusion due to significant enlargement of the cranium.

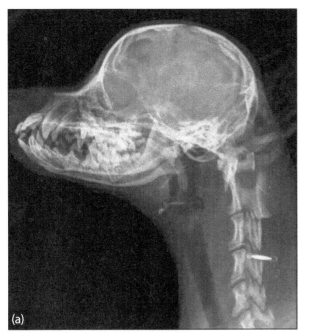 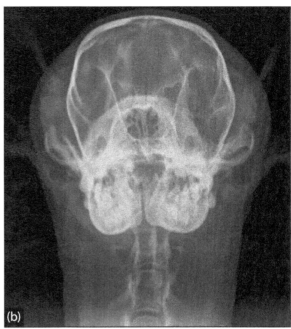

Fig. 5.7a, b Radiographs of a normal puppy of similar size to the puppy in Fig. 5.6.

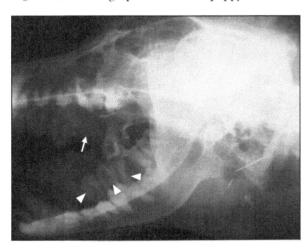

Fig. 5.8 Radiopaque foreign body (broken needle) in the throat area. Additional findings on this radiograph are: missing maxillary fourth premolar tooth (arrow), resorption in ipsilateral mandibular premolars three and four as well as in the mesial root of the first mandibular tooth (arrowheads). Because the sides were not assigned while exposing the radiograph, it is impossible to define them radiographically; however, the missing maxillary fourth premolar can act as the landmark.

- Generalized problems affecting larger anatomic regions (**Figures 5.6–5.7**).
- Suspicion and/or confirmation of presence of foreign bodies (**Figure 5.8**).
- Prior to 3D imaging to predefine areas of interest (**Figure 5.9**).
- Any skeletal deformities and defects present in the oral cavity and maxillofacial part of the head (**Figure 5.10**).

- Cephalometric and orthodontic assessment to evaluate skull symmetry in dogs and cats (**Figure 5.11**).
- As part of the diagnostic plan for orofacial pain, masticatory muscle disorders, malfunction of the temporomandibular joint (TMJ), and nasal problems (**Figure 5.12**).
- In small mammals it is standard to obtain entire skull radiographs (see Chapter 9).

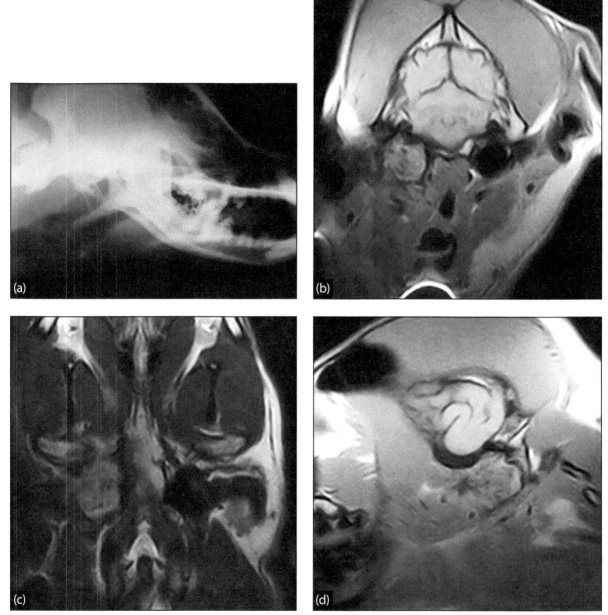

Fig. 5.9 A Golden retriever with pain on yawning and eating. (a) Radiograph taken with a regular x-ray system reveals radiopacity in the area of the right tympanic bulla. There was no crepitation on temporomandibular joint (TMJ) manipulation. (b) MR image of the TMJ area and tympanic bullae showing a mass filling the right bulla. It can be seen that the lesion is affecting the TMJ. The degree of involvement was only appreciated on the horizontal projection (c) not on the lateral projection (d). Biopsy and histhopathology diagnosed squamous cell carcinoma.

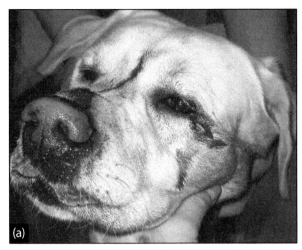

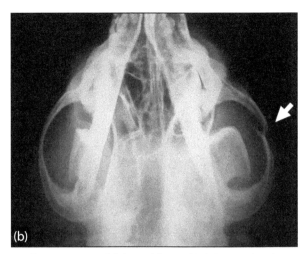

Fig. 5.10 (a) Wound and swelling of the left periorbital area after a motor vehicle accident. (b) A DV projection radiograph revealed a fracture of the zygomatic arch (arrow).

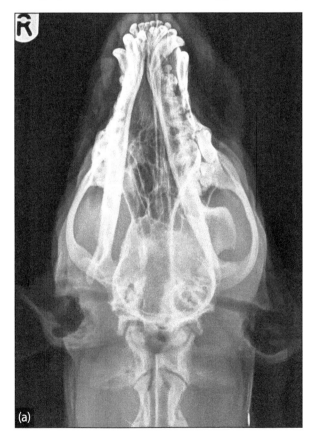

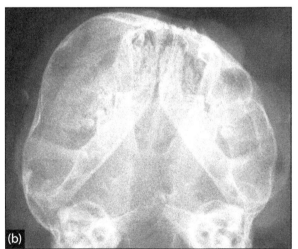

Fig. 5.11 VD (a) and DV (b) projections of the head confirming skeletal malocclusion caused by significant asymmetry in position, orientation, shape, and length of the mandibles in a dog (a) and significant skull asymmetry in a longhaired cat (b). The head of the animal was positioned as ideally as possible in both cases. Due to the asymmetry of the skull the ideal positioning was not achievable.

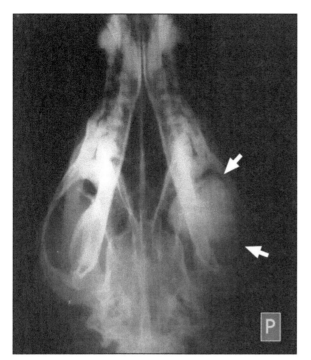

Fig. 5.12 **DV radiograph of a dog with exophthalmos and an inability to open its mouth. A radiopaque mass is present at the caudal part of right mandible (arrows).**

PROJECTIONS AND VIEWS OF THE HEAD

Ventrodorsal and dorsoventral projections

Whether to use a ventrodorsal (VD) or a dorsoventral (DV) projection will depend on which part (dorsal or ventral) of the head is to be imaged (**Figure 5.13**). According to the fundamental rules of radiography, the area of interest should be as close as possible to the film/sensor.[1] The body should be in sternal recumbency for a DV projection and in dorsal recumbency for a VD projection. The x-ray beam is perpendicular to the film. The position of the head must be symmetrical.

DV views should be easier to obtain as the mandible naturally positions the head for this view, provided the mandible is normal and symmetrical. VD views require stabilization of the entire body with sandbags, V-trays, or compression bands. These positions allow for evaluation of head symmetry, which is a part of the orthodontic assessment. With this evaluation, the endotracheal tube may interfere with the radiographic interpretation and therefore it is best to expose them prior to intubation (**Figure 5.14**).

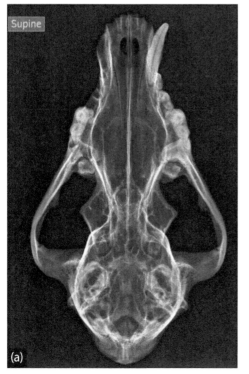

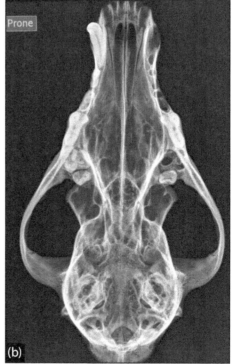

Fig. 5.13 **VD (a, dorsal) and DV (b, sternal) projections, which will depend on which part (dorsal or ventral) of the head is to be imaged. The area of interest should be located closer to the film/sensor.**

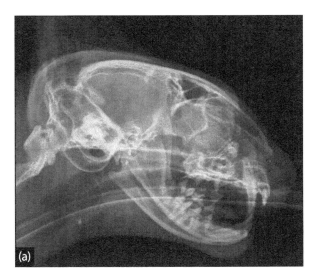

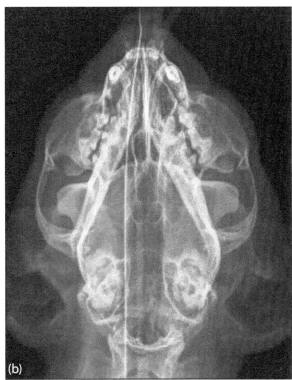

Fig. 5.14 Endotracheal tube interfering with an image of the head on both lateral (a) and VD (b) projections. It is better to expose head radiographs prior to intubation if possible.

What can be seen

Symmetry of the skull; TMJs, condyle shapes, outline of articular spaces and their symmetry; zygomatic arches, buccal and lingual margins of mandibular body, tympanic bullae, and a part of the nasal cavity.

Lateral projection

The head should be laid laterally with the nose slightly elevated (something radiolucent can be placed under the nose to provide parallelism between the film and the long axis of the head (**Figure 5.15**).

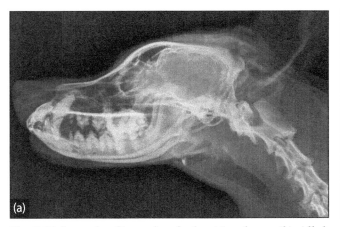

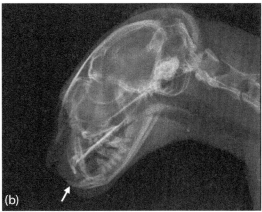

Fig. 5.15 Lateral radiographs of a dog (a) and a cat (b). All the structures that need to be evaluated in this projection are visible. Additionally, the position of the mandibular premolars and the length of the mandibles is shown in both symmetric positions. In (b) malposition of the mandibular canine tooth (without discrepancy in length of mandibles) is shown (arrow indicates a rostrally malpositioned right mandibular canine tooth).

This projection is rarely used alone, especially since it is not easy to obtain an ideal view. It is necessary to lift the nose and position the head in the best plane to obtain a lateral view of the maxillary or mandibular part of the head, and sometimes it is

necessary to repeat the exposure. When evaluating the frontal sinuses and nasal cavity, an additional frontal projection will be required to determine which side is affected.

What can be seen
The outline of the palatal bone, the nasal structures, the margin of the maxillary and frontal bone, and the frontal sinus. The ventral margins of the mandibles are often superimposed and therefore it is difficult to distinguish left from right. In addition, most oral structures are superimposed and render the radiograph of very limited value.

Left and right oblique lateral
This should be performed with the mouth both open and closed. It is important to mark which side is which either on the radiograph or, preferably, with a radiodense marker on the tooth (**Figures 5.16, 5.17**).

With open-mouth lateral projections it is easier to expose the caudal part of mandible and/or evaluate the TMJ in different functional situations. Radiopaque markers must be used to determine which side of the head is which. Props (plastic tubes) to keep the mouth open should be radiolucent, and it is important to avoid overstretching the jaws when placing the mouth gag or prop. This is particularly important in cats because

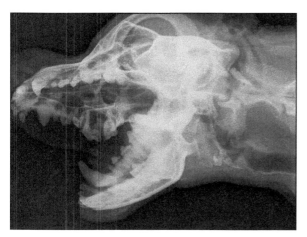

Fig. 5.16 Open-mouth oblique projections with different orientations will expose the maxillary and mandibular dentition in quasi parallel projection. If such a radiograph is exposed without marking right and left sides, it will be impossible to determine right from left. By convention, if the nose is to the left, the right maxillary dental arch will be visible, but markers should still be be present to avoid confusion.

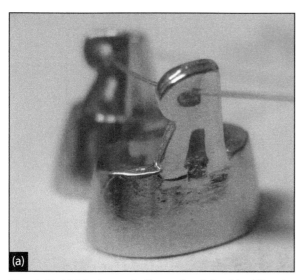

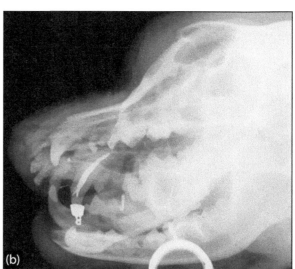

Fig. 5.17 (a) Marker to indicate the right side. The ring makes it possible to insert the marker on the canine crown. A radiograph with markers is easier to interpret and orientate. Note: In some countries it is a legal requirement to mark the sides on the radiograph. (b) In this radiograph, an additional landmark is an endodontically treated canine tooth. (Radiograph courtesy Dr. Seth Wallack.)

mouth gags were identified as a potential risk factor for cerebral ischemia and blindness in cats.[2]

Open-mouth oblique projections with different orientations will expose the maxillary dentition in quasi parallel projection as well as possibly the mandibular dentition. In a full-mouth series, this projection is used for both maxillary and mandibular dentition.

An oblique lateral view may also be helpful to use in emergency situations as the survey image.

What can be seen

TMJ articular space (one side better than the other) (see Chapter 6); one side of the mandibular dentition; ventral margin of the mandibles; general outline of the head. Dentition can be well exposed with an appropriate angle. In general, the angle is approximately 30 degrees, but may differ with breeds and type of skull.

Open-mouth extraoral projections: VD or DV

These projections are used to visualize the frontal sinus, the TMJs, the nasal cavity, and the tympanic bullae (**Figures 5.18–5.20**).

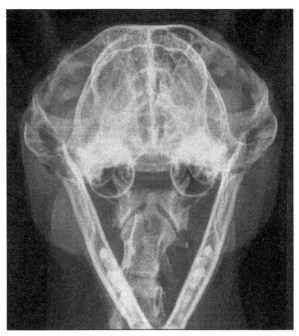

Fig. 5.18 **Open-mouth extraoral frontal projection in a cat. Visible are the TMJs, the tympanic bullae, and the nasal cavity from a frontal aspect. Note: The side marker was deleted when this radiograph was cropped.**

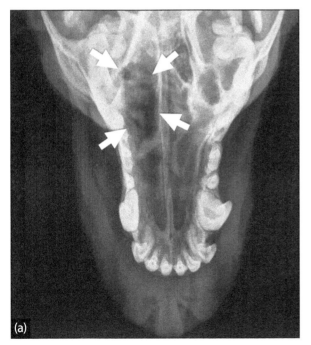 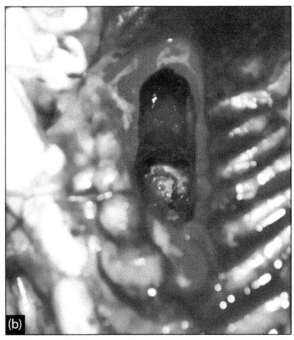

Fig. 5.19 **Open-mouth extraoral VD projection of the upper jaw and nasal cavity. (a) There is loss of structure clarity in the caudal part of the left nasal cavity (arrows). (b) Transpalatal rhinotomy of the left nasal cavity revealed necrotic infected masses. Note: The side marker was deleted when this radiograph was cropped.**

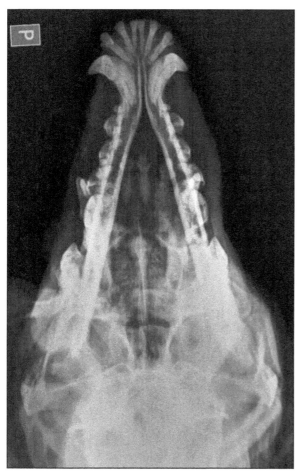

Fig. 5.20 **Open-mouth extraoral DV projection** showing the rostral part of the mandible. This is not a very practical projection. It is easier to perform an intraoral occlusal VD projection of the mandible.

Open-mouth extraoral frontal projection

The patient should be in dorsal recumbency with the jaws wide open. The x-ray beam is directed at the caudal aspect of the mouth with the maxilla perpendicular to the film. The open mouth enables exposure of the tympanic bullae.

What can be seen

A frontal view of the nasal cavities and the frontal sinus, the tympanic bullae, and the TMJs (**Figure 5.18**).

Open-mouth extraoral VD projection

The x-ray beam is directed at the palate with the patient in dorsal recumbency. The maxilla is parallel to the film.

What can be seen

The structures of the nasal cavity (compare the left and right cavity), the vomer bone, the TMJs, and the palatal and buccal aspects of the maxillary dentition (**Figure 5.19**).

Open-mouth extraoral DV projection

The x-ray beam is directed at the mandible with the patient in ventral recumbency. The mandible is parallel to the film.

What can be seen

The mandibular canine and incisor teeth, the mandibular symphysis, the lingual and buccal surfaces of the mandibular body, and the lingual and buccal aspects of the mandibular dentition (**Figure 5.20**).

Frontal projection

The position for a frontal projection is similar to that for the open-mouth extraoral frontal projection (see above), but the maxilla is angulated to the film and the central beam is directed at the frontal bone. In some breeds (Chihuahua, Pug) or in specific pathologies (hydrocephalus) it can be difficult or even impossible to obtain this view. Radiography of the nasal cavities and sinuses is discussed in Chapter 7.

Temporomandibular joint projections

Lateral oblique, DV, VD, and other projections for the TMJ are described in Chapter 8.

FULL-MOUTH RADIOGRAPHS

To obtain full-mouth radiographs and visualize the entire dentition using large format screens, it is necessary to have at least six projections (two maxillary oblique, two mandibular oblique, one VD or DV maxillary, and one DV or VD mandibular). For diagnostic quality x-rays it is necessary to expose additional radiographs, in particular for maxillary dentition. All of these projections can be made extraorally (**Figures 5.21, 5.22**), but it is easier to make the latter two intraorally with the cassette inserted into the mouth. Such a projection is called occlusal.

In small dogs and cats, it is possible to use size 4 dental films extraorally instead of films

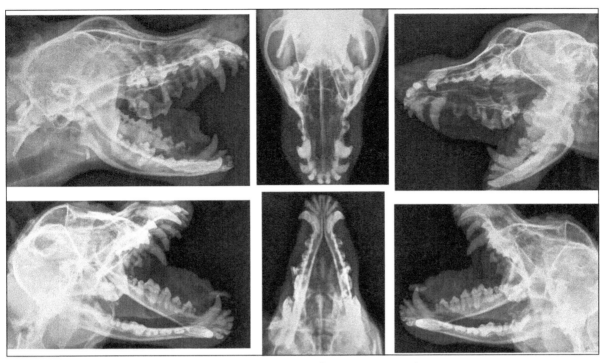

Fig. 5.21 Full-mouth radiography performed with extraoral projections in a dog.

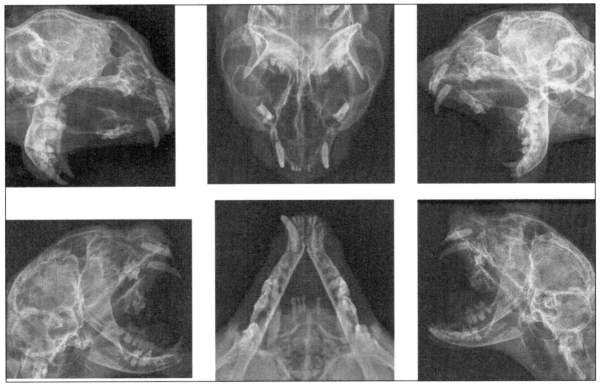

Fig. 5.22 Full-mouth radiography performed with extraoral projections in a cat, mounted as appropriate for assessment.

in cassettes, which improves the quality of the image. In addition, with dental films it is possible to expose intraoral projections of the mandible and maxilla. With extraoral techniques, obtaining ideal images is more complicated than with intraoral projections and it is advisable to use these projections only for survey images. Using them for more complex procedures such as endodontic treatment is not advised.

In some conditions conventional 2D radiography cannot provide an accurate diagnosis. For congenital defects of the cranium, only 3D imaging is diagnostic (**Figure 5.23**).

All the extraoral views and projections (**Figures 5.24–5.38**) were taken with the use of models. Most of the examples show the veterinary view from a distance (focal film distance) and x-ray beam perspective.

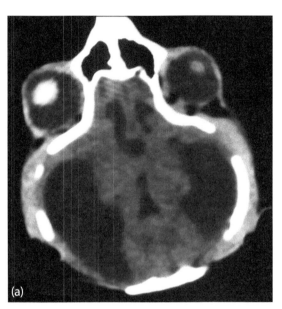
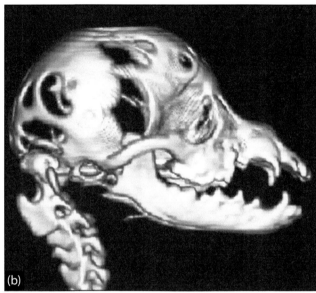

Fig. 5.23 **A 4-month-old Yorkshire terrier puppy with severe neurologic deficits and no accurate radiographic evidence of lesions was referred for CT examination, which revealed numerous defects in the cranial bones (a). A 3D reconstruction provided an accurate picture of the condition (b).**

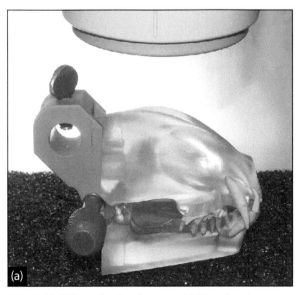
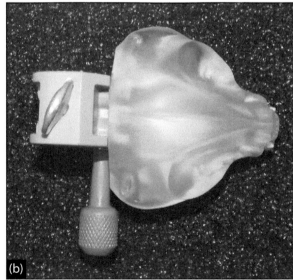

Fig. 5.24 **DV projection in a cat. (a) Veterinarian perspective, (b) x-ray beam perspective.** *(Continued)*

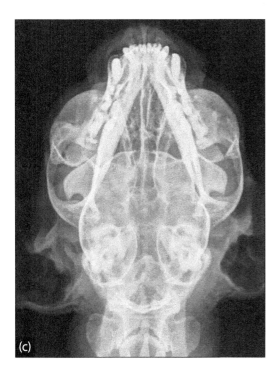

Fig. 5.24 *(Continued)* **DV** projection in a cat. (c) Image example.

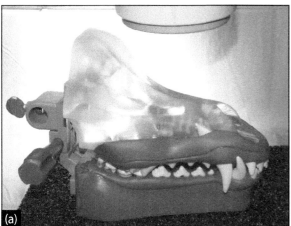

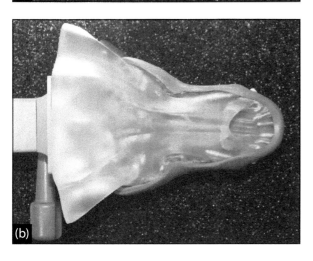

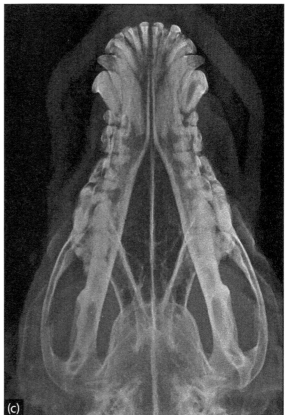

Fig. 5.25 **DV** projection in a dog. (a) Veterinarian perspective, (b) x-ray beam perspective, (c) image example.

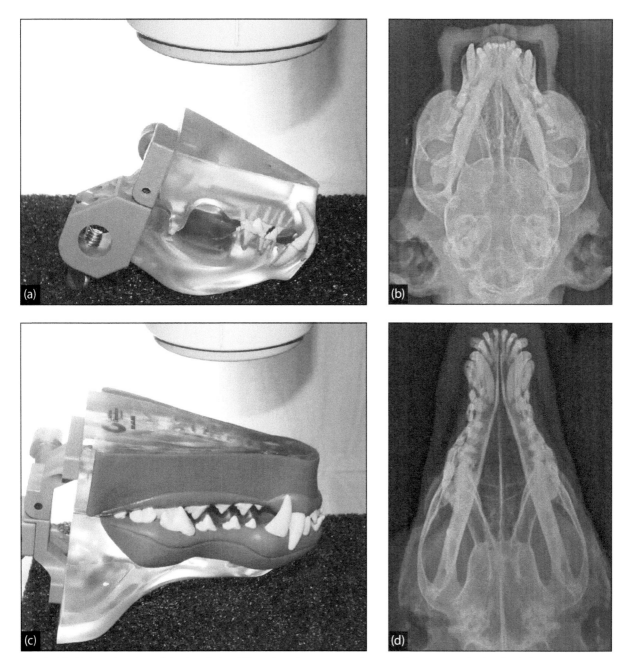

Fig. 5.26 VD projection of the head. (a, c) Veterinarian perspective: cat, dog, respectively; (b, d) image examples: cat, dog, respectively.

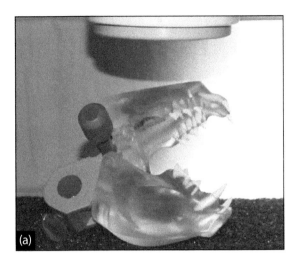

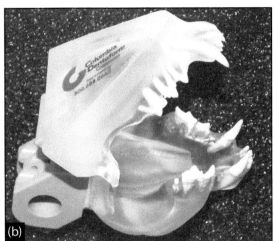

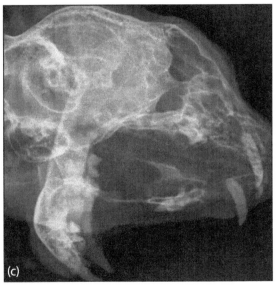

Fig. 5.27 Lateral oblique projection in a cat focused on the maxillary dentition. (a) Veterinarian perspective, (b) x-ray beam perspective, (c) image example.

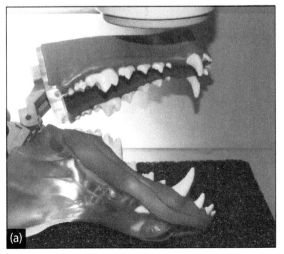

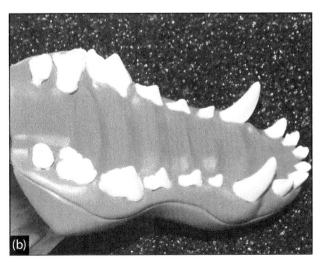

Fig. 5.28 Lateral oblique projection in a dog focused on the maxillary dentition. (a) Veterinarian perspective, (b) x-ray beam perspective. *(Continued)*

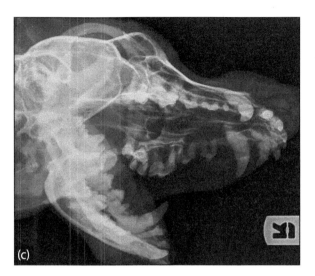

Fig. 5.28 *(Continued)* Lateral oblique projection in a dog focused on the maxillary dentition. (c) Image example.

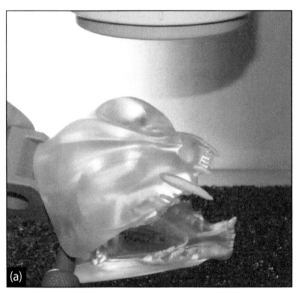

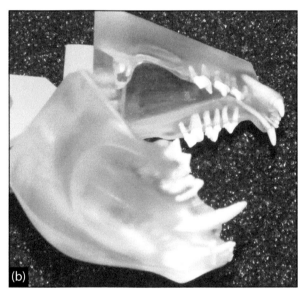

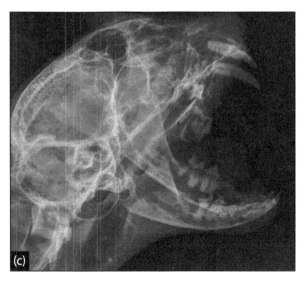

Fig. 5.29 Lateral oblique projection in a cat focused on the mandibular dentition. (a) Veterinarian perspective, (b) x-ray beam perspective, (c) image example.

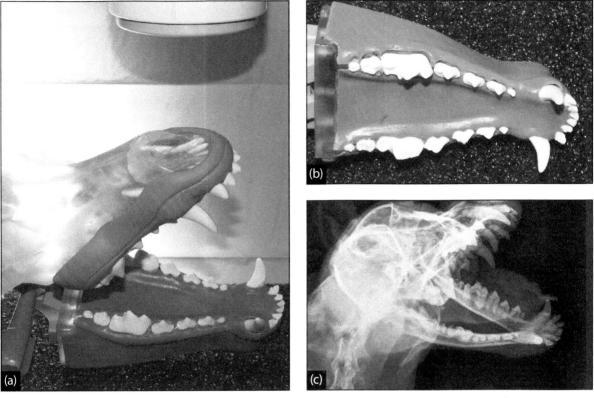

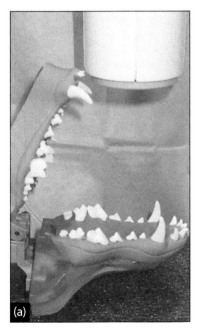

Fig. 5.30 Lateral oblique projection in a dog focused on the mandibular dentition. (a) Veterinarian perspective, (b) x-ray beam perspective, (c) image example.

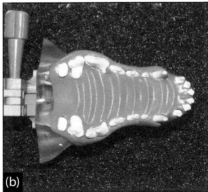

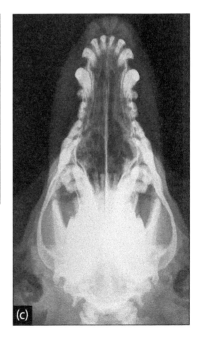

Fig. 5.31 Open-mouth extraoral VD projection of the upper jaw and nasal cavity in a dog. (a) Veterinarian perspective, (b) x-ray beam perspective, (c) image example.

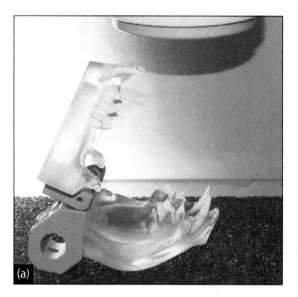

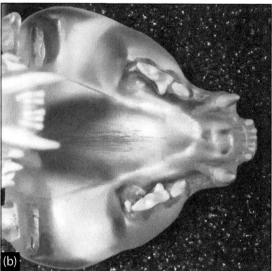

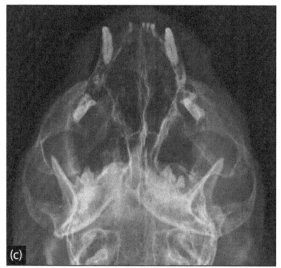

Fig. 5.32 Open-mouth extraoral VD projection of the upper jaw and nasal cavity in a cat. (a) Veterinarian perspective, (b) x-ray beam perspective, (c) image example.

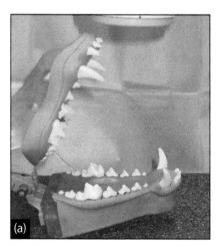

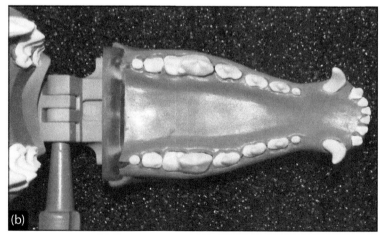

Fig. 5.33 Open-mouth extraoral DV projection of the lower jaw in a dog. (a) Veterinarian perspective, (b) x-ray beam perspective. *(Continued)*

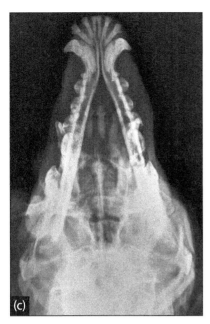

Fig. 5.33 *(Continued)* Open-mouth extraoral DV projection of the lower jaw in a dog. (c) Image example.

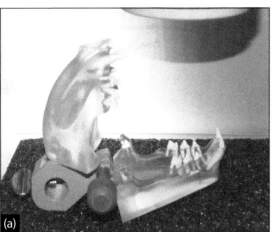

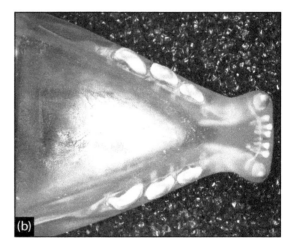

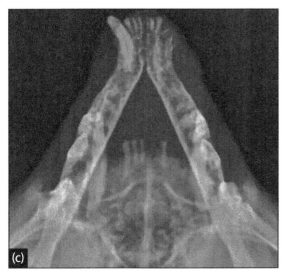

Fig. 5.34 Open-mouth extraoral DV projection of the lower jaw in a cat. (a) Veterinarian perspective, (b) x-ray beam perspective, (c) image example.

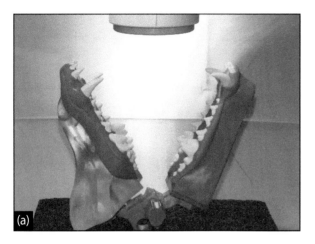

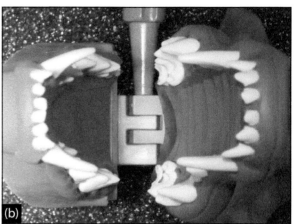

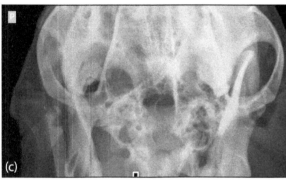

Fig. 5.35 Open-mouth extraoral frontal projection in a dog focused on the tympanic bullae. (a) Veterinarian perspective, (b) x-ray beam perspective, (c) image example.

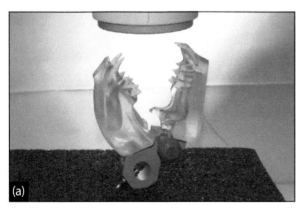

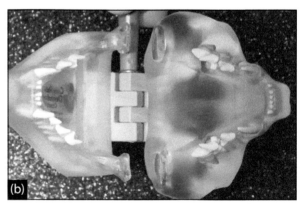

Fig. 5.36 Open-mouth extraoral frontal projection in a cat focused on the tympanic bullae. (a) Veterinarian perspective, (b) x-ray beam perspective. *(Continued)*

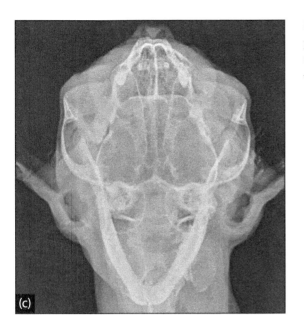

Fig. 5.36 *(Continued)* **Open-mouth extraoral frontal projection in a cat focused on the tympanic bullae. (c) Image example. Note: The side marker was deleted when this radiograph was cropped.**

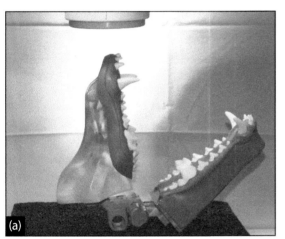

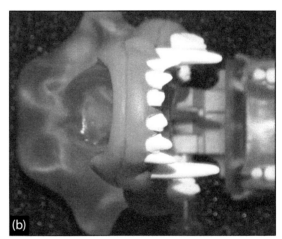

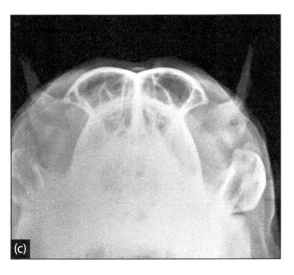

Fig. 5.37 **Open-mouth extraoral frontal projection in a dog focused on the nasal cavity and sinuses. (a) Veterinarian perspective, (b) x-ray beam perspective, (c) image example. It is not necessary to use an open-mouth projection to obtain this view. Note: The side marker was deleted when this radiograph was cropped.**

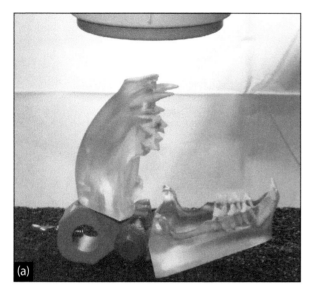

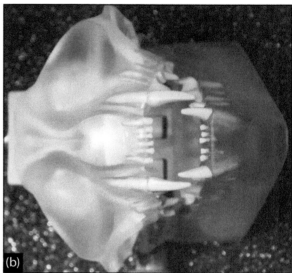

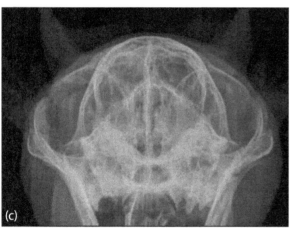

Fig. 5.38 Open-mouth extraoral frontal projection in a cat focused on the nasal cavity and sinuses. (a) Veterinarian perspective, (b) x-ray beam perspective, (c) image example. It is not necessary to use an open-mouth projection to obtain this view. **Note:** The side marker was deleted when this radiograph was cropped.

REFERENCES

1 Douglas SW Williamson HD (1978) Radiographic factors which influence radiological interpretation. In: *Veterinary Radiological Interpretation.* (eds. SW Douglas, HD Williamson) Lea & Febiger, Philadelphia, pp. 1–13.

2 Stiles J, Weil AB, Packer RA *et al.* (2012) Post-anesthetic cortical blindness in cats: twenty cases. *Vet J* **193(2):**367–373.

CHAPTER 6

DEVELOPING/PROCESSING DENTAL RADIOGRAPHS

Brook A. Niemiec

INTRODUCTION

Although dental radiography is definitely trending towards digital technology, standard 'analog' films are certainly still diagnostic and require less initial investment. Standard dental radiographs can be developed by hand or by automatic dental film processors. It is important to note that standard (full-body) radiograph automatic processors should *not* be used for developing dental films. Standard films require different chemicals than those used for dental film, negatively affecting the quality of the radiographs. In addition, they will not archive well.[1,2] For automatic dental processing, refer to the operating manual for that particular piece of equipment. Step by step instructions for hand developing will be covered in this chapter. Investing in a new automatic dental film developer is unjustified at this time with the prices of digital systems dropping and becoming more accessible.

STEP 1: CREATING A LIGHT SAFE ENVIRONMENT[1,3–6]

Hand dental film processing can be performed in a dark room using household cups or bowls. However, it is recommended to use a chairside developer in the dental suite. A chairside developer unit (chairside darkroom) holds the chemicals for developing and fixing the film as well as water for rinsing. The film and solutions are visualized through a colored filter, while the hands are placed through a light safe aperture (**Figure 6.1a**). Chairside developing has several advantages, such as no requirement for a dark room, time efficiency, and allowing for continual patient monitoring by the technician during the development process. Amber filters are used for 'D' speed films and red is correct for 'E' and 'F' speeds (**Figure 6.1b**).[1,6]

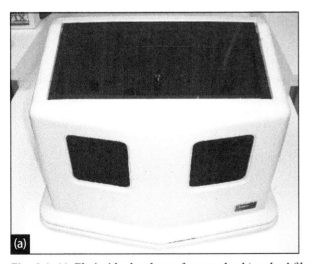

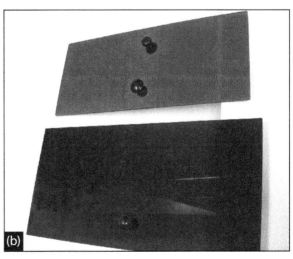

Fig. 6.1 **(a) Chairside developer for standard 'analog' films with a colored filter for viewing and light safe apertures for the hands to pass through for developing. (b) Light safe filters: top, amber; bottom, red.**

STEP 2: REMOVAL OF FILM FROM THE PROTECTIVE PACKET[1,4]

Carefully open the package by grasping the supplied tag. Once opened, three components will be revealed: the film, a piece of black paper, and a lead sheet (**Figure 6.2**). The paper is either in front of the film or wrapped around the film entirely. The lead sheet is behind the film, to control and minimize back-scatter. These all feel very different. Remove the contents and separate the film from the other pieces. Grasp only the very corner of the film to avoid finger print artifacts.[3] In addition, place the film clip on the film prior to separation to help avoid touching the film.[3] The clip should be placed on the edge of the film and ideally near the embossed dot to decrease artifacts (**Figure 6.3**).

DEVELOPMENT AND FIXING[1–3,6,7]

Developing the film by hand via chemicals is similar to dip tank developing methods used for standard (whole-body) films.

Hand developing methods utilize one of two different techniques to correctly produce an image on the film: (1) time/temperature or (2) sight.[4] Each technique is best performed when the chemicals (developing and fixing solutions) are at room temperature. Acceptable temperature range is between 60 and 75°F (15 and 24°C), with 70°F (21°C) being ideal.[3,8] Both methods ideally use a two-step rapid development solution. The solutions designed for standard radiographs are a poor substitute, since the time of development (not including fixing) will be greatly increased (4.5–5 minutes compared with approximately 15 seconds for rapid dental film developing solutions).[2,6] Furthermore, the quality of development and fixation will also be inferior if standard x-ray chemicals are used.[1]

Time/temperature development is performed by continually monitoring the temperature of the developing solution and determining the required development time by consulting the manufacturer's recommendations (**Figure 6.4**).[4,6] This is the most scientifically correct method of development, but it can be cumbersome.[4,7] In addition, it becomes less accurate as the chemicals age.

Sight development is accomplished by dipping the film in the developer for a short time, removing it, and then examining the film with a safe light

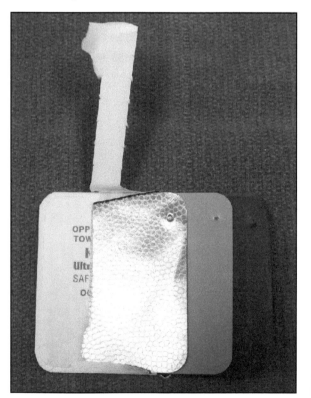

Fig. 6.2 **Opened size 4 film packet revealing from left: lead, film, paper.**

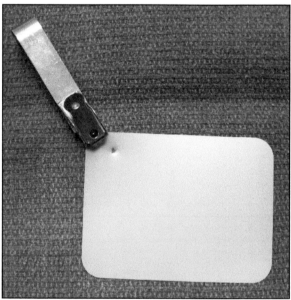

Fig. 6.3 **Film clip applied to the corner of a radiographic film.**

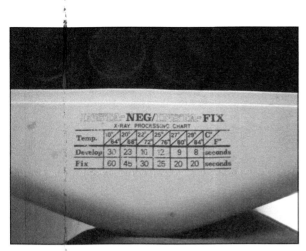

Fig. 6.4 Processing chart for time/temperature development (located on most chairside developers).

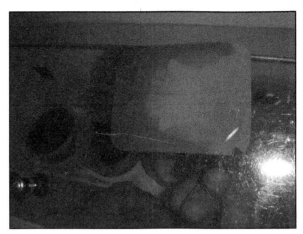

Fig. 6.5 A dental radiograph viewed through the light safe filter. This appearance indicates that development is completed and rinsing/fixing can commence.

or through the filter (**Figure 6.5**).[1,7] This process is repeated until the *very first hint* of an image appears, indicating the film is properly developed.[1] Sight development has some significant advantages over the time/temperature technique:[4]

- Continuous temperature monitoring is not necessary. Solution temperatures typically rise during the day, which speeds up development. When using time/temperature development this will result in overdeveloped films unless frequent temperature readings are taken.
- Time measurement becomes inaccurate as the chemicals become exhausted, leading to underdeveloped films.
- The biggest advantage of sight developing is that minor technique errors can be corrected by slightly over- or underdeveloping the film. This will not compensate for major errors, but will avoid some retakes.

Once the film is removed from the packet, it can be placed directly into the developer solution; however, some authors recommend an initial short placement in water.[6] If the latter option is performed, make sure to use a water bath that is separate from the rinsing bath so as not to contaminate the undeveloped film. To ensure full development, make sure the cups are full and take care to submerge the entire film until it is developed. This is most important when using size 4 dental films, as these barely fit in the supplied cups (**Figures 6.6a, b**).[4] Following proper development, the film is rinsed by agitating in water for 1 minute (some authors recommend distilled water for this step[6]), and then placed in the fixer. After the film has been fixed for 1 minute, it can removed from the dark room and quickly interpreted.[1,9] However, in order to archive the film for later viewing, it should be replaced in the fixer for a minimum of 10 minutes and ideally for 30 minutes, depending on the condition of the fixer. In fact, films will not be adversely affected if they stay in the fixer for prolonged periods.

It is critical for the films to be thoroughly rinsed after completing the fixation process. Adequate rinsing requires the film to be placed in the water rinse for a minimum of 10 minutes, but true archival quality requires a 30 minute rinse time. In order to avoid fixer solution dripping down from the clip and ruining the image, the film should be transferred to a clean clip and quickly rinsed or agitated again before drying.

Note: 'Dry' films are superior for interpretation compared with wet films, and therefore images should be re-evaluated following complete drying. However, it is not generally realistic to wait for full fixing and drying during the anesthetic procedure.

Radiographs must be completely dried prior to evaluation and storage or the films will stick together, resulting in significant film damage. Drying can be

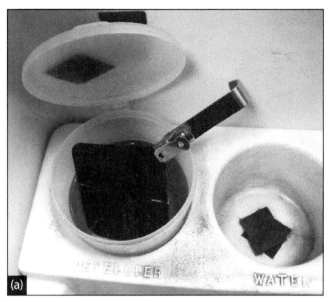 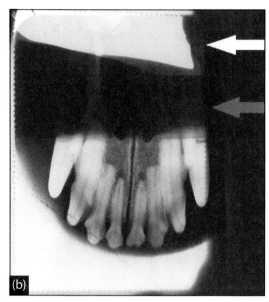

Fig. 6.6 **Proper film development. (a) Ensuring that size 4 films are fully immersed in the developing solution is important for quality films. (b) Example of not fully immersing films. The bottom part of the film was properly developed and fixed, revealing a quality image. However, the middle part of the film was not placed fully in the fixer, resulting in a darkened unreadable radiograph (red arrow). The top part was not immersed in either solution, resulting in an undeveloped area (white arrow). The radiograph, although properly positioned and exposed, was ruined by improper developing technique.**

accomplished with a dental film dryer or hair dryer, or the radiographs may be hung to air dry. If the air-drying method is used, a full 24 hours should be allowed for complete drying. When drying multiple radiographs, they can be transferred to a multifilm clip (**Figure 6.7**). Once completely dry, the radiographs are stored in an envelope labeled with the patients name and date (**Figure 6.8**). Envelopes can be kept in an index box system or in the individual patient's medical chart.

When using small cups, the chemicals used in hand development must be replaced frequently.[3] A six-ounce (170 ml) volume of developer will generally develop 10–15 size 4 films, or a larger number of smaller size 2 films, before replenishment is necessary.[10]

Regardless of the quality of development, fixing, and rinsing, some degradation of the radiographic

quality is expected over time.[4] Therefore, it is recommended that high-quality digital photos of the radiographs should be taken and stored in a folder on a computer that is routinely backed-up (**Figure 6.9**). This, in essence, is a permanent copy of the radiograph and will also facilitate telemedicine with specialists or other veterinarians. For instructions on how to take quality digital images of dental radiographs see Chapter 3 or go to www.vetdentalrad.com and click on 'How to prepare files' and then 'Digital camera'.

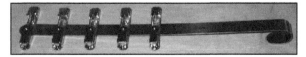

Fig. 6.7 **Multifilm clip for drying dental films.**

Fig. 6.8 **Envelope for storage of dental films.**

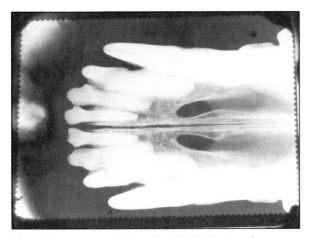

Fig. 6.9 **Proper technique for 'digitizing' analog dental radiographs. A light safe area was created on the radiograph viewer where the film is placed. Taking an image of this radiograph will produce a digital image of the film.**

PROCESSING ERRORS[1,3,4,6,11]

There are numerous opportunities for errors in the development of dental radiographs. These errors typically result in poor quality or unreadable films. Common errors include:

- Underdeveloping. Underdeveloped (or underexposed) radiographs will appear washed out or 'light' and can result from insufficient exposure or developing time, as well as exhausted developer solution (**Figure 6.10**). This issue can usually be corrected by increasing the development time or exposure. If this does not resolve the issue, the solution should be replaced.
- Overdeveloping. Overdeveloped (or overexposed) film results in a radiograph that is 'dark' (**Figure 6.11**). This problem is

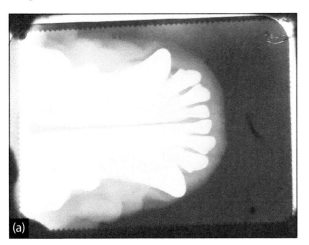
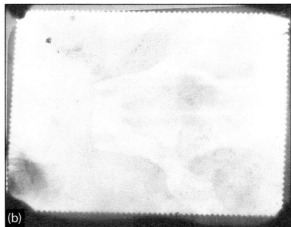

Fig. 6.10 **Underexposed/developed images in a dog (a) and cat (b). Note the washed out appearance and lack of detail and contrast. Interpretation is significantly limited.**

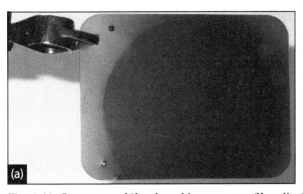
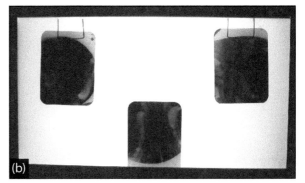

Fig. 6.11 **Overexposed/developed images on a film clip (a) and dental radiograph viewer (b). These images are too dark to be diagnostic.**

corrected by decreasing the exposure time, but occasionally decreasing the development time utilizing the 'sight' technique may be effective.

- Underfixing. Extreme underfixing will cause the film to turn black prior to viewing (**Figure 6.12**). This can be avoided by leaving the film in the fixer for at least 1 minute before initial viewing. Slight underfixing will cause the radiograph to yellow over time. Films can only achieve long-term stability (archival quality) by fixing for at least 10 minutes.

- Under-rinsing. Insufficient rinsing may not cause adverse effects initially, but the consequences will manifest later. Fixer that

remains on the film over time will turn the film brown (**Figure 6.13**), resulting in an unreadable image. Adequate rinsing requires 30 minutes in a container or several minutes under running tap water. Unfortunately, if errors of underfixing and rinsing are not discovered at the time of the procedure, they cannot be corrected later and the radiographs will be irreplaceable.

- Light exposure. Fogged or unclear radiographs (**Figure 6.14**) can occur secondary to a variety of problems and these may be frustrating to identify and correct. The most common causes of fogging are:
  - Old/exhausted chemical solutions.
  - Old film.
  - Poor radiographic technique.
  - Light exposure.
  - Improper light filter or developer type.
- Scratches.
- Bending during processing to fit small containers.
- Poor placement of the film clip over pathology.

Troubleshooting through this list should elucidate the cause. Light fogging (due to leakage) in a dark room can be confirmed by placing a coin on an opened film for a few minutes and then developing the film.[3] If the coin is visible, there is a light leak. Finally, if the wrong color safelight/filter is being used, overexposure and nondiagnostic

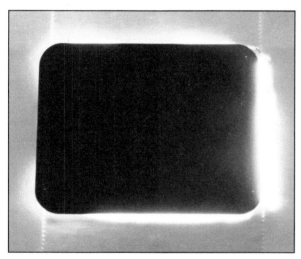

Fig. 6.12 **Extreme underfixing resulting in a black film, which is unreadable.**

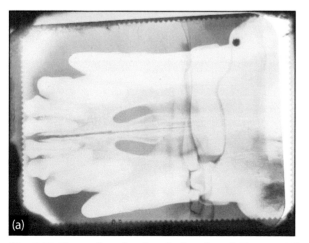

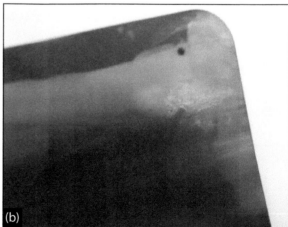

Fig. 6.13 **Examples of under-rinsing dental films. (a) This is a slightly under-rinsed film, which is slightly brown and has some chemical interference. (b) This is a severely under-rinsed film, which is completely unreadable.**

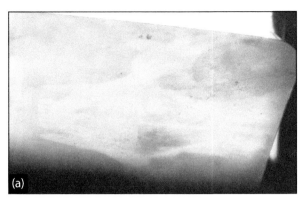
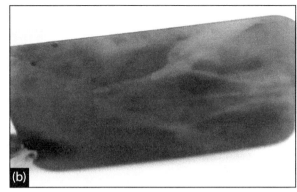

Fig. 6.14a, b **Examples of unclear or fogged films, which can occur from a number of conditions.**

films can result.[12] Light fogging can occur with chairside developers if exposed to bright/direct sunlight.

KEY POINTS

- Standard medical film automatic processors are not recommended.
- Ensure there are no light leaks.
- Make sure to separate all three components of the film prior to developing.
- Avoid touching the film with fingers, as this will create artifacts.
- Ensure that the processing chemicals are fresh.
- Make sure film is completely covered by solutions to avoid undeveloped areas.
- Films can be viewed after 1 minute of fixing, but optimal resolution is possible only after drying.
- A minimum of 10–30 minutes of fixing is needed for archiving.
- Films must be completely dry prior to storage.
- Digital photographs of radiograph are recommended to preserve images indefinitely.

REFERENCES

1 Niemiec BA, Sabitino D, Gilbert T (2004) Developing dental radiographs. *J Vet Dent* **21(2):**116–21.
2 Oakes A (2000) Radiology techniques. In: *An Atlas of Veterinary Dental Radiology*. (eds. DH DeForge, BH Colmery BH) Iowa State University Press, Ames, pp. xxi–xxiv.
3 Mulligan TW, Aller MS, Williams CA (1998) Technical errors and troubleshooting. In: *Atlas of Canine and Feline Dental Radiography*. Veterinary Learning Systems, Trenton, pp. 45–64.
4 Niemiec BA (2010) Veterinary dental radiology. In: *Small Animal Dental, Oral and Maxillofacial Disease: A Color Handbook*. (ed. BA Niemiec) Manson Publishing, London, pp. 63–87.
5 Woodward TM (2009) Dental radiology. *Top Companion Anim Med* **24(1):**20–36.
6 Bellows J (2008) Dental radiography. In: *Small Animal Dental Equipment, Materials, and Technique: A Primer*. Wiley-Blackwell, Ames, pp. 63–104.
7 Wiggs RB, Lobprise HB (1997) Dental and oral radiology. In: *Veterinary Dentistry: Principles and Practice*. Lippincott–Raven, Philadelphia, pp. 140–66.
8 Langland OE, Langlais RP, Preece JW (2002) Processing and film mounting procedures. In: *Principles of Dental Imaging*. Lippincott, Williams, and Wilkens, Baltimore, pp. 139–54.
9 Mulligan TW, Aller MS, Williams CA (1998) Basic equipment needs. In: *Atlas of Canine and Feline Dental Radiography*. Veterinary Learning Systems, Trenton, pp. 7–14.
10 Holmstrom SE, Frost P, Eisner ER (1998) *Veterinary Dental Techniques*, 2nd edn. WB Saunders, Philadelphia.
11 Eisner ER (2000) Film artifacts, visual illusions, and technical errors. In. *An Atlas of Veterinary Dental Radiology*. (eds. DH DeForge, BH Colmery) Iowa State University Press, Ames, pp. 201–14.
12 Tutt C (2006) *Small Animal Dentistry: A Manual of Techniques*. Wiley-Blackwell, Ames, pp. 97–98.

CHAPTER 7

COMMON ERRORS OF DENTAL RADIOGRAPHY PROJECTION

Brook A. Niemiec

INTRODUCTION

There are several errors that can be made in veterinary dental imaging. These include:

- Placing the film/sensor in backwards.
- Errors of vertical angulation.
- Errors or horizontal angulation.
- Under- or overexposure.
- Missing the desired tooth/root on the film/sensor.
- Cone cut.

This chapter will cover each of these issues by discussing the reasons behind the error, showing how each one would appear radiographically, and finally demonstrating how to correct them.

PLACING THE FILM/SENSOR IN BACKWARDS

When utilizing standard film, there is an embossed dot (or 'dimple') on one corner of the film, which can be felt on the white side of the film packet (**Figure 7.1a**). The convex side should be placed towards the x-ray beam. With most films, this side is pure white and the opposite (or 'back') side of the film is colored. For digital radiography (DR) sensors, the cord will exit on the 'back' side of the sensor and this side goes away from the tube head. For photostimulable phosphor (PSP) plates, the side with writing on it is placed away from the tube head.

If standard film is placed backwards in the mouth, it will be underexposed with a grid pattern. This is because the lead has absorbed the x-ray beam (**Figure 7.1b**). If a DR sensor is placed backwards, the image will be one of electronics (**Figure 7.1c**). A PSP plate *can* be imaged with either side facing the

tube head, but this will affect the ability to determine right from left on the image that is created. Make sure to place the correct side towards the tube head as indicated by the manufacturer.

ERRORS OF VERTICAL ANGULATION

This is the most common error in dental radiography, and generally occurs when using the bisecting angle technique. If the calculated or approximate angle is incorrect, the resulting image will be distorted, showing teeth/roots that are longer or shorter than the true object being radiographed. The best way to visualize this concept is to think of a shadow of a building outside in the sun. The building (tooth root) is at a 90-degree (right) angle to the ground (film). In this case, the bisecting angle would be 45 degrees.

Early and late in the day, the sun is at an acute angle to the ground and casts a long shadow. In dental radiography, this occurs when the angle of the x-ray beam to the film/sensor is too small (or the tube head is placed too parallel to the film/sensor [**Figure 7.2a**]). This improper angle creates '*elongation*' of the image (i.e. the imaged roots are longer than they truly are [**Figure 7.2b**]). To correct this mistake, the tube head should be rotated so that it is more perpendicular to the film/sensor (**Figures 7.2c, d**).

As the sun travels higher in the sky, the shadow shortens. In dental radiology, this occurs when the angle of the x-ray beam to the object is too great (or when the tube head is placed too perpendicular to the film/sensor [**Figure 7.2e**]). This is known as '*foreshortening*' of the image (i.e. the imaged roots are shorter than they truly are [**Figure 7.2f**]). To fix this error, the tube head should be rotated more parallel to the film/sensor, which will lengthen the image of the roots (**Figures 7.2c, d**).

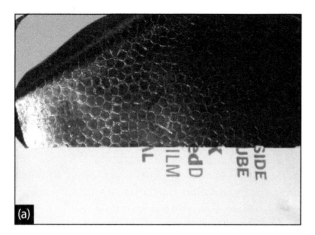

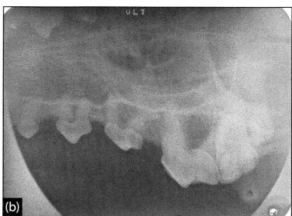

Fig. 7.1 Placing the film/sensor in backwards. (a) In the film packet, there is a lead sheet behind the film to decrease back-scatter. (b) When the film is placed in backwards (i.e. colored side toward the tube head), the image will be negatively affected by the dimpling effect of the lead. (c) If a sensor is placed in backwards, the electronics will be visualized.

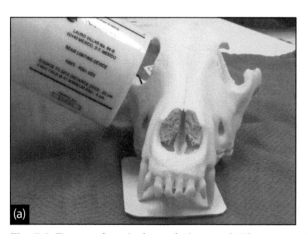

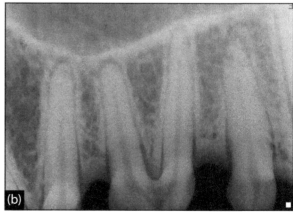

Fig. 7.2 Errors of vertical angulation. (a–d) Elongation. When the x-ray beam is placed too parallel to the film/plate/sensor (a), the roots are elongated (b). This is corrected by placing the the beam more perpendicular to the film/plate/sensor (c), which will produce the desired image (d). (e, f) Foreshortening. When the x-ray beam is placed too perpendicular to the sensor (e), the roots are shortened (f). This is corrected by placing the beam more parallel to the sensor (see c), which will give the desired image (see d). *(Continued)*

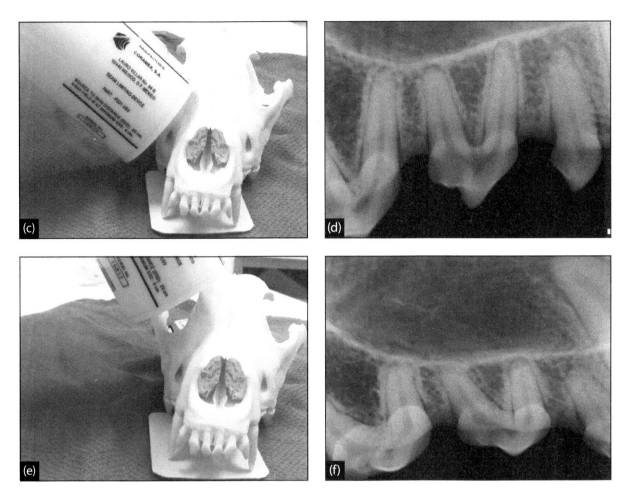

Fig. 7.2 *(Continued)*

ERRORS OF HORIZONTAL ANGULATION

This is a fairly uncommon issue. The most common reason for this complication is when performing the mesial or distal tubeshift technique to separate the mesial roots of the maxillary fourth premolar (**Figure 7.3**). To properly perform this technique, the tube head is rotated approximately 30 degrees from perpendicular to the maxilla. This should separate the mesial roots with minimal distortion. If the angle is greater than 30 degrees, the roots become elongated horizontally. If elongation occurs, the tube head should be rotated back more perpendicular to the maxilla. If the angle is insufficient, the roots will not be effectively separated. This problem is corrected by rotating the tube head further from perpendicular to the long axis of the maxilla.

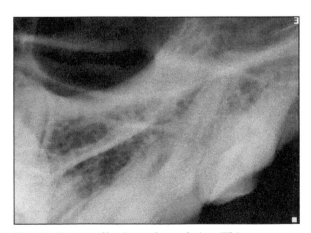

Fig. 7.3 **Errors of horizontal angulation. This error typically occurs when attempting to 'split the roots' of the maxillary fourth premolar. If the tube head is acutely angled, it will image the mesial roots over the third premolar. To fix this, bring the tube head back more perpendicular to the sensor in the horizontal plane.**

The only other scenario involving this type of error is when imaging the maxillary canine. In this case, if the tube head is not rotated sufficiently, the canine tooth root is superimposed on the first and second premolars. This is corrected by rotating the beam further to the side (i.e. more perpendicular to the long axis of the maxilla).

UNDEREXPOSURE AND OVEREXPOSURE

These errors are caused by either incorrect settings on the machine or having the tube head too far away from the film/sensor.

If a manual setting machine is being used, the time can be adjusted with the up and down arrows. If the image is too dark (overexposed) (**Figure 7.4a**), push the down arrow button a few times to decrease the exposure, and retake the image. Repeat until the exposure is correct. Conversely, if the image is too light (underexposed) (**Figure 7.4b**), push the up arrow to increase exposure.

If utilizing the computer-controlled settings, select the patient size, target tooth, and system type (digital versus analog). Because of the significant differences in the exposure needs of different digital systems, this author prefers to use the time setting option.

Most direct digital sensors (DR systems) have a very narrow exposure range, therefore a small movement (0.5–1.0 cm) away from the sensor often requires an increase in exposure time. This is especially true in the maxillary premolar and molar area of dogs. This is due to the lateral expansion of the zygomatic arch (**Figures 7.4c–e**). Note that older dental x-ray generators provide a very limited range of exposure times, which means even the lowest

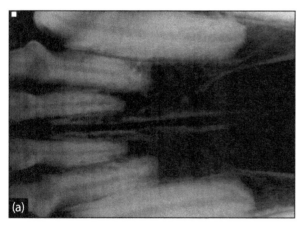

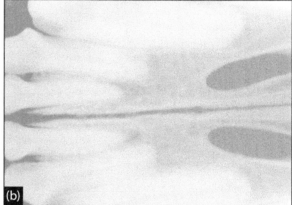

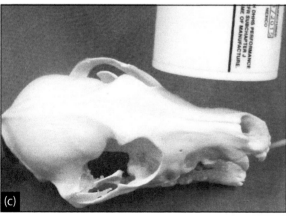

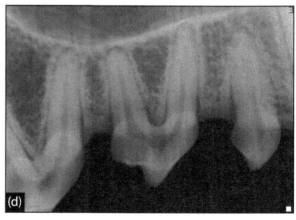

Fig. 7.4 **Examples of overexposure (a) and underexposure (b). On occasion, moving from one tooth to another can affect exposure based on distance from the tube head to the sensor/film or increased tissue density. When imaging the premolars the tube head can be placed very close to the teeth, therefore minimal exposure is needed (c, d).**

(Continued)

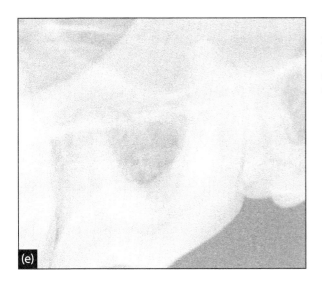

Fig. 7.4 *(Continued)* When moving back to the fourth premolar and molars, the tube head moves away from the sensor due to zygomatic arch interference, resulting in an underexposed film (e). The exposure time will need to be increased for this image.

setting can overexpose modern sensors because they require lower exposures. When purchasing second-hand equipment, be sure to confirm that the x-ray generator and sensor are compatible.

MISSING THE INTENDED STRUCTURE ON THE IMAGE

If the tooth/area of interest is not on the image, the sensor/film is not in the right position (**Figure 7.5**). The film/sensor should be moved in the direction of the missing area to ensure the entire structure is imaged. This issue occurs most commonly when imaging large breed dogs with a size 2 sensor. It is

important to note that not all of the canine teeth or carnassial teeth of large breed dogs can be imaged on one view.

CONE CUT

This issue is most commonly encountered when using a size 4 film or photostimulable phosphor (PSP) plate. Cone cut occurs when the tube head is not placed in the correct position to expose the entire film/sensor, resulting in a 'white' area on the image (**Figure 7.6**). This can be corrected by moving the tube head in the direction of the missed sensor area to cover the whole sensor/film. Cone cut errors can be avoided

Fig. 7.5 Missing the tooth/area of interest on the image. This is due to misplacement of the sensor/film and is a common issue when imaging canine and mandibular first molars in large breed dogs. If the structure is not on the image, move the sensor in that direction.

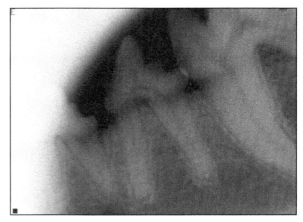

Fig. 7.6 Cone cut. This occurs when the tube head is not centered on the sensor, resulting in part of the sensor not being exposed. If this occurs, move the tube head so that it centers over the sensor.

by looking down the tube head, like a rifle scope, to make sure the whole film/sensor is covered.

Cone cut errors are particularly problematic when using size 4 (or larger) films/PSP plates. To image the entire plate, the tube head will need to be moved away from the object/film. When this adjustment is made, the x-rays are divergent (like a flashlight beam) and cover the entire film/PSP plate. This adjustment also increases the focal film distance, and therefore the exposure time must also be increased.

KEY POINTS

- If the tooth roots are short, rotate the tube head more parallel to the film/sensor.
- If the tooth roots are long, rotate the tube head more perpendicular to the film/sensor.
- If the film is too dark, decrease the exposure or development time.
- If the film is too light, increase the exposure or development time.
- If the structure of interest is not on the image, move the film/sensor to accommodate the objects.

- If there is a large area of white (cone cut), move the tube head to cover the entire sensor/film.

FURTHER READING

Bellows J (2008) Dental radiography. In: *Small Animal Dental Equipment, Materials, and Technique: A Primer*. Wiley-Blackwell, Ames, pp. 63–104.

Eisner ER (2000) Film artifacts, visual illusions, and technical errors. In: *An Atlas of Veterinary Dental Radiology*. (eds. DH DeForge, BH Colmery) Iowa State University Press, Ames, pp. 201–214.

Mulligan TW, Aller MS, Williams CA (1998) Technical errors and troubleshooting. In: *Atlas of Canine and Feline Dental Radiography*. Veterinary Learning Systems, Trenton, pp. 45–64.

Niemiec BA (2010) Veterinary dental radiology. In: *Small Animal Dental, Oral and Maxillofacial Disease: A Color Handbook*. (ed. BA Niemiec) Manson Publishing, London, pp. 63–87.

Niemiec BA, Sabitino D, Gilbert T (2004) Equipment and basic geometry of dental radiography. *J Vet Dent* **21:**48–52.

Woodward TM (2009) Dental radiology. *Top Companion Anim Med* **24(1):**20–36.

CHAPTER 8

DENTAL RADIOGRAPHIC INTERPRETATION

PART A

EVALUATION OF DENTAL RADIOGRAPHS AND DETERMINING THE TYPE, AGE, AND SIZE OF THE TEETH IMAGED

Jerzy Gawor

INTRODUCTION

Evaluation of dental radiographs starts with appropriate orientation of the image according to established standards. The current standard is labial mounting, which gives the viewer the perspective of 'outside looking in'. In other words, your eyes are the x-ray beam (**Figures A8.1, A8.2**).

The first step in radiographic interpretation is determining which teeth have been imaged. This requires a thorough knowledge of oral anatomy as well as the nature of dental films and digital systems. Digital systems with veterinary templates do not require this step as long as the images are properly placed; however, do not assume it was done correctly. Always consult the owner's manual for instructions for use of your particular system.

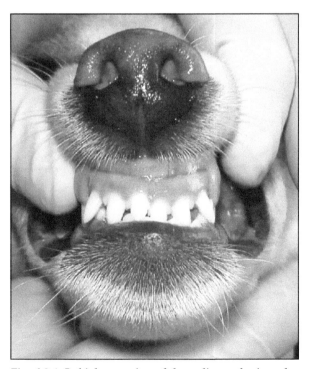

Fig. A8.1 Labial mounting of the radiograph gives the viewer the perspective of outside looking in.

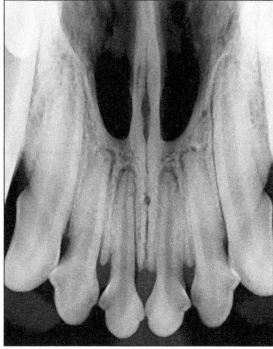

Fig. A8.2 Labial mounting of the maxillary incisors. The radiograph give the viewer the perspective of outside looking in.

The key to properly identifying the imaged teeth on standard (analog films) radiographs is the embossed dot, which is near one corner of the film. When exposing a radiograph on standard radiographic films, the convex surface points towards the radiographic tube head when the film is properly positioned. It is not possible to obtain a diagnostic radiograph with the film in backwards, because of the lead sheet on the back side of the film. Therefore, when exposing the film, the embossed dot must be facing out of the mouth.

ORIENTATION

Interpreting dental radiographs starts with the appropriate orientation. First, place the convex side of the dot towards you. This means you are looking at the teeth as if your eyes are the x-ray beam. (This step is done for you on most digital systems). The dot should always be located in such a way that it is not superimposed on structures being imaged. When chemical development is performed, place the clip to hold the film adjacent to the dot (**Figures A8.3, A8.4**). This will provide an area of interest free of interfering artifacts. Next, rotate the film so that the roots are in their natural position (pointing up on maxillary views and down on mandibular) (**Figures A8.5–A8.8**).

When this is done, it is necessary to determine if it is the left or right side of the patient. For lateral oblique projections (canine, premolar, and maxillary molar teeth) or parallel projections (mandibular molar teeth), the side of the film where the more mesial teeth are located indicates the side that was imaged. In other words, if the mesial teeth are on the right side of the film, it is an image of the right side of the patient (**Figure A8.8**). With other projections, such as dorsoventral (DV) or ventrodorsal (VD) images (i.e incisors or canines), the right side of the mouth is on the left side of the film and vice versa for the left side of the mouth. This is similar to a VD image of the abdomen.

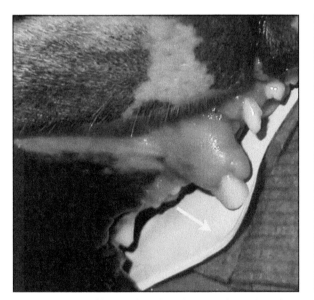

Fig. A8.3 **The film is placed in the mouth so that the dot (arrow) does not interfere with interpretation of the radiograph.**

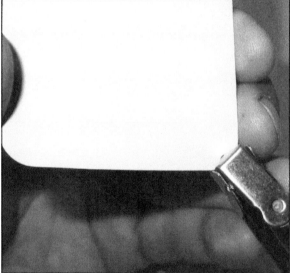

Fig. A8.4 **The clip used to hold the film during processing is attached near the dot.**

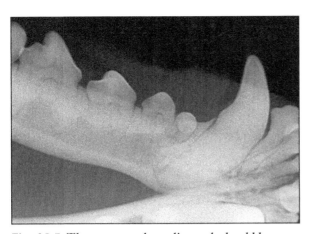

Fig. A8.5 The roots on the radiograph should be placed in their natural position (up on maxillary view and down on mandibular view). Here the tooth roots of the mandibular premolars and the canine roots point down on this correctly orientated radiograph.

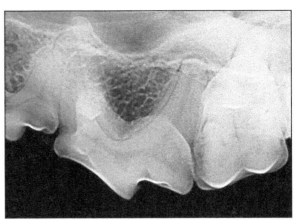

Fig. A8.6 The roots of the maxillary premolars and molar point up on this correctly orientated radiograph.

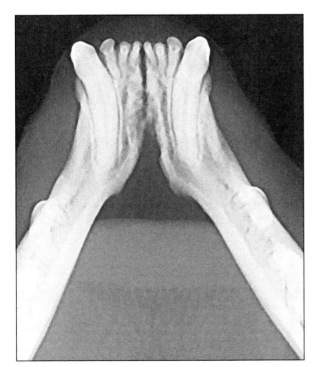

Fig. A8.7 The roots of the mandibular incisors, canines, and premolars point down on this correctly orientated radiograph.

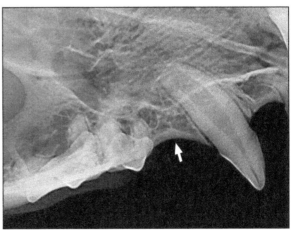

Fig. A8.8 The roots of the maxillary incisors, canines, premolars, and molar point up on this correctly orientated radiograph. Note the missing right maxillary second premolar (106) (arrow). The mesial tooth (canine) is on the right side, which means it is a radiograph of the right maxilla.

This orientation technique does not refer to radiographs in cassettes, as there is no embossed dot on these images. Therefore, it is important to mark the film during exposure. In some countries it is legal requirement to label all radiographs other than intraoral dental films.

MANDIBULAR AND MAXILLARY IMAGES

To distinguish between mandibular and maxillary images, certain landmarks should be evaluated.

Mandible

- The presence of the mandibular canal, mental foramina, mandibular symphysis and ventral mandibular margin (cortex).
  - The most rostral mental foramen is located in the second incisor area, the middle at the level of apex of the second premolar, and the caudal is at the level of the third premolar.[1]
- In dogs, the mandibular second, third, and fourth premolars and the first and second molars should have two roots.
- In cats there are normally only three teeth caudal to the canine.
- There are obviously exceptions to these rules (e.g. third root in a molar, fused roots or the presence of the second premolar in cats, and supernumerary teeth) (**Figures A8.9–A8.11**).

Maxillary

- The presence of palatine fissures, incisive canal; the conchal crest rostrally and pterygopalatine fossa caudally.
- The radiopaque line running across the canine root and just dorsally to the roots of the premolars and molars is the nasal surface of the alveolar process of the maxilla (**Figure A8.12**).
- Nasal structures are visible above the conchal crest with symmetric turbinate details (**Figure A8.13**).
- Typical structures for the nasal cavity are the palatine fissures and incisive foramen (**Figure A8.14**).
- In dogs, the fourth premolar as well as two maxillary molars normally have three roots; however, the second molar often has fused roots.
- In cats, the zygomatic arch is typically superimposed on the maxillary cheek teeth. To avoid this interference, an extraoral projection is performed, which changes the position of the zygoma on the radiograph (**Figure A8.15**).

In some breeds, it can be difficult to produce a diagnostic image of the entire tooth, due to the patients/tooth size, shape, and/or position as well as anatomic features. The maxillary canines in brachycephalic dogs are an example. To obtain a

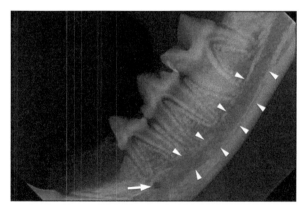

Fig. A8.9 **Feline left mandible. In cats there are normally only three teeth behind the canine and all have two roots. The mandibular canal (arrowheads), mental caudal foramen (arrow) and ventral margin of the mandible (cortex) are visible. Note that for diagnostic purposes the distal root of the molar tooth should have further distance from the edge.**

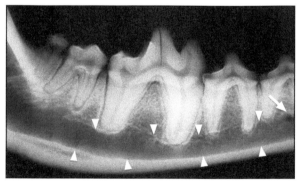

Fig. A8.10 **Canine right mandible: the fourth premolar as well as the first and second molars should have two roots, and the third molar one root. Visible on the radiograph: mandibular canal (arrowheads), caudal mental foramen (arrow), and cortex of the mandible. This radiograph was exposed on a dry skull. The drying process caused cracks on the molar tooth.**

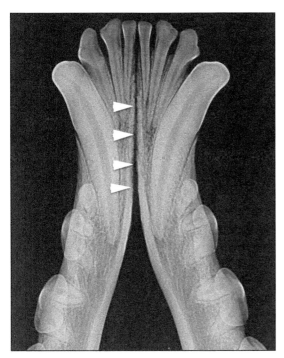

Fig. A8.11 Canine mandibular symphysis (arrowheads). Intraoral VD projection.

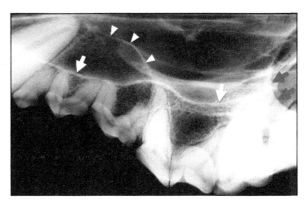

Fig. A8.12 A lateral oblique left maxillary canine radiograph. The conchal crest rostrally and the pterygopalatine fossa (red arrows) caudally are visible. The nasal structures visible above the conchal crest (arrowheads) are also normal anatomy. The opaque line running across the canine root and just dorsal to the roots of the premolars and molars (white arrows) is the nasal surface of the alveolar process of the maxilla. In dogs, the fourth premolar as well as the two maxillary molars are normally three rooted; however, the second molar quite often has fused roots.

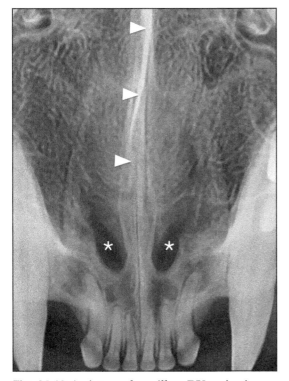

Fig. A8.13 An intraoral maxillary DV projection. Visible are the palatine fissures (asterisks) and nasal structures divided into two cavities by the nasal septum, which is ventrally articulated to the vomer (arrowheads).

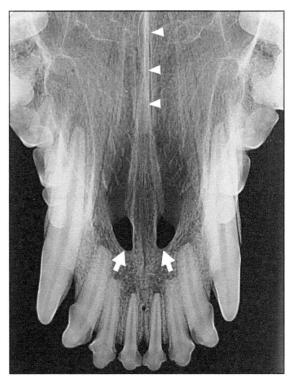

Fig. A8.14 Intraoral canine maxillary DV projection. This provides an image of the palatine fissures (arrows), the vomer (white arrowheads), and the incisive canal present between the apices on the first incisors (red arrowhead).

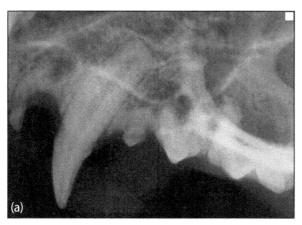

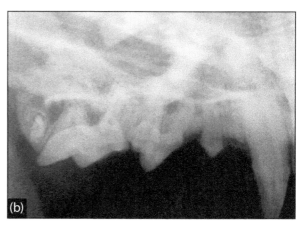

Fig. A8.15 **In cats, the zygomatic arch is often superimposed on maxillary cheek teeth. (a) A left maxillary intraoral projection showing the zygomatic arch overlapping the left maxillary third and fourth premolars (207 and 208) and the left maxillary molar (209). (b) To avoid this superimposition, an extraoral projection has been performed, which has changed the orientation of the film.**

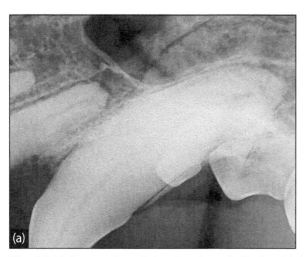

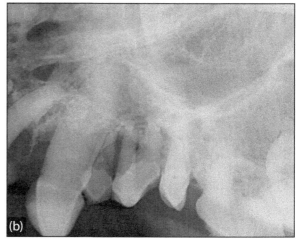

Fig. A8.16 **In some breeds (e.g. brachycephalic dogs) it is very difficult to obtain an appropriate image of the entire maxillary canine. Diagnostic images of the maxillary canine of a boxer (a) and a pug (b) are shown. Note the superimposition of the left maxillary first premolar (205) on the image of the canine tooth in (a). Note the horizontal bone loss affecting areas of 203, 204, 205, and 206 and rotation of 207.**

diagnostic image of the maxillary canine in a boxer or pug, several radiographs are often required (**Figure A8.16**). There also may be limitations created by the size of the oral cavity. Rigid size 2 sensors may be too large to provide a parallel view of the mandibular dentition in small cats and dogs (especially pediatric patients) (**Figure A8.17**). The best way to obtain diagnostic images in this situation is to use a small sized sensor or a photostimulable phosphor plate (**Figure A8.18**).

DETERMINING THE AGE AND SIZE OF THE PATIENT

Determining the approximate age and size of a patient, as well as defining the exact tooth, are helpful in forensic medicine and in evaluation of rescued or found animals.

For example, a foreign body was found in a dog's food bowl and the author was asked to determine if this specimen was a tooth and if so, what age, size,

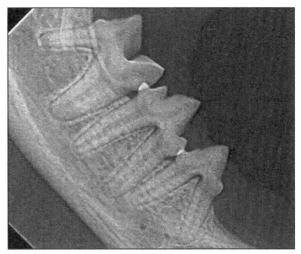

Fig. A8.18 **The result using a size 1 sensor in the same cat as Fig. A8.17, which improved the visibility of dental structures, although the mesial root of the right mandibular third premolar (407) should still have at least a 3 mm area from the edge to fulfill diagnostic requirements.**

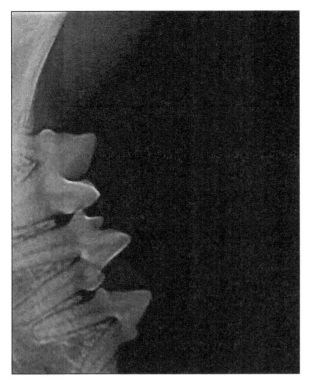

Fig. A8.17 **An attempt to obtain a parallel projection of the mandibular teeth in a small cat using a size 2 sensor.**

and species of animal it could have belonged to. The investigation showed it was most likely canine dentition, right maxillary second molar (110), in a dog 8–10 years old, weight 18–25 kg, with periodontal disease. Later it was discovered that the owner also had a 9-year-old boxer with periodontal disease, who was missing that tooth (**Figure A8.19**). The dog owner claimed that the specimen was present in the original pet food pack, but based on the investigation performed, such a claim is unlikely.

Another situation was a request from the police department to determine the age of a German shepherd dog that had been offered for sale as a supposedly young animal – approximately 1 year of age (**Figure A8.20**). Based on the clinical evaluation of the dentition, followed by radiographic assessment of the root canals and pulp chambers of the entire dentition, the estimated age was 5–7 years.

The size and shape of the crown is defined before eruption begins. In contrast, the root(s) change their dimensions during eruption and it is not until eruption is complete that the tooth will develop its final size and shape. The odontoblast layer within the pulp first produces primary dentin during eruption then, after eruption is complete, secondary dentin. This growth causes deposition of consecutive layers of secondary dentin in the pulp chamber/root canal as the odontoblast layer moves towards the center of the pulp cavity. At the same time, the lumens of the root canal and pulp chamber become progressively narrower. The rate of production of human dentin during the early period of tooth development is 4.5 µm a day.[2] After eruption is completed, the rate of dentin deposition gradually decreases.

Size of dentition

Some dogs from the group II classification of the Fédération Cynologique Internationale (FCI – World Canine Organization), called molossoid breeds, have relatively small teeth with shorter crowns and curved canines. These are boxers, Dogue de Bordeaux, and bulldogs. Fox terriers normally have relatively large dentition with long canine crowns, which make determining the bisecting angle for these teeth more difficult. When a dog belonging to a breed that is supposed to have proportionally large dentition presents with small teeth it is called microdontia.[3] Microdontia also describes

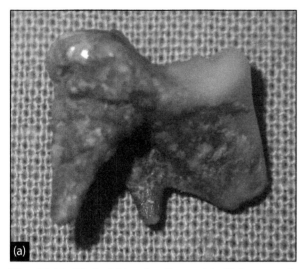
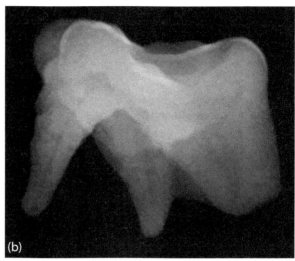

Fig. A8.19 Clinical (a) and radiographic (b) images of a tooth found in a dog's feeding bowl.

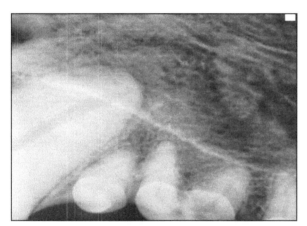
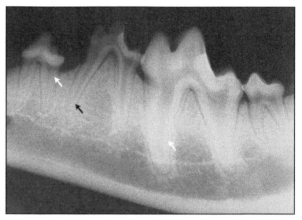

Fig. A8.20 Intraoral projection of the maxillary canine (204) of a German shepherd dog that was offered for sale as a supposedly young animal of approximately 1 year of age. Based on the clinical evaluation of the dentition followed by radiographic assessment of the root canals and pulp chambers of the entire dentition the estimated age was 5–7 years.

Fig. A8.21 Parallel projection of the left mandibular premolars and molars of an 18-month-old retriever. The following teeth can be identified, starting from the left (or rostrally): left mandibular third premolar (307) (white arrow), deciduous left mandibular fourth premolar (708) (black arrow), left mandibular first molar (309) (white arrowhead) and left mandibular second molar (310) (black arrowhead). Tooth 708 is a persistent deciduous tooth, which had no permanent successor.

small teeth found adjacent to teeth of normal size (see Chapter 8, Part E).

Deciduous teeth differ significantly from permanent teeth. They have relatively smaller crowns as well as more divergent, thinner, and longer roots than their permanent successors. The pulp chamber and root canal are relatively larger in deciduous dentition than in permanent dentition (**Figure A8.21**).

There are also single rooted and multirooted teeth. The distribution of root numbers in deciduous and permanent dentition is shown in *Table A8.1*. Supernumerary roots in dogs are most common in the maxillary third premolar (**Figure A8.22**)[4] and

Table A8.1 **Distribution of root numbers in deciduous and permanent dentition**

SPECIES	SINGLE ROOTED TEETH	TEETH WITH TWO ROOTS	TEETH WITH THREE ROOTS
Canine deciduous (28 teeth)	12 incisors (501, 502, 503, 601, 602, 603, 701, 702, 703, 801, 802, 803) 4 canine (504, 604, 704, 804)	8 premolars: second maxillary, second, third and fourth mandibular premolars (506, 606, 706, 707, 708, 806, 807, 808)	4 premolars: third and fourth maxillary (507, 508, 607, 608)
Canine permanent (42 teeth)	12 incisors (101, 102, 103, 201, 202, 203, 301, 302, 303, 401, 402, 403) 4 canine (104, 204, 304, 404) 4 first premolars (105, 205, 305, 405) 2 last mandibular molars (311, 411)	10 premolars (106, 107, 206, 207, 306, 307, 308, 406, 407, 408) 4 molars (309, 310, 409, 410)	2 maxillary fourth premolars (108, 208) 4 maxillary molars (109, 110, 209, 210)
Feline deciduous (26 teeth)	12 incisors (501, 502, 503, 601, 602, 603, 701, 702, 703, 801, 802, 803) 4 canine (504, 604, 704, 804) 2 premolars (506, 606)	4 mandibular premolars (707, 708, 807, 808) 2 maxillary premolars (507, 607)	2 maxillary premolars (508, 608)
Feline permanent (30 teeth)	12 incisors (101, 102, 103, 201, 202, 203, 301, 302, 303, 401, 402, 403) 4 canines (104, 204, 304, 404) 2 second maxillary premolars (106, 206) (most often they have two roots)	6 premolars (107, 207, 307, 308, 407, 408) 4 molars (109, 209, 309, 409) (occasionally 109 and 209 have one fused root)	2 maxillary fourth premolars (108, 208)

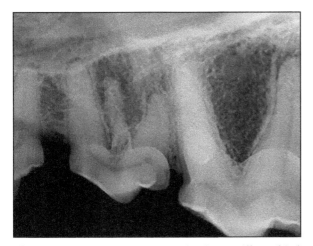

Fig. A8.22 **Supernumerary root in the maxillary third premolar of a dog.**

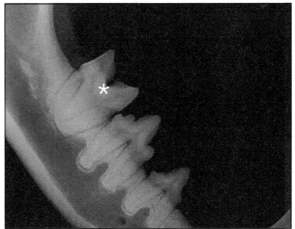

Fig. A8.23 **Parallel projection of the right mandibular premolars and molar tooth in a cat, revealing fused roots of the right first molar tooth (409) (asterisk).**

mandibular first molar, while fused roots are most common in the mandibular second premolars and second molars in both jaws.[5] However, this phenomenon is seen in other teeth as well as in cats (**Figure A8.23**).

Age of patient

It is possible to estimate the age of the patient based on dental radiographs. The first important landmark for maturation assessment is the period and order of changing the dentition, which normally lasts from

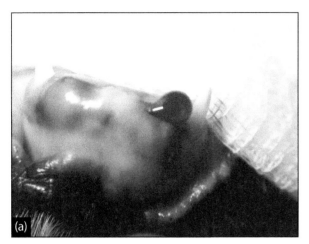

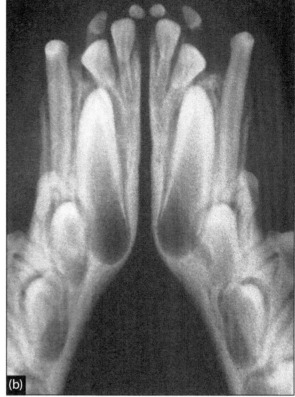

Fig. A8.24 A 10-week-old Tibetan terrier with unerupted deciduous incisor teeth. (a) After incising the operculum, the liquid from an eruption cyst was evacuated. (b) The radiograph additionally reveals missing incisors (both deciduous and permanent) as well as missing left and right mandibular first premolars (305 and 405).

4.5 to 7 months of age, depending on the breed. In small breeds, this period may last longer and eruption may be delayed. In some breeds, delayed eruption appears to be a genetic problem (e.g. in Tibetan terriers) (**Figure A8.24**).[6] The first permanent teeth to erupt are the incisors, followed by the canines, premolars, and the molars.[7] By 8 weeks of age all the deciduous teeth should be in their correct position, and by 6 months of age all the permanent teeth should have erupted.[8] The first premolars and molar teeth have no deciduous predecessor. The second important time point is when the apex closes. This process should be completed by between 9 and 11 months of age. The mandibular molars are the first to close and the maxillary canines last.[9] Secondary dentin is produced following complete eruption and apexogenesis and causes the pulp chamber and root canal to become progressively narrower. This process may be accelerated by pulpitis (e.g. due to tooth wear) or other chronic traumatic conditions that may

stimulate odontoblasts to produce more dentin than normal (**Figure A8.25**). Deposition of dentin is terminated when the pulp dies.[10] The width of the pulp chamber in nonvital teeth can suggest the age when the pulp necrosis occurred (**Figure A8.26**).

The age and respective radiographic features of dogs and cats are described in *Tables A8.2* and *A8.3*, respectively.

Size of the patient

Based on radiographs, some information about the size of the animal is available. The ratio of the height of the mandibular first molar tooth (crown and root) to the adjacent bone height is significantly increased in smaller dogs and gradually decreases with increasing size (**Figure A8.27**).[11] This feature predisposes the mandible of small and especially toy breed dogs to pathologic fractures when the mandibular first molar is affected by periodontal and/or endodontic disease (**Figure A8.28**).

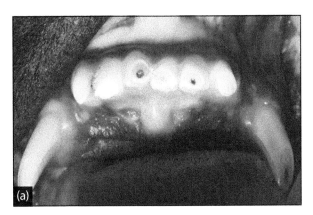

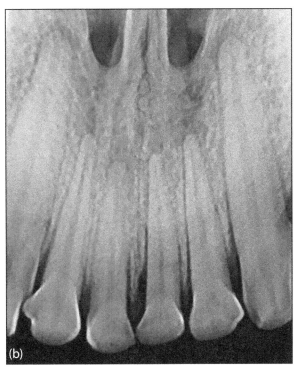

Fig. A8.25 An 18-month-old Staffordshire terrier with a habit of chewing hard objects and a very tight occlusion (teeth in occlusion contact one another very tightly and not only on the occlusal surfaces). (a) Worn teeth with direct pulp exposure are visible (right maxillary first incisor [101], left maxillary second incisor [202], and left maxillary canine [204]. (b) Radiographically, the root canals of these incisors are relatively narrower than in a dog of the same age with normally used teeth.

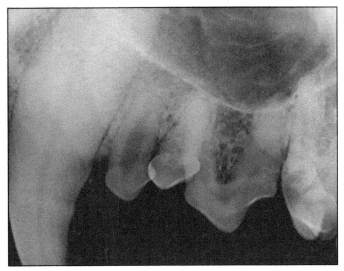

Fig. A8.26 A 6-year-old boxer with a supernumerary left maxillary first premolar (205). The rostral supernumerary 205 has a wide pulp chamber and root canal whereas the caudal one has very narrow ones. The termination of dentin deposition (likely caused by death of the pulp) probably happened around 1 year of age. Note the periapical rarefaction in the non-vital 205.

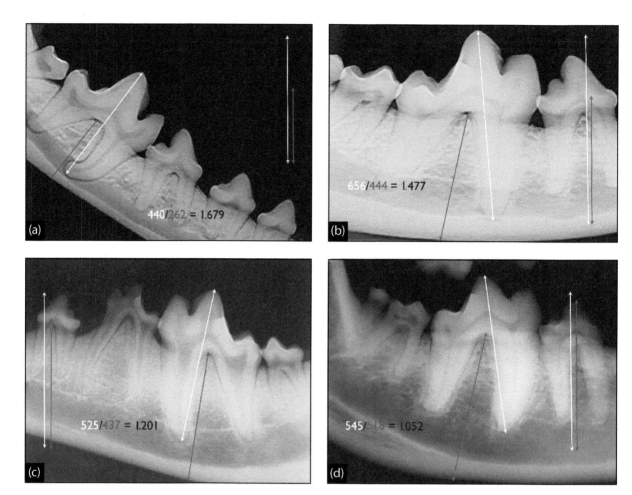

(a) 440/262 = 1.679

(b) 656/444 = 1.477

(c) 525/437 = 1.201

(d) 545/516 = 1.052

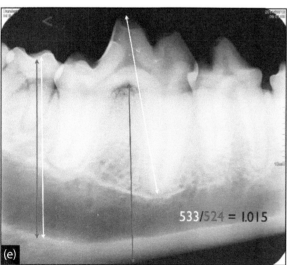

(e) 533/524 = 1.015

Fig. A8.27 **Radiographs showing the ratios of the height of the mandibular first molar tooth (crown and root = white line) to the adjacent bone height (red line). The distances in the calculated ratios were digital and measured the number of pixels. (a) 2.7 kg Yorkshire terrier = 1.679 despite the fact that the molar tooth is dilacerated, which reduced the tooth height. (b) 8 kg West Highland White terrier = 1.477. (c) 20 kg retriever = 1.201. (d) 30 kg Labrador = 1.052. (e) 55 kg Mastiff = 1.015.**

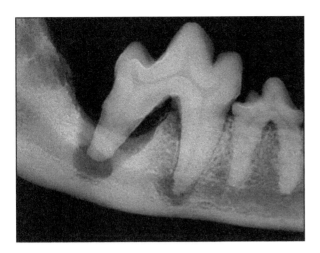

Fig. A8.28 Eleven-year-old Dachshund with a severe class II perio-endo lesion of the right mandibular first molar (409). Extraction of this tooth needs to be performed carefully.

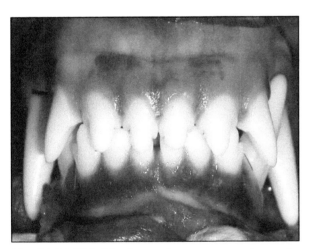

Fig. A8.29 This 8 kg fox terrier represents a 'strong' type of dentition with large crowns in relation to jaw width, and tight solid occlusion.

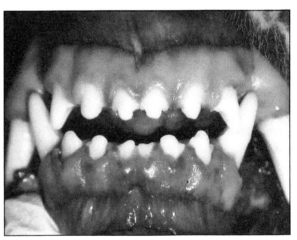

Fig. A8.30 This 45 kg Tatra shepherd dog has relatively smaller teeth compared with the dog in Fig. A8.29. The crowns are smaller in relation to jaw width; alignment and occlusion is looser.

Some software allows for measuring and this helps determine the size of the radiographed tooth. One should take into account that some breeds have 'strong' dentition (e.g. terriers) while others have small teeth (e.g. certain brachycephalic breeds) (**Figures A8.29, A8.30**).

The dimensions of the endodontic system are a good guide for evaluating age provided that the dentition is normal, the pulp is vital, and there are no coexisting factors that may influence dentin production. The canine and feline aging process is shown in **Figures A8.31** and **A8.32**, respectively.

Table A8.2 **Age and respective radiographic features of dogs (Figure A8.31)**

AGE	FEATURE
4 months	Mixed dentition. Erupted deciduous: canines, third incisors, premolars, and permanent molar; nonerupted permanent: canines, third incisors, and premolars (**A8.31[1]**)
6 months	Erupted permanent dentition, open apices (**A8.31[2]**)
9 months	Closed apices (**A8.31[3]**)
18 months	Comparable width of dentin layer in root and crown (**A8.31[4]**)
3 years	Pulp chamber and root canal narrower than on previous radiographic recording at 18 months (**A8.31[5]**)
6 years	Root canal narrower than pulp chamber in M1 (**A8.31[6]**)
12 years	Pulp chamber wider than root canal (**A8.31[7]**)
16 years	Root canal hardly visible (**A8.31[8]**)

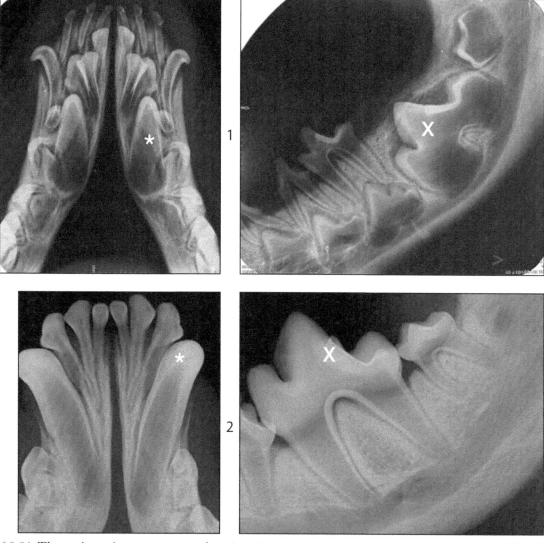

Fig. A8.31 The canine aging process. x, molars; *, canines.   (*Continued*)

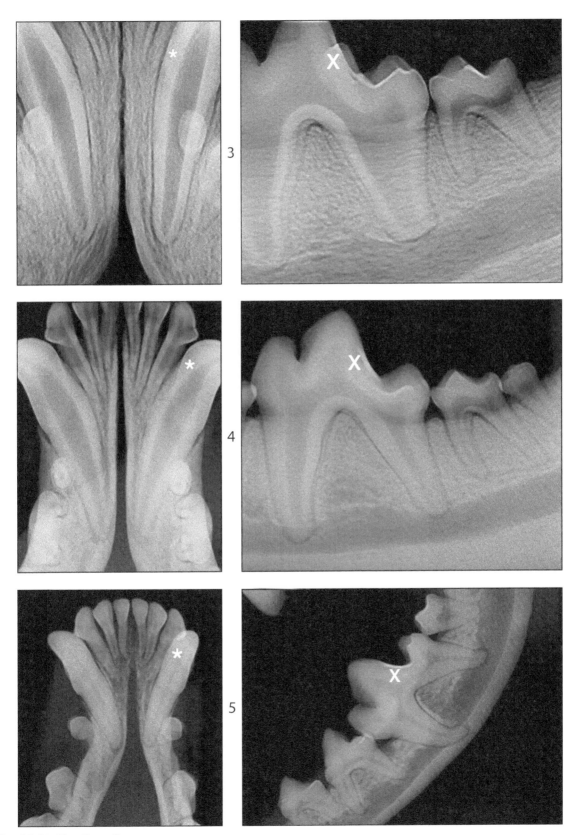

Fig. A8.31 *(Continued)*

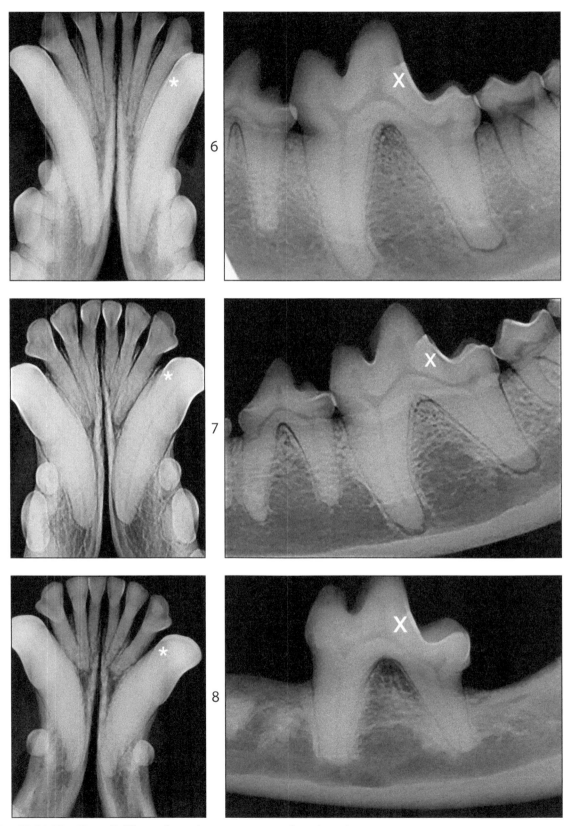

Fig. A8.31 *(Continued)* The canine aging process. x, molars; *, canines.

Table A8.3 **Age and respective radiographic features of cats (Figure A8.32)**

AGE	FEATURE
4 months	Mixed dentition. Erupted deciduous: third incisors, canines, premolars, and permanent molar; nonerupted permanent: third incisors, canines, and premolars (**A8.32[1]**)
6 months	Erupted permanent dentition, open apices (**A8.32[2]**)
9–11 months	Closed apices (**A8.32[3]**)
18 months	Comparable width of dentln layer in root and crown (**A8.32[4]**)
3 years	Pulp chamber and root canal narrower than on previous radiographic recording at 18 months (**A8.32[5]**)
6 years	Root canal narrower than pulp chamber in M1 (**A8.32[6]**)
12 years	Pulp chamber wider than root canal; note alveolar bone expansion in 304 (**A8.32[7]**)
16 years	Root canal hardly visible; note 307 affected by tooth resorption (left radiograph) and horizontal alveolar bone loss (right radiograph) (**A8.32[8]**)

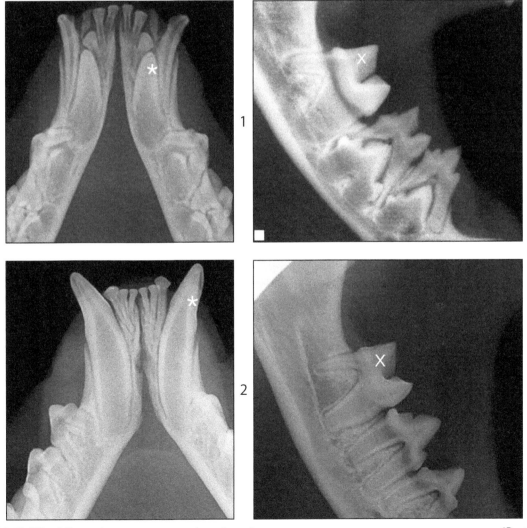

Fig. A8.32 The feline aging process. x, molars; *, canines.

(Continued)

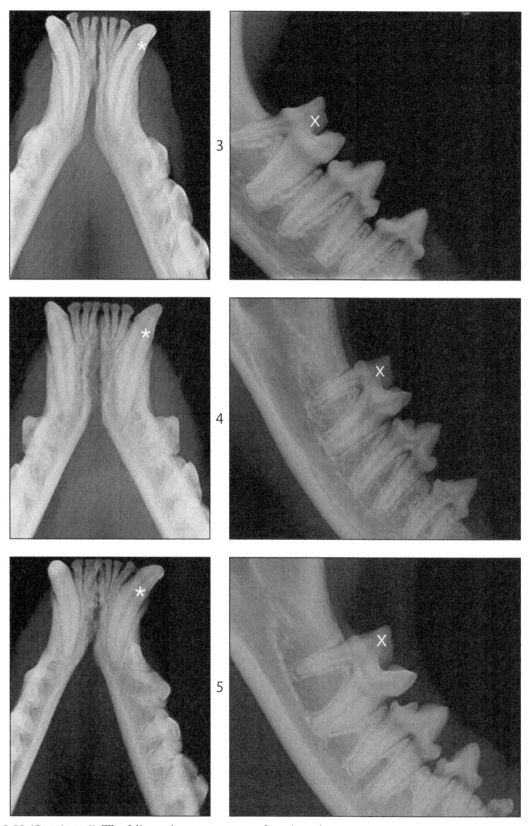

Fig. A8.32 (Continued) The feline aging process. x, molars; *, canines.

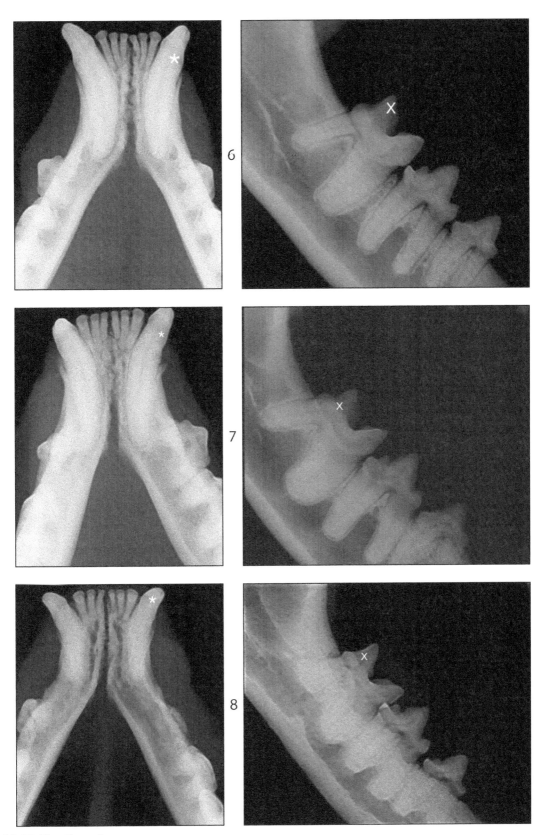

Fig. A8.32 *(Continued)*

REFERENCES

1 Mulligan WT, Aller MS, Williams CA (1998) Normal radiographic anatomy. In: *Atlas of Canine and Feline Dental Radiography*. Veterinary Learning Systems, Trenton, p. 68.

2 Kawasaki K, Tanaka S, Ishikawa T (1979) On the daily incremental lines in human dentine. *Arch Oral Biol* **24:**939–943.

3 Verheart L (2007) Developmental oral and dental conditions. In: *BSAVA Manual of Canine and Feline Dentistry*. (eds. C Tutt, J Deeprose, DA Crossley) British Small Animal Veterinary Association, Gloucester, pp. 77–95.

4 DuPont GA, DeBowes LJ (2008) Developmental dental abnormalities. In: *Atlas of Dental Radiography in Dogs and Cats*. Saunders/Elseveir, St. Louis, pp. 195–207.

5 Bannon K (2013) Clinical canine dental radiography. *Vet Clin North Am Small Anim Pract* **43:**507–532.

6 Ackerman LJ (2011) *The Genetic Connection: A Guide to Heath Problems in Purebred Dogs*, 2nd edn. American Animal Hospital Association Press, Lakewood, p. 41.

7 Evans HE, de Lahunta A (2013) The digestive apparatus and abdomen. In: *Miller's Anatomy of the Dog*, 4th edn. Elsevier, St. Louis, p. 286.

8 Fulton A, Fiani N, Verstreate F (2014) Canine pediatric dentistry. *Vet Clin North Am Small Anim Pract* **44:**303–324.

9 Gracis M (2007) Orodental anatomy and physiology. In: *BSAVA Manual of Canine and Feline Dentistry*. (eds. C Tutt, J Deeprose, DA Crossley) British Small Animal Veterinary Association, Gloucester, pp. 1–21.

10 DuPont GA, DeBowes LJ (2008) Intraoral radiographic anatomy of the dog. In: *Atlas of Dental Radiography in Dogs and Cats*. Saunders/Elsevier, St. Louis, pp. 5–80.

11 Gioso M, Shofer P, Barros P *et al.* (2001) Mandible and mandibular first molar tooth measurements in dogs: relationship of radiographic height to body weight. *J Vet Dent* **18(2):**65–68.

PART B

NORMAL RADIOGRAPHIC ANATOMY

Brook A. Niemiec

INTRODUCTION

There are numerous structures within the oral cavity that can mimic pathologic states. This is especially true with certain projections and techniques. A firm grasp of normal radiographic anatomy is helpful to avoid overinterpretation (or misinterpretation).[1-7]

BONE

Normal alveolar bone (**Figure B8.1**) appears gray and relatively uniform throughout the dental arch. It is slightly more radiopaque (darker) than tooth roots. It is also slightly but regularly mottled. In general, maxillary alveolar bone is less dense than mandibular bone. The bone should be at a constant level across the dental arch. The bone becomes denser with age, so older patients will demonstrate increased bone density. There should be no radiolucent areas in normal bone (with the exception of the normal anatomic structures listed below).

TEETH

The crowns of the teeth are covered with a thin layer of enamel. Enamel is the most radiodense structure in the body, because it is 97% mineralized. Therefore, it is seen as a thin white line covering the crowns of the teeth (**Figure B8.2**).

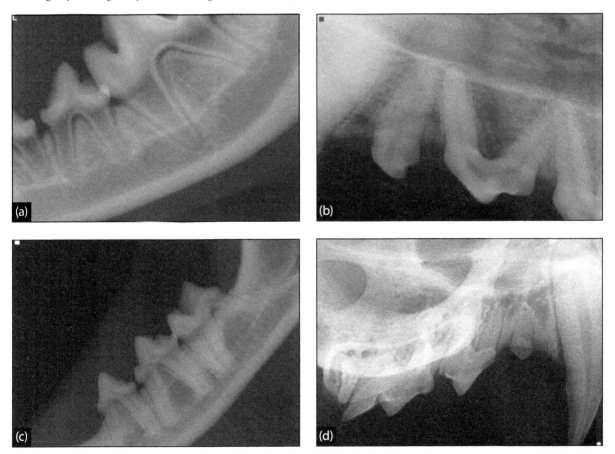

Fig. B8.1 **Radiographic appearance of normal dental arches. (a) Mandibular first molar area in a young dog. (b) Maxillary premolar area in a middle aged dog. (c) Mandible of a middle aged cat. (d) Maxillary cheek teeth of a normal cat.**

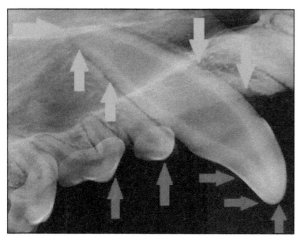

Fig. B8.2 **The enamel is the thin bright white line over the crowns of the teeth (red arrows). The rest of the teeth will appear whiter and more regular than bone (blue arrows).**

The rest of the hard tooth structure (dentin and cementum) is slightly more radiodense than bone. This means the teeth will appear whiter than bone on radiographs and also slightly more regular than bone (**Figure B8.2**). The roots of multirooted teeth should be slightly divergent (**Figure B8.3**).

The root canals should appear regular and smooth. Root canals should all appear similar in width in relation to the size of the tooth. Suspicious differences in the width of a root canal should be compared against surrounding as well as contralateral teeth. Surrounding (adjacent) teeth can often be seen on the same film with the 'lesion'. The contralateral view should be taken at the same angle as the original view. It is important to note that root canals are not exact cylinders (especially in canine teeth) (**Figure B8.4**) (i.e. a lateral view may show a very different canal width (wider) compared with a ventrodorsal [VD] view).

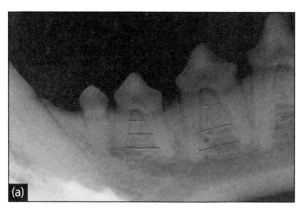

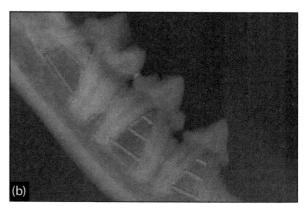

Fig. B8.3 **The tooth roots in multirooted teeth tend to be apically divergent (lines). (a) Mandible of a dog; (b) mandible of a cat.**

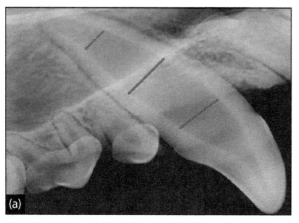

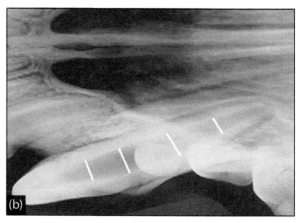

Fig. B8.4 **Lateral (a) and more DV (b) projection intraoral dental radiographs of a maxillary canine. The root canal appears wider on the more lateral view (a, red lines) than it does on the DV view (b, white lines). If the angulation of the views is not similar, this may lead to an incorrect interpretation of a nonvital tooth.**

TOOTH/BONE INTERFACE

The alveolar bone should completely fill the area between the roots (called the furcation), ending at or within 2 mm of the cementoenamel junction (CEJ).[8] A regular thin dark line (periodontal ligament space) should be visualized around the roots. The width of the periodontal ligament generally decreases with age. The area of bone surrounding the periodontal ligament is more dense and regular and therefore will be seen as a white line surrounding the teeth. This is the lamina dura (**Figure B8.5**).

The periodontal ligament should be of uniform width around the tooth (**Figures B8.6a, b**). A widened and/or uneven area (especially at the apex of tooth) is generally diagnostic for endodontic

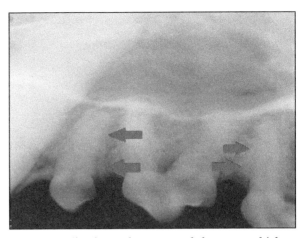

Fig. B8.5 **The denser bone around the roots, which show up more radiodense on the radiograph (arrows). This is the lamina dura.**

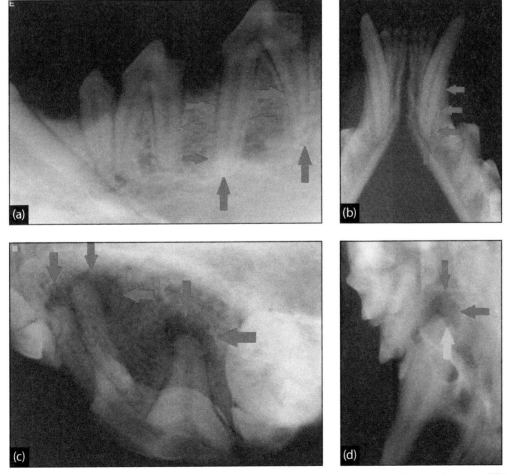

Fig. B8.6 **The periodontal ligament is seen as a thin black line around the entire root surface (red arrows). This is shown in the mandible of a dog (a) and a cat mandibular canine (b). A widening of the periodontal ligament (especially at the apex) (red arrows) is indicative of probable endodontic disease. This is shown on the maxillary fourth premolar of a dog (c) and maxillary canine of a cat (d). In (d) note that the apex of the root is undergoing resorption (blue arrow).**

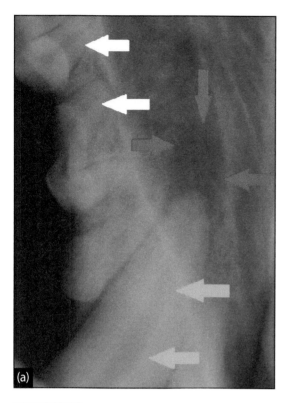

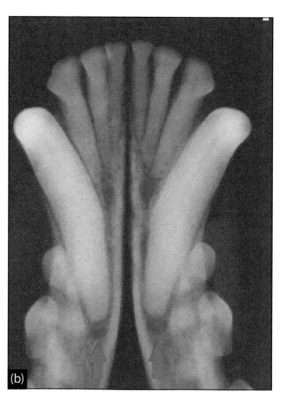

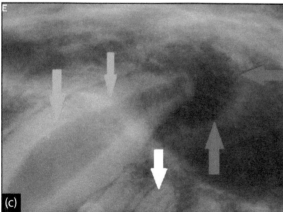

Fig. B8.7 **The chevron effect. (a) Intraoral dental radiograph of the right maxillary canine (104) in a dog. The regular lucency at the apex of this tooth (red arrows) is a 'chevron' effect and not a true periapical lucency associated with endodontic disease. The endodontic system of the canine (blue arrows) is of similar size relative to the premolars (white arrows). The most accurate assessment is to the contralateral canine, and this should be performed as well as a complete oral examination to rule out infection. (b) Chevron effect of the mandibular canines (red arrows). (c) Dental radiograph of a left maxillary canine in a dog with periapical rarefaction indicative of an endodontic infection (red arrows). The more round appearance is indicative of infection. In addition, the root canal of the canine (blue arrows) is significantly wider than the premolar teeth seen on the same image (white arrow).**

disease (**Figures B8.6c, d**). However, a slight widening of the periodontal ligament at the apex of the canine teeth (especially the maxillary) is normal (**Figures B8.7a, b**). This is called a 'chevron effect'. This may appear to be a periapical lesion, but can be differentiated from pathology because (1) it is very smooth and regular and (2) it is V-shaped as opposed to irregular and round (**Figure B8.7c**).

Any suspicious periapical lucency (especially in the area of the mandibular premolars) should be evaluated with an additional film exposed at a slightly different angle, either in the horizontal or

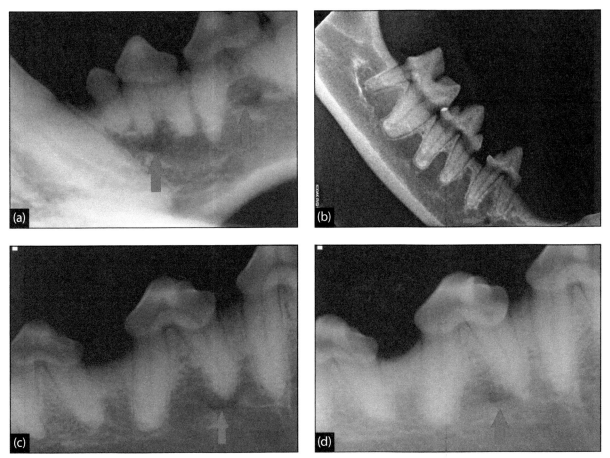

Fig. B8.8 Mental foramina. (a) The middle and caudal mental foramina in a dog (arrows). (b) The caudal mental foramina in a cat (arrow). (c, d) Caudal mental foramina masquerading as periapical rarefaction. In (c) the foramina is centered on the distal root (arrow). This may be mistaken for an endodontic lesion. However, when the image is taken at a slightly different angle (d) the lucency moves off the apex (arrow), revealing the lucency as 'artifact'. Also note that it is rare to have a lucency on one root of a multirooted tooth.

vertical plane. If the lucency is still centered on the apex, it is likely real. If the lesion moves off the apex or disappears on the comparison views, it is an artifact (typically a mental foramina) (**Figure B8.8**).

There are several normal anatomic findings that are commonly misinterpreted in dental images as being pathologic, including findings affecting the maxilla and the mandible.[9]

Maxilla

- A radiodense line running across the root of the maxillary canine and then just above the roots of the maxillary premolars is the lateral aspect of the floor of the nasal cavity. This is where the bones of the maxilla merge with the palatine process (**Figure B8.9b**).
- The radiodense line on the midline of the palate is the vomer bone (**Figure B8.10**).
- In the rostral maxillary region there are paired radiolucent areas caudal to the second incisors on each side, which are the palatine fissures (**Figure B8.10**).
- The radiodense structure running over the maxillary third and fourth premolars and first molar in cats (as well as in many brachycephalic dogs) is the zygomatic arch (**Figure B8.11**).
- On images of the maxillary fourth premolar in dogs, it is common for the furcational bone between the mesial and distal roots to

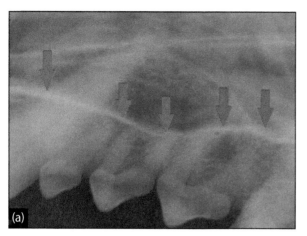

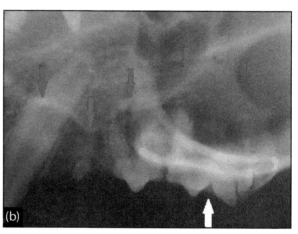

Fig. B8.9 The radiodense line running across the root of the maxillary canine and then just above the roots of the maxillary premolars is the lateral aspect of the floor of the nasal cavity (red arrows: a, dog; b, cat). In (b) the white arrow is pointing to the maxillary fourth premolar.

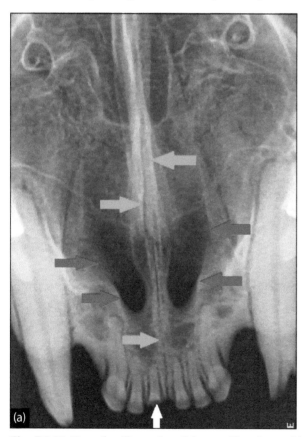

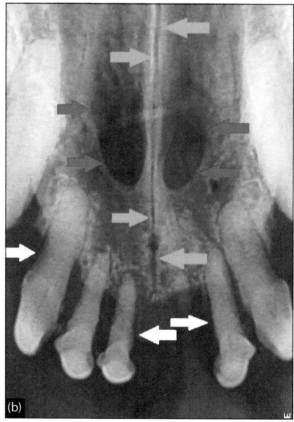

Fig. B8.10 Dental radiographs of the maxilla of a cat (a) and a dog (b) demonstrating the vomer bone (blue arrows) and palatine fissures (red arrows). These are normal findings. In (a) there is also a fractured and retained root of the right first incisor (101) (white arrow). In (b), the incisors have advanced horizontal alveolar bone loss (white arrows).

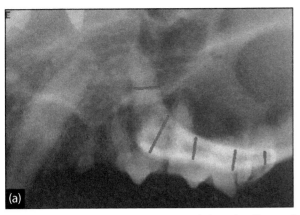

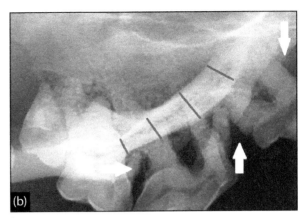

Fig. B8.11 **Zygomatic arch. Intraoral dental radiographs of the zygomatic arch (lines) in a cat (a) and a dog (b).
In (b), the teeth have advanced horizontal alveolar bone loss (arrows).**

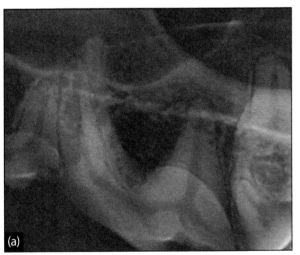

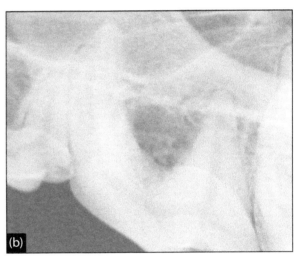

Fig. B8.12 **The influence of exposure on the furcational area of the maxillary P4. (a) In this image there appears
to be a significant class 3 furcation exposure. However, the image is overexposed. (b) In this additional image
with less exposure the bone is shown to be present.**

be 'burnt out' and not be seen on radiographs
(**Figure B8.12a**). This is due to the significant
difference between the density of the
superimposed mesial roots and the large distal
root in comparison with the relatively thin
area of bone in the furcational area. If this is
seen, a second image should be made with a
shorter exposure time to properly view this area
(**Figure B8.12b**).

Mandible

On radiographs of the mandibular cheek teeth, a
wide, horizontal radiolucent line courses parallel to

and just dorsal to the ventral cortex of the mandible.
This is the mandibular canal. The ventral cortex is
the relatively thin radiodense structure just below
the mandibular canal. Below the ventral cortex, the
radiograph should be black (**Figure B8.13**).

- There are one or two circular radiolucent
  areas seen in the area of the apices of the
  rostral mandibular premolars (**Figure B8.8**).
  These are the mental foramina (middle and
  caudal).
- On rostral mandibular views for the canines
  (**Figure B8.14**), a radiolucent line is typically

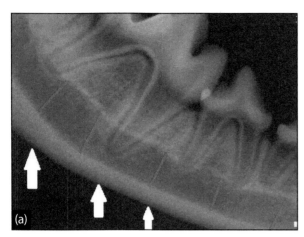
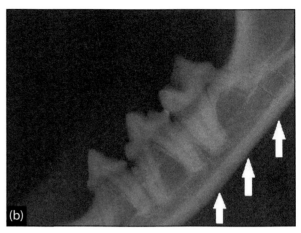

Fig. B8.13 **Intraoral dental radiograph of a normal mandible in a dog (a) and a cat (b). The radiolucent line (red lines) is the mandibular canal. The radiodense structure apical to this is the ventral cortex (white arrows).**

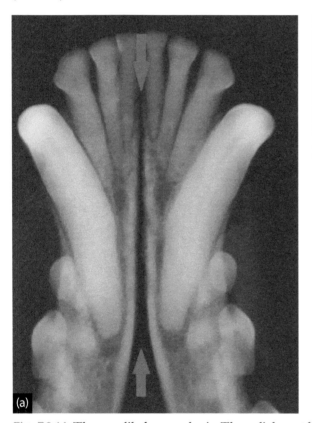
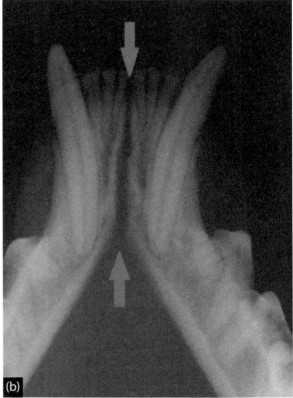

Fig. B8.14 **The mandibular symphysis. The radiolucent line between the incisors (arrows) is the fibrocartilagenous synchrondrosis known as the mandibular symphysis. This is demonstrated in a dog (a) and a cat (b).**

present between the central incisors, extending between the mandibles. This fibrocartilagenous synchrondrosis is known as the mandibular symphysis.

- A 'double periodontal ligament' may be seen along the furcational side of the mandibular first molar in dogs (especially the mesial root) (**Figure B8.15**).[10] This is a normal groove in the teeth.[11]

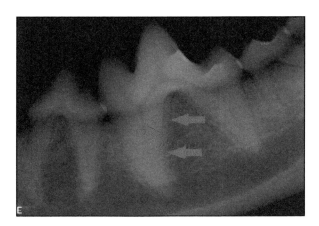

Fig. B8.15 A 'double periodontal ligament' is seen along the furcational side of the mandibular first molar in dogs (arrows), which is a normal groove in the teeth.

REFERENCES

1 Niemiec BA (2005) Dental radiographic interpretation. *J Vet Dent* **22(1)**:53–59.

2 Niemiec BA (2010) Veterinary dental radiology. In: *Small Animal Dental, Oral and Maxillofacial Disease: A Color Handbook*. (ed. BA Niemiec) Manson Publishing, London, pp. 63–87.

3 Aller MS (2000) Normal feline oral radiographic anatomy. In: *An Atlas of Veterinary Dental Radiology*. (eds. DH DeForge, BH Colmery) Iowa State University Press, Ames, 117–134.

4 DeBowes LJ, DeForge DH, Kesel ML et al. (2000) Normal canine intraoral radiographic anatomy. In: *An Atlas of Veterinary Dental Radiology*. (eds. DH DeForge, BH Colmery) Iowa State University Press, Ames, 3–14.

7 Bellows J (2008) Dental radiography. In: *Small Animal Dental Equipment, Materials, and Technique: A Primer*. Wiley-Blackwell, Ames, pp. 63–104.

6 Mulligan TW, Aller MS, Williams CA (1998) Normal radiographic anatomy. In: *Atlas of Canine and Feline Dental Radiography*. Veterinary Learning Systems, Trenton, pp. 68–90.

7 Bellows J (2010) Radiology. In: *Feline Dentistry: Oral Assesment, Treatment, and Preventative Care*. Wiley-Blackwell, Ames, pp. 39–83.

8 Gawor J (2013) Dental radiology for periodontal disease. In: *Veterinary Periodontology*. (ed. BA Niemiec) Wiley-Blackwell, Ames, pp. 107–128.

9 Gracis M (1999) Radiographic study of the maxillary canine tooth in four mesaticephalic cats. *J Vet Dent* **16(3)**:115–128.

10 Niemiec BA (2012) *Dental Extractions Made Easier*. Practical Veterinary Publishing, Tustin.

11 Woodward TM (2009) Interpretation of dental radiographs. *Top Companion Anim Med* **24(1)**:37–43.

PART C

PERIODONTAL RADIOGRAPHY

Jerzy Gawor

"Bone loss is always greater than is seen in the radiograph."

Fermin A. Carranza

INTRODUCTION

Periodontal disease is the number one health problem in small animal patients[1], therefore appropriate diagnosis has become very important.[2] The periodontium is a three-dimensional group of different tissues, structures, and substances that represent different levels of radiographic density (**Figure C8.1**). A clinical evaluation of the periodontium is always performed first, followed by the radiographic study. These two examinations are complementary[3], therefore the gold standard of veterinary oral health care includes a thorough clinical assessment of all teeth (periodontal probing) as well as full-mouth radiography.[4]

The value of radiographic evaluation in veterinary patients was proven in studies that found that 27.8% of clinically important lesions in dogs and 41.7% in cats would be missed without radiography (**Figures C8.2, C8.3**).[5,6]

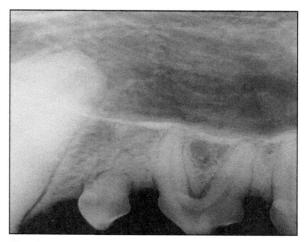

Fig. C8.2 This malformed root in the left maxillary first molar (205) is not detectable on clinical examination. Without radiography this problem would have been missed. Knowledge of the root morphology is important prior to extraction or endodontic or orthodontic treatment.

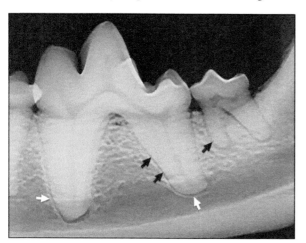

Fig. C8.1 In this radiograph the most radiopaque periodontal structure is the lamina dura (white arrows) and the least radiopaque is the periodontal ligament space (black arrows). Alveolar bone is present between the teeth and the roots. Note the horizontal alveolar bone loss at the area of 310.

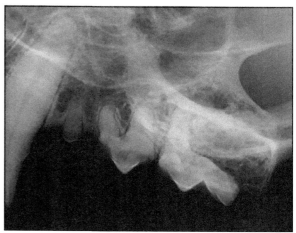

Fig. C8.3 The resorbed distal root of the left maxillary fourth premolar (208) in this cat, as well as resorption of left maxillary third premolar (207), were diagnosed incidentally on routine full-mouth radiography. Note the presence of remnants of resorbed left maxillary molar (209).

Periodontal disease is more common in older animals[7], therefore full-mouth radiography, which is an obligatory part of the diagnostic plan, is even more important in older animals or in those more prone to periodontal disease (small and toy breed dogs) as well as in other predisposed breeds (e.g. greyhounds or poodles) (**Figures C8.4, C8.5**).[8]

The clinical appearance of the evaluated area often does not correlate completely with the radiographic appearance (**Figures C8.6, C8.7**).[9] One study revealed that the clinical and radiographic examinations differ and this difference is increased when utilizing histometric measurements. The disparity between these two evaluations was between 14% and 60%.[10]

Although radiographic evaluation is a very important part of the diagnostic and therapeutic plans in the management of periodontal disease, it does have certain limitations:

- Dental radiographs will not show bony changes until more than 30–60% mineral resorption has occurred.[11] Therefore, dental radiographs will always *underestimate* the level of bone loss.
- The early stage of periodontal disease (gingivitis), as well as class 1 furcation involvement, are not radiographically evident (**Figures C8.8, C8.9**). On the other hand, furcation lesions are often overestimated radiographically (especially on overexposed films)

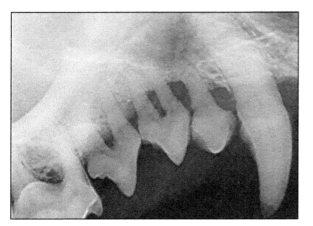

Fig. C8.4 **Radiograph of a 7-year-old Yorkshire terrier with horizontal alveolar bone loss around the right maxillary canine and premolars (104, 105, 106, 107). Note the calculus present on 104, 105, and 106.**

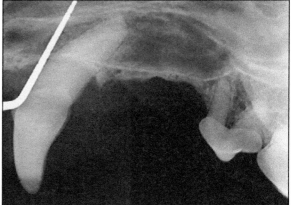

Fig. C8.5 **Radiograph of a 10-year-old dachshund with nasal discharge. The periodontal probe has entered the nasal cavity from the palatal side of the left maxillary canine tooth (204). Dolichocephalic breeds (e.g. greyhounds, poodles, dachshunds) often develop significant periodontal disease on the palatal aspect of the canines, which leads to oronasal fistula formation.**

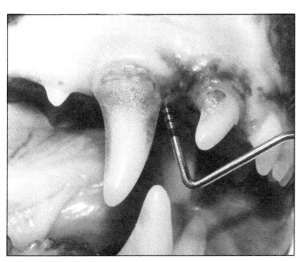

Fig. C8.6 **Periodontal probing with the use of a UNC 15 probe reveals a periodontal pocket in the right maxillary canine tooth (104). The depth of the periodontal pocket (10 mm) is recorded.**

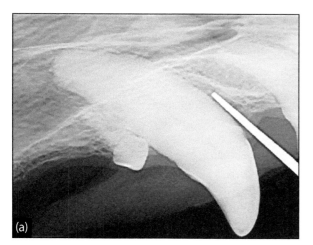
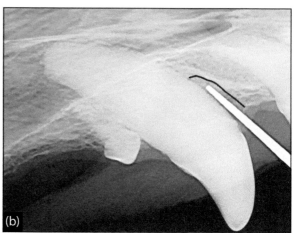

Fig. C8.7 Radiographs of the probing presented in Fig. C8.6. Radiographic assessment reveals the deeper extent of the pathology. Pressure on the probe during examination should be gentle so as not to rupture the soft periodontal tissue. (a) Note that the probe does not reach the apical end of the periodontal pocket. (b) The black line shows the radiographic appearance and extension of the periodontal pathology.

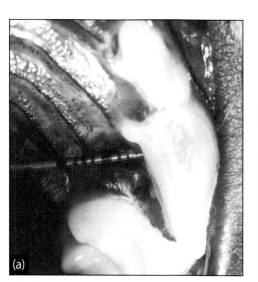
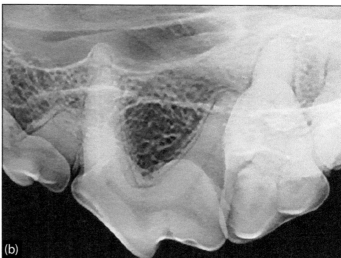

Fig. C8.8 (a) Periodontal probing of the left maxillary fourth premolar (208) of this dog reveals class 1 furcation involvement. The probe has entered the furcation area, but not gone deeper than one-third of the horizontal depth. (b) This radiograph does not show any evidence of periodontal disease or grade 1 furcation. Dental radiographs will not show changes until more than 30–60% bone resorption has occurred.

and it is necessary to return and probe the tooth again to rule out artifacts.

- Radiography cannot be relied on to identify if bone loss occurs only on the lingual or buccal/palatal aspect of the alveolus (**Figure C8.10**).[12]
- 2D evaluation of the results of regenerative periodontal treatment does not provide accurate information about the entire volume of treated space, nor does it accurately depict areas of ankylosis present on the buccal or lingual/palatal surface.

Appropriate radiographic evaluation depends on the quality of exposure, which requires correct

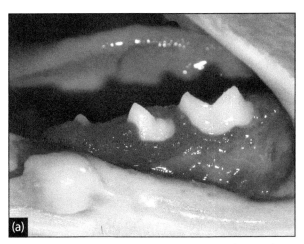
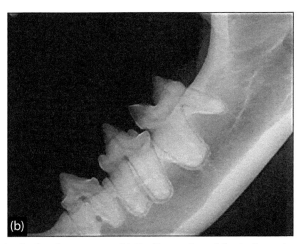

Fig. C8.9 (a) Severe gingivitis in a cat with significant gingival enlargement. (b) Radiography of the inflamed area does not show pathologic changes comparable with the clinical appearance. Note the horizontal bone loss at the left mandibular third premolar (307) and flattening of the interproximal alveolar margin between 307/308.

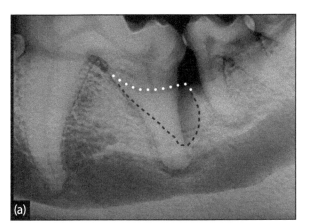
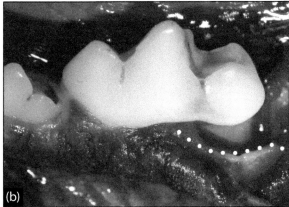

Fig. C8.10 (a) Radiograph demonstrating alveolar bone loss. The white dots indicate the affected alveolar crest and the black dashes the bottom of the periodontal pocket. The bone loss along the root surface is not easily seen. (b) Tooth 309 during periodontal surgery and after extraction of 310. The flap is exposing the distal root of the tooth and the alveolar bone loss (white dots).

positioning and exposure conditions. Under- and overexposed radiographs, as well as malpositioned radiographs, are nondiagnostic (**Figures C8.11, C8.12**). In general, dental radiographs for periodontal assessment should be made slightly underexposed to provide optimal presentation of periodontal structures.[13]

Before any radiographs are taken, it is useful to clean the teeth, as dental calculus is radiodense and can obscure pathologic lesions on a radiograph (**Figure C8.13**).[14]

The best radiographic technique for avoiding image distortion is the direct lateral view (parallel technique) (see Chapter 4).[15] This is where the film is parallel to the object and the tube head is perpendicular to both the film and the tooth roots. If these conditions are not fulfilled, the diagnostic value of the image is compromised (**Figure C8.14**).

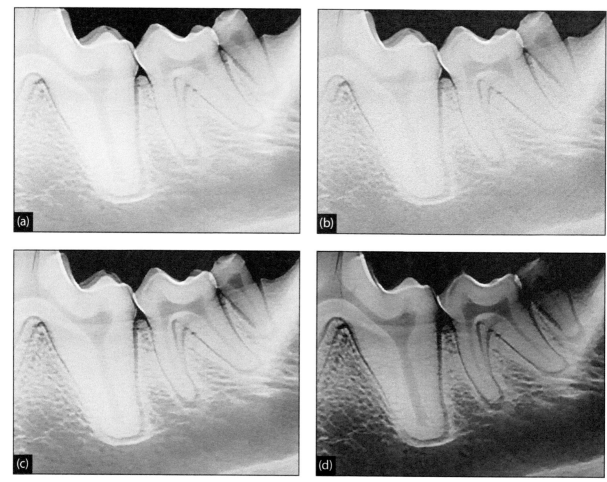

Fig. C8.11 **These under- (a) and overexposed (d) radiographs are nondiagnostic. The slightly underexposed (b) and hard dental tissue (c) radiographs yield a radiograph that will enable evaluation of the soft tissues. Note that other structures on the overexposed radiograph (a), such as the root canal and apical third of the distal root, are visualized better than on the underexposed radiograph (b).**

The radiographic appearance of periodontal structures and normal anatomic features refers to both the deciduous and permanent dentition. The radiopaque periodontal tissues are:

- The alveolar bone with increased density of the lamina dura.
- The alveolar process, which is comprised of cancellous bone that shapes the interalveolar septa and interradicular area.
- The alveolar margin as well as the buccal and lingual (palatal) surfaces, which consist of compact bone (**Figure C8.15**).

The radiolucent zone between cementum and lamina dura is the periodontal ligament (PDL) space (**Figure C8.1**). In most teeth, the PDL space is radiographically linear. Some tooth roots (particularly the mandibular first molars of dogs) show a double radiolucent line. This is created by the presence of the developmental radicular grooves, which strengthen the resistance to twisting movements (**Figure C8.16**).[16]

The process of creation of the periodontal structures occurs during root development and subsequent eruption. This process is discussed and illustrated in Chapter 8b.

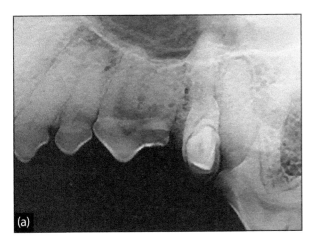

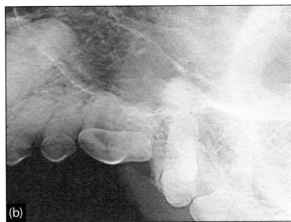

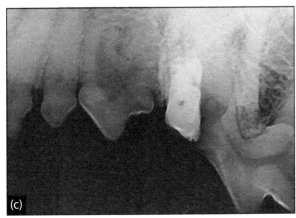

Fig. C8.12 Correct positioning is very important.
(a) The optimal position is the isometric (bisecting angle) technique. Malpositioned projections have limited to no diagnostic value. Foreshortened (b) and elongated (c) objects do not allow for proper evaluation.

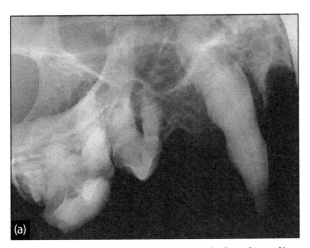

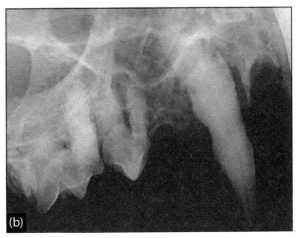

Fig. C8.13 Radiographs before (a) and after (b) scaling of a bulk of calculus from a right maxillary fourth premolar (108).

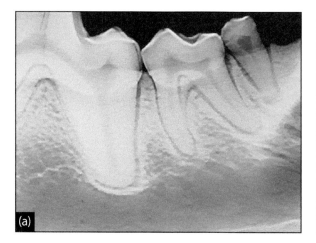

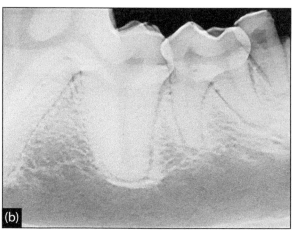

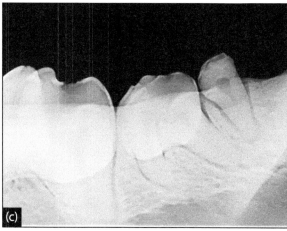

Fig. C8.14 (a) Lateral radiographic view (parallel technique). (b) Incorrect placement of the radiographic beam will directly affect the quality of the image. This horizontal oblique shift has caused overlapping of the crowns and adjacent structures. (c) Errors of vertical angulation have caused the cementoenamel junction to overlap the roots and obscure part of the radiographed object.

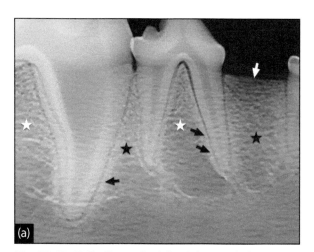

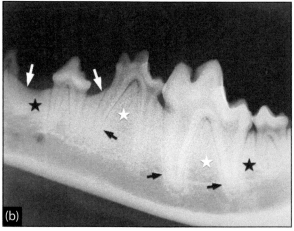

Fig. C8.15 (a) Radiograph of the right mandible of a dog with a missing mandibular third premolar (407). (b) Radiograph of the left mandible of a dog missing its second and fourth premolars (306 and 308) with persistent deciduous second and fourth premolars (706 and 708). The radiopaque periodontal tissues are alveolar bone with increased density of the lamina dura (black arrows); the alveolar process, which is comprised of cortical and cancellous bone that shape the interalveolar septa (black stars) and interradicular area (white stars); the alveolar wall and margin (white arrows) as well as the buccal and lingual (palatal) surfaces, which consist of compact bone.

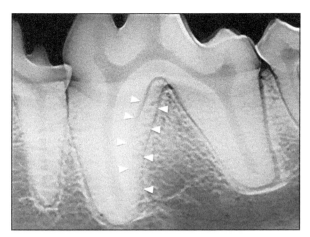

Fig. C8.16 **Radiograph showing the periodontal ligament space appearing as a double radiolucent line. This is created by the presence of the developmental radicular grooves (arrowheads), which strengthen the resistance to twisting movements.**

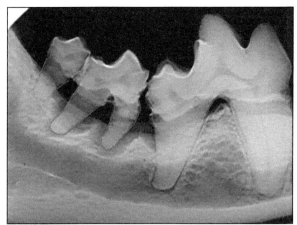

Fig. C8.17 **Radiograph indicating parts of the roots (red lines) that have no lamina dura in their adjacent alveolar bone and significantly widened periodontal ligament space. Both features indicate periodontal disease.**

RADIOGRAPHY IN PERIODONTAL DISEASE

Numerous mechanical, metabolic, inflammatory, and microbiologic factors influence the quality, density, and structure of periodontal tissues, resulting in radiographic changes. Proper classification of periodontal defects is critical as it is strongly associated with prognosis and treatment options.[17] All the possible types of periodontal lesions listed below can be combined on one tooth. Radiographic interpretation of periodontal structures is focused on the following features:

- The lamina dura should normally be visible, continuous, linear, and smooth. In periodontal disease, the lamina dura loses its anatomic character (**Figure C8.17**).
- The interalveolar septa edges lose their sharpness in periodontal disease. This is a very important early sign of periodontal disease in humans (**Figure C8.18**).[18]
- The PDL space becomes widened and irregular in periodontal disease (**Figure C8.19**).
- Vertical (angular) bone loss occurs when there is one area of recession with the surrounding tissue being higher and closer to the cementoenamel junction.[19] Vertical bone loss lesions include one-, two-, three-, and four-wall pockets. One- and two-wall pockets have poorer prognoses than three-and four-wall pockets.

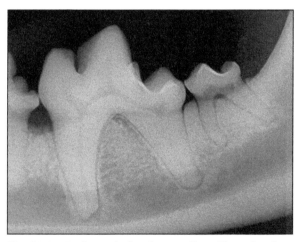

Fig. C8.18 **Radiograph showing an affected interalveolar septum between the left mandibular fourth premolar and first molar (308 and 309) and normal appearance of the interradicular septa in 309 and 310 as well as interalveolar septum between 309 and 310. Note missing 311.**

The prognosis for treatment is related not only to the class of periodontal defect, but also to clinical attachment loss, endodontic status, adjacent teeth, and tooth mobility (**Figures C8.20, C8.21**).

- Furcation involvement appears as a loss of density and lack of substance at the coronal aspect of the interradicular bone. Clinically, it has three grades (grade 0 = no furcation involvement):
  - Grade 1 – the periodontal probe may be inserted into the furcation area but the

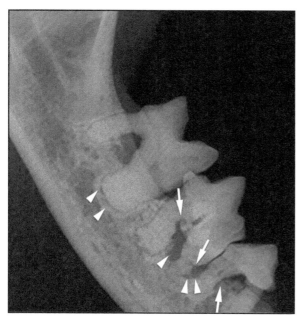

Fig. C8.19 **This 10-year-old cat has periodontal disease with horizontal and vertical bone loss and an irregular locally widened periodontal ligament space (arrowheads). The right mandibular third and fourth premolars (407, 408) have type 1 tooth resorptions (arrows).**

destruction is less than one-third of the horizontal width (**Figure C8.8**).
- Grade 2 – the probe enters the furcation more than one-third of the width of the tooth, but does not pass all the way through (**Figure C8.22**).
- Grade 3 – total involvement; the probe passes through the furcation from one side to the other (**Figure C8.23**).[20]

- Radiographic appearance of calculus: visible subgingival deposits and calculus bridges joining adjacent teeth can mimic other pathology and camouflage hard tissue defects (**Figure C8.24**).
- Horizontal bone loss (**Figure C8.25**) is defined as an osteolytic process leading to a decreased height of the alveolar ridge and root exposure at a similar level over all or part of a dental arch.[21]
- Dentoalveolar ankylosis appears as the lack of a PDL space. The alveolar bone and root substance have no significant border line. Resorption of cementum is

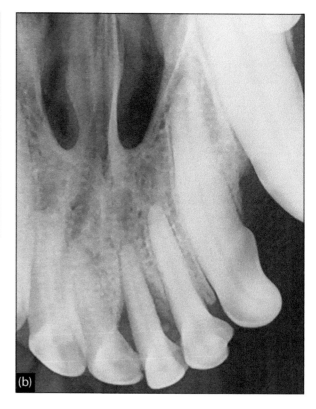

Fig. C8.20 **Clinical (a) and radiographic (b) images of a two-wall defect involving the left maxillary first incisor (201). This condition has a poor prognosis and requires either an apically repositioned flap or extraction.**

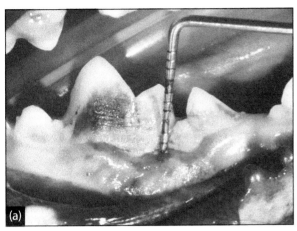

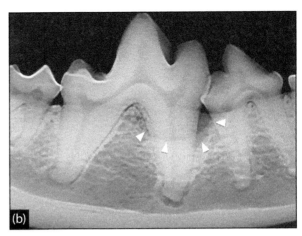

Fig. C8.21 (a) Probing of this right mandibular first molar (409) revealed an 8-mm periodontal pocket. (b) Radiographically there is 25–50% bone loss in the mesial root of 409 (arrowheads). This is a three-wall bony pocket; the defect is defined by the root as one wall and three surfaces of the alveolar bone. It carries a fair to good prognosis for periodontal treatment.

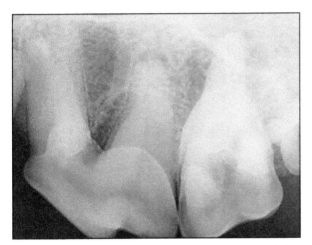

Fig. C8.22 Grade 2 furcation involvement in the left maxillary fourth premolar (208) of a dog associated with a vertical pocket on the mesial aspect of the distal root.

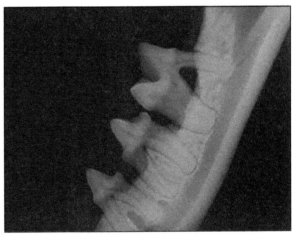

Fig. C8.23 Grade 3 furcation involvement (total exposure), in this case in the left mandibular first molar (309). This radiograph demonstrates horizontal and vertical bone loss affecting all imaged teeth.

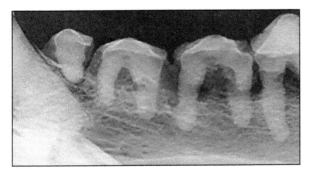

Fig. C8.24 Radiographic appearance of calculus covering the coronal half of the left mandibular premolar teeth. In this case it is very likely associated with horizontal bone loss, which is partially camouflaged by dental calculus.

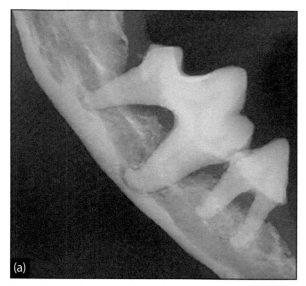

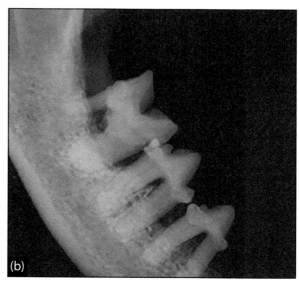

Fig. C8.25 **Horizontal bone loss in a dog (a) and a cat (b). Note how similar they look.**

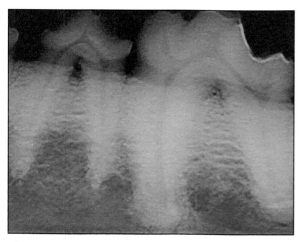

Fig. C8.26 **The left mandibular fourth premolar and first molar (308, 309) in a dog with ankylosed roots. Ankylosis of the tooth to the bone appears as the lack of a periodontal ligament space. The alveolar bone and root substance have no significant differentiation.**

often followed by replacement with bone (**Figure C8.26**).[22]

- Toothless incisive bone after extraction. Cancellous bone has filled the pre-existing alveoli of maxillary incisors (**Figure C8.27**). In humans, the edentulous areas typically undergo atrophy.
- Chronic periodontitis may cause osteomyelitis of the entire maxilla or mandible (**Figure C8.28**).

This is a serious complication of periodontal disease, which significantly influences the quality of life of the patient. Proper diagnosis requires histopathologic evaluation of the affected bone in addition to radiographs. (See also Chapter 8, Part G.)

- Tooth luxation due to periodontal disease. The tooth is extruded from the alveolus (**Figure C8.29**).
- Combination of periodontal and endodontic lesions. Endo-perio lesions (class I) have primarily an endodontic involvement with subsequent periodontal involvement. Perio-endo lesions (class II) have a primarily periodontal character with secondary endodontic involvement. Class III lesion, the true combined lesion, is a problem comprising both periodontal and endodontic causes (**Figures C8.30–C8.32**).
- Complete loss of periodontal attachment and level III mobility (**Figure C8.33**). A high degree of mobility of the tooth can be caused by loss of attachment as well as by a root fracture or neoplastic process. Radiographic assessment is necessary for a definitive diagnosis. Histopathology should be considered if there is any doubt as to the cause of the bone loss.

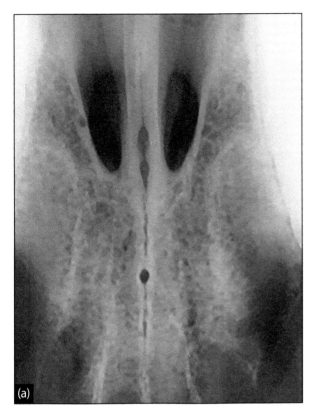

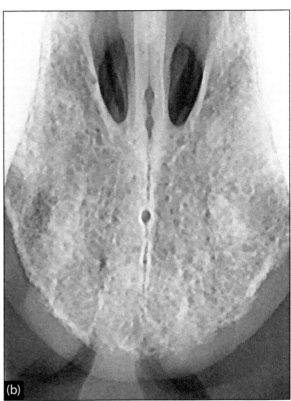

Fig. C8.27 **Radiographs of the incisive area immediately after extraction (a) and 2 years postoperatively (b). Cancellous bone has replaced pre-existing interalveolar septa and alveoli; no bone atrophy is observed.**

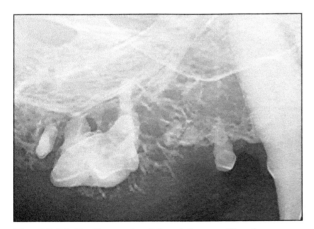

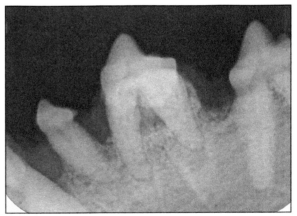

Fig. C8.28 **Radiograph of the right maxilla of a 10-year-old cat with chronic periodontitis and secondary osteomyelitis. Histopathologic evaluation of the affected bone is mandatory to rule out neoplasia, which may have a similar radiographic appearance.**

Fig. C8.29 **Tooth extrusion of the left mandibular second premolar (406) of a dog due to advanced periodontal disease. The tooth is pushed out from the alveolus.**

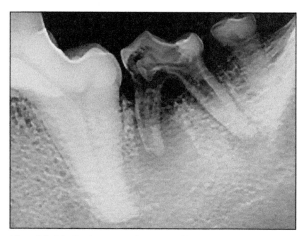

Fig. C8.30 **Endo-perio lesions (class I) have primarily endodontic with subsequent periodontal involvement. In this case, the cause of the pulp disease in the left mandibular second molar (310) is tooth resorption.**

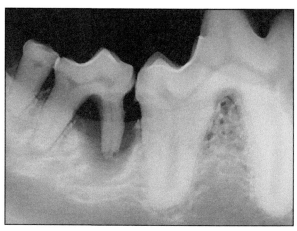

Fig. C8.31 **Perio-endo lesions (class II) have primarily periodontal character with secondary endodontic involvement. This image shows an affected right mandibular second molar (410).**

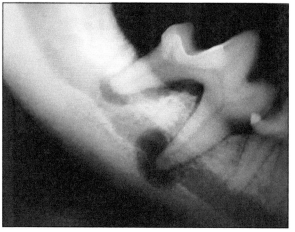

Fig. C8.32 **Class III lesion in the right mandibular first molar tooth (409). Note the missing molar teeth.**

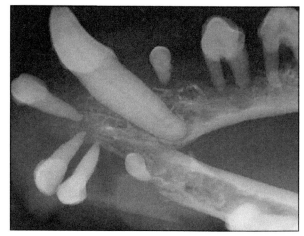

Fig. C8.33 **Radiograph showing complete loss of periodontal attachment and grade III mobility of all imaged teeth (mandibular incisors and premolars). Part of the attachment remains in the canine tooth and mesial root of 308.**

Periodontal tissues are affected in numerous conditions discussed in other chapters. Inflammatory, neoplastic, metabolic, genetic, hormonal, or traumatic conditions, separately or in combination, influence the appearance of alveolar bone, cementum, PDL space, and clinical attachment.[8] Therefore, an indication for radiography is associated with all oral problems. To obtain diagnostic images for periodontal tissue interpretation it is often necessary to expose a series of images with specific conditions and positioning. Proper periodontal radiographic technique and interpretation is of particular importance for extractions and orthodontic and endodontic treatment, as well as implantology. In all these applications it is necessary to obtain diagnostic images both preoperatively and postoperatively (**Figures C8.34–8.37**).

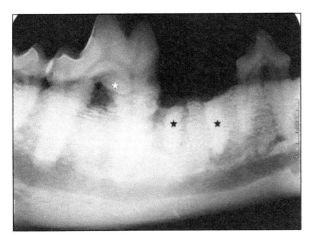

Fig. C8.34 Radiograph showing alveolar bone loss on the mesial root of the right mandibular first molar (409). In addition, the tooth also has furcation involvement and ankylosis. The retained roots of the right mandibular fourth premolar (408) are both ankylosed and have periapical rarefaction (black asterisks). Note an unusual radiopacity in 409 furcation, which was identified as calculus (white asterisk).

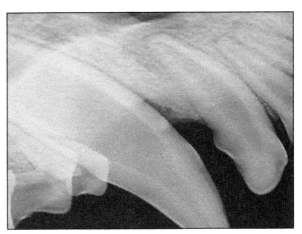

Fig. C8.35 Orthodontic treatment requires assessment of the periodontal tissues of target as well as the anchorage teeth. Utilizing digital radiography, it is easier to record and measure distances and progress in the treatment. This patient presents with teeth crowding and a narrowed diastema between the right maxillary third incisor (103) and canine (104). In this patient, the right mandibular canine (404) is linquoversed and cannot fit into the space between 103 and 104. The orthodontic plan includes interceptive orthodontics, including extraction of the right maxillary first premolar (105) and active orthodontic treatment aiming to expand the diastema between 103 and 104, followed by tipping 404 buccally to the appropriate position.

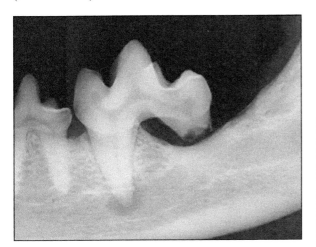

Fig. C8.36 Before performing root canal treatment it is important to evaluate the condition of the entire tooth and plan treatment accordingly. Following examination of this radiograph, the only treatment option for the left mandibular first molar tooth (309) was either root canal treatment of its mesial root followed by resection and extraction of the distal portion, or extraction of the entire tooth. Note that the remaining molar teeth are missing.

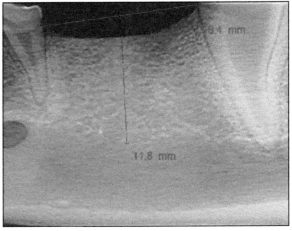

Fig. C8.37 Implant planning starts with radiographic evaluation and accurate tissue measurements, as shown in this radiograph.

REFERENCES

1   Harvey CE, Emily PP (1993) Periodontal disease. In: *Small Animal Dentistry*. (eds. CE Harvey, PP Emily) Mosby, St. Louis, pp. 89–144.

2   Hoffman S (2006) Diagnostic imaging in veterinary dental practice. Focal advanced periodontal disease. *J Am Vet Med Assoc* **228(11):**1683–1684.

3   Ivanusa T, Babic A, Petelin M (1997) Diagnostic systems for assessing alveolar bone loss. *Stud Health Technol Inform* **43(Pt B):**478–481.

4   Colmery B (2005) The gold standard of veterinary oral health care. *Vet Clin North Am Small Anim Pract* **35:**781–787.

5   Verstraete FJ, Kass PH, Terpak CH (1998) Diagnostic value of full-mouth radiography in dogs. *Am J Vet Res* **59(6):**686–691.

6   Verstraete FJ, Kass PH, Terpak CH (1998) Diagnostic value of full-mouth radiography in cats. *Am J Vet Res* **59(6):**692–695.

7   Gawor J, Reiter A, Jodkowska K *et al.* (2006) Influence of diet on oral heath in cats and dogs. *J Nutr* **136(7):**20215–20235.

8   Gawor J (2013) Dental radiology for periodontal disease. In: *Veterinary Periodontology*. (ed. BA Niemiec) Wiley-Blackwell, Ames, pp. 107–128.

9   Smith MM, Zontine WJ, Willits NH (1985) A correlative study of the clinical and radiographic signs of periodontal disease in dogs. *J Am Vet Med Assoc* **186(12):**1286–1290.

10 Yun JH, Hwang SJ, Kim CS *et al.* (2005) The correlation between the bone probing, radiographic and histometric measurements of bone level after regenerative surgery. *J Periodontal Res* **40(6):**453–460.

11 Verstraete FJ (1999) *Self Assesment Colour Review of Veterinary Dentistry*. Manson Publishing, London, p. 194.

12 Tutt C (2007) Radiographic differentiation between vertical and horizontal bone loss. *Proc 16th Ann Conf ECVD*, The Hague, p. 44.

13 DuPont GA, DeBowes LJ (2008) *Atlas of Dental Radiography in Dogs and Cats*. Saunders/Elsevier, St. Louis, pp. 134–135.

14 Gorrel C (2008) *Small Animal Dentistry*. Saunders/Elsevier, St. Louis, pp. 22–68.

15 DuPont GA, DeBowes LJ (2008) *Atlas of Dental Radiography in Dogs and Cats*. Saunders/Elsevier, St. Louis, p. 232.

16 Tutt C (2006) Radiography. In: *Small Animal Dentistry*. Blackwell Publishing, Oxford, pp. 120–121.

17 Wiggs RB, Lobprise H (1997) *Veterinary Dentistry: Principles and Practice*. Lippincott-Raven, Philadelphia, pp. 203–204.

18 Różyło KT, Różyło-Kalinowska I (2007) *Radiologia Stomatologiczna*. Wydawnictwo Lekarskie PZWL, Warszawa, p. 175.

19 Niemiec BA (2005) Dental radiographic interpretation. *J Vet Dent* **22(1):**53–59.

20 Theuns P (2013) Furcation involvement and treatment. In: *Veterinary Periodontology*. (ed. BA Niemiec) Wiley-Blackwell, Ames, pp. 289–295.

21 Morgan JP, Miyabayashi T, Anderson J *et al.* (1990) Periodontal bone loss in the aging beagle dog. A radiographic study. *J Clin Periodontol* **17(9):**630–635.

22 Arnbjerg J (1996) Idiopathic dental root replacement resorption in old dogs. *J Vet Dent* **13(3):**97–99.

PART D

RADIOGRAPHIC INTERPRETATION FOR ENDODONTIC DISEASE

Brook A. Niemiec

INTRODUCTION

Endodontic disease may be diagnosed radiographically in several ways.[1-14] An individual tooth may have one, some, or all of the various signs described below. However, only one of these signs needs to be present to establish a presumptive diagnosis of endodontic disease. These radiographic findings may be broken into two broad classifications: (1) changes in the surrounding bone; and (2) changes within the appearance of the tooth itself.

BONY CHANGES

The classic and easiest finding to identify is periradicular bone rarefaction. This appears as a radiolucent (or at least less radiopaque) area surrounding the apex of a root (**Figure D8.1**). On rare occasions, there may be a mid-root area of lucency due to a lateral canal, but these will virtually always be seen in conjunction with periapical disease. Other changes include a widened periodontal ligament (PDL) space, a thickened or discontinuous lamina dura, or even periradicular sclerosis (**Figure D8.2**).

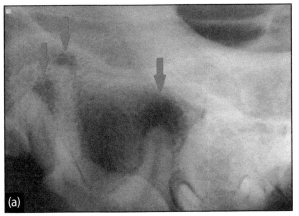
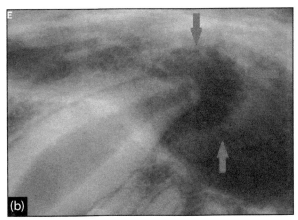

Fig. D8.1 **Periapical rarefaction (arrows), which is indicative of endodontic infection, in a maxillary fourth premolar (a) and canine (b) of a dog.**

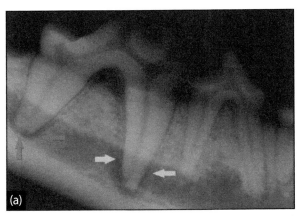
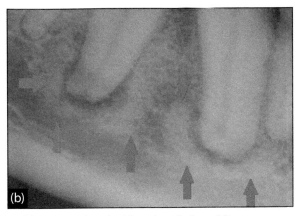

Fig. D8.2 **(a) Discontinuous lamina dura on the mesial root (blue arrows) and widened periodontal ligament space on both roots (shown as red arrows on distal root) on the mandibular first molar of a dog. (b) Periradicular sclerosis (arrows) on a mandibular first molar of a dog. Note that this tooth also has mild periapical rarefaction.**

It is critical that the clinician is aware of the possibility of artifacts, which are created by superimposed lucencies. These structures (e.g. mental foramina) can be superimposed over an apex and falsely appear as periapical rarefaction (**Figure D8.3a**). There are several clues that these lucencies are not real periapical rarefaction. First, superimposed artifacts are typically seen on only one root, whereas it is rare to find a true periapical lesion on only one root of a multirooted tooth. In addition, artifacts tend to be regular/smooth in appearance, whereas true periapical lesions tend to be ragged or irregular. If any area is in question, it is best to expose an additional film with a slightly different x-ray beam angle. If the lucency is still centered over the apex, it is likely real and not an artifact (**Figures D8.3b, c**).

Another common radiographic finding that is misdiagnosed as endodontic disease is a slight widening of the periapical PDL space, which is typically elliptical in shape.[15] This demonstrates an increase in size of the apical vascular network, and is most common on the canines (especially maxillary) and mandibular premolars and molars (especially the mandibular first molars) (**Figure D8.4**).[16] This is more pronounced when the apex is within the mandibular canal. It has been postulated that this may improve the 'shock-absorber' function of the periodontal ligament.[15] When this finding occurs in the canine teeth, it is commonly called the 'chevron effect'.[2] These changes may be differentiated from pathology because they are very regular and bilateral. Furthermore, on canine teeth, the radiolucent area is V-shaped, as opposed to irregular and round. It is important to compare the apex with that of the contralateral tooth. If the lucency is bilateral, it is more likely to be anatomic (i.e. the chevron effect) as opposed to pathologic. Finally, if there are no other

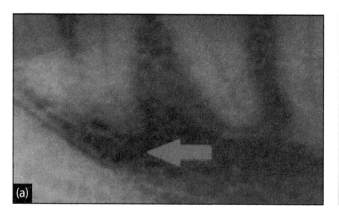

(a)

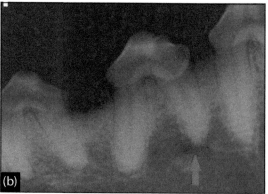

(b)

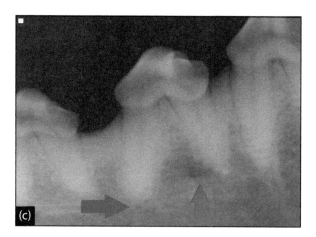

(c)

Fig. D8.3 (a) The middle mental foramen is imaged over the mesial root of the second premolar (arrow). This could be mistaken as a sign of endodontic disease. (b) In this image the caudal mental foramina is centered on the distal root of the third premolar (arrow). This could easily result in a misdiagnosis of endodontic infection in this tooth. (c) When the beam is moved in the *horizontal* plane, the lucency moves off the apex (red arrow), confirming that this suspected infection is actually a normal anatomic feature. The other sign that this tooth is likely not infected is that no lucency exists on the mesial root (blue arrow). It is exceedingly rare (although possible) to have a periapical lucency on one root of a multirooted tooth.

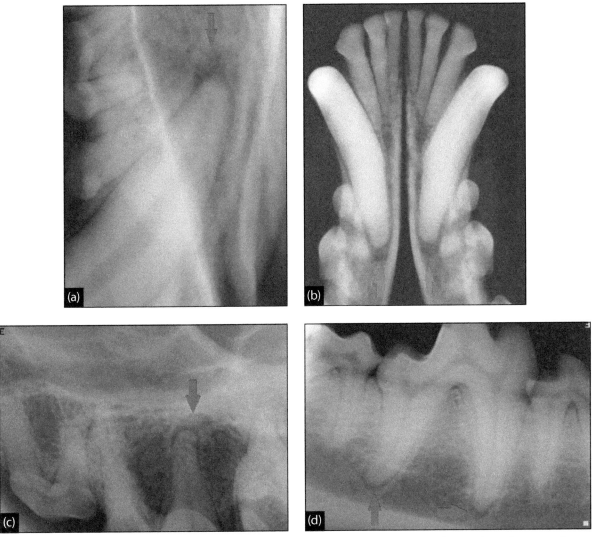

Fig. D8.4 The 'chevron' effect, or normal widening of the periodontal ligament (arrows), at the apex of a maxillary (a) and mandibular (b) canine, the distal root of a maxillary fourth premolar (c) and both roots of a mandibular first molar (d). These small, regular areas of radiolucency are normal anatomic variations and not signs of endodontic disease. Note, however, that a complete oral examination for clinical signs of disease (including transillumination) should be performed on these teeth prior to dismissing the radiolucent lesions. In addition, look for other signs of endodontic disease (e.g. widened endodontic systems or internal/external resorption).

clinical signs of nonvitality (fracture/intrinsic staining), the tooth is likely vital. However, any questionable teeth should be monitored radiographically on a regular basis.

Diagnosis of endodontic disease in deciduous teeth is generally confined to periapical rarefaction (**Figure D8.5**). This is due to the fact that deciduous teeth are not typically in the mouth long enough

to develop the tooth changes other than potentially external resorption.

TOOTH CHANGES

The most common change within the tooth itself, secondary to endodontic disease, is a root canal with a different diameter. As the tooth matures,

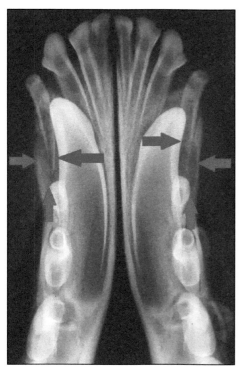

Fig. D8.5 This radiograph demonstrates bilateral endodontic infection of the deciduous mandibular canines. There is periapical rarefaction (red arrows) as well as external root resorption at the apex (blue arrows).

secondary dentin production causes a decrease in canal width. When a tooth dies, this development stops. Consequently, nonvital teeth typically have wider root canals than the surrounding or contralateral vital teeth (**Figure D8.6**). A tooth with width discrepancy can be compared with any tooth (taking the size of tooth into consideration), but it is most accurate to compare it with the contralateral tooth (**Figure D8.7**).

It is important to note that on rare occasions pulpitis may result in increased dentin production (dystrophic calcification), leading to an endodontically diseased tooth with a *smaller* root canal (**Figure D8.8**). This finding is especially common in teeth that are also periodontally diseased or undergoing pulpitis (intrinsically stained).[2] This could potentially lead to a misdiagnosis of the endodontically diseased tooth as healthy, and vice versa with the contralateral tooth. Hence, it is important to evaluate the adjacent teeth as well as the contralateral tooth.

It is also important to remember that the endodontic system in canine teeth is not perfectly cylindrical in most cases.[17] It is oval and wider in the rostrocaudal direction than in the lateromedial

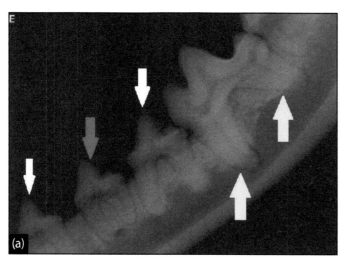

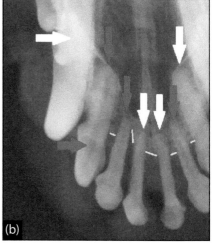

Fig. D8.6 (a) Intraoral dental radiograph of the left mandible of a dog. In this image, the endodontic system of the third premolar (red arrow) is wider than the surrounding teeth (white arrows). This is an indication that this tooth is nonvital. The endodontic system is about the same width as the much larger first molar (yellow arrows). (b) Intraoral dental radiograph of the maxillary incisors of a dog. Both second as well as the left third incisors (red arrows) have much larger endodontic systems than the other imaged teeth (white arrows). This is an indication that these teeth are nonvital. This image also shows evidence of significant horizontal bone loss (yellow lines), indicating advanced periodontal disease.

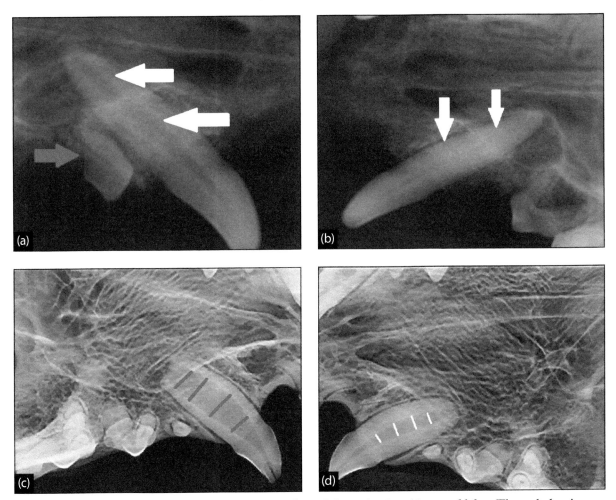

Fig. D8.7 (a) Intraoral dental radiograph of the maxillary right canine in a 10-year-old dog. The endodontic system of the canine (white arrows) is much wider than the first premolar (red arrow). This leads to a presumptive diagnosis of a nonvital canine. However, there is a significant size difference in these teeth, therefore comparing the size of the endodontic system of the contralateral tooth is more accurate. (b) Intraoral dental radiograph of the left canine of the same dog, which has a significantly smaller endodontic system (arrows) than the right canine. This confirms the nonvitality of the right maxillary canine. (c) Intraoral dental radiograph of the maxillary right canine in a 3-year-old cat. The endodontic system of the canine (lines) is much wider than the other teeth in this dental arch. This leads to a presumptive diagnosis of a nonvital canine. However, there is a significant size difference in these teeth and the angle is not the same, therefore comparing the size of the endodontic system of the contralateral tooth is more accurate. (D) Intraoral dental radiograph of the left canine of the same cat, which has a significantly smaller endodontic system (lines) than the right canine. This confirms the nonvitality of the right maxillary canine.

direction. Therefore, the radiographic projection will affect the size of the canal, particularly in young, large breed dogs (**Figure D8.9**). Consequently, it is important to obtain contralateral comparative images at exactly the same angle.

Note that this difference tends to decrease as a patient ages.

Finally, root resorption can be a sign of endodontic disease. Radiographic manifestations can demonstrate both internal and external resorption.

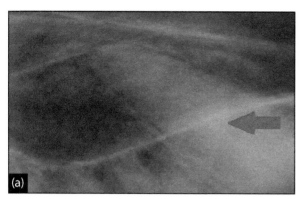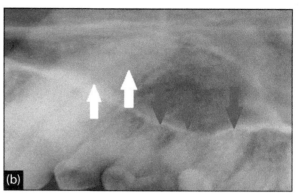

Fig. D8.8 (a) Intraoral dental radiograph of the maxillary right canine in a 7-year-old dog. The endodontic system of the canine (arrow) is very small, even smaller than the surrounding premolars (which are just on the edge of the image). This would lead one to believe that this tooth is vital. (b) Intraoral dental radiograph of the left canine of the same dog. This canine has a wider endodontic system (white arrows) than the right canine, which is more in alignment with the premolars, which are seen better on this view (blue arrows). This leads to a presumptive diagnosis of nonvitality of the right maxillary canine.

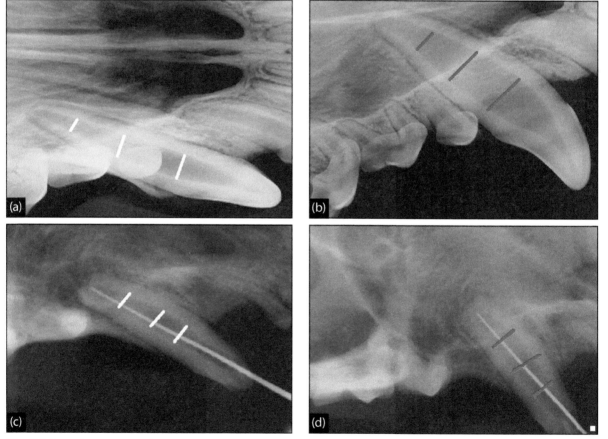

Fig. D8.9 In these intraoral dental images of the maxillary right canine in a dog (a, b) and a cat (c, d), the variation of the endodontic diameter can be clearly seen. In (a) and (c), the image was created with a much more DV projection and thus the endodontic system appears narrower (white lines) than when the same tooth is imaged from a more lateral aspect (b, d) (red lines). This is important knowledge to ensure that the canal width of the canine is properly interpreted.

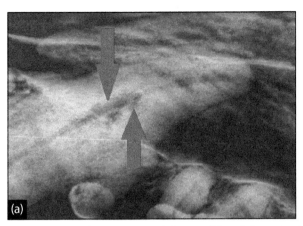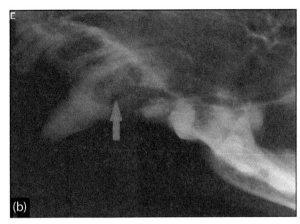

Fig. D8.10 **In these images of the maxillary left canine in a dog (a) and a cat (b) there is an area of internal resorption, which is indicative of endodontic infection (arrows).**

Internal resorption results from osteoclastic activity within the root canal system due to pulpitis. These changes create an irregular, enlarged region within an area of the root canal system (**Figure D8.10**). External root resorption appears as a defect of the external surface of the root, generally accompanied by a loss of bone in the area (**Figure D8.11**). External resorption occurs most often at the apex of the tooth in companion animals, and is quite common in cats with chronic endodontic disease (**Figure D8.12**).

USING DENTAL RADIOGRAPHY TO MONITOR ENDODONTIC DIAGNOSIS AND THERAPY

Dental radiography is absolutely critical for monitoring potentially diseased or endodontically treated teeth. This is because animal patients rarely show clinical signs of infection or treatment failure, but they definitely suffer regardless. All endodontically treated teeth, as well as those with *possible* disease, should be monitored on a regular basis. The ideal interval is 6–9 months, but annual rechecks are more commonly done with animal patients.[6,18,19]

Treated teeth

Examples of treated teeth that require regular monitoring are: vital pulp therapy, standard root canal therapy, and surgical root canal therapy (**Figure D8.13**).[19–21]

Radiographic monitoring of vital pulp therapy is absolutely critical, as the long-term success rate of this procedure is lower than that of standard root canal therapy.[18,20–24] This is especially true with fractured teeth when the root canal has been exposed for more than 48 hours are treated with vital pulp therapy.[24] There are several radiographic indications of vitality, as listed above, but two findings of particular interest should be a lack of periapical rarefaction and canals that continually decrease in size. Ideally, the contralateral tooth is used for comparison. Previously, the presence of a dentinal bridge below the pulpotomy was considered a sign of continued vitality. However, it is now known that the dentinal bridge does not form a bacteria-tight seal, and therefore it is not unusual to find that teeth with thick dentinal bridges are nonvital (**Figure D8.14**).[25]

When monitoring standard endodontic therapy, the main diagnostic clue for success or failure is the size of the periapical rarefaction (see **Figures D13a–d**).[5] These are nonvital teeth, therefore the size of the canal will not change. Keep in mind also that internal resorption is rare in an endodontically treated tooth. A novel periapical rarefaction on recheck radiographs is obvious evidence of failure of standard endodontic therapy. When periapical rarefaction exists at the time of treatment, monitoring can be a little more challenging. If the lucency grows, this is obvious evidence of endodontic failure. The strict criteria for success would be

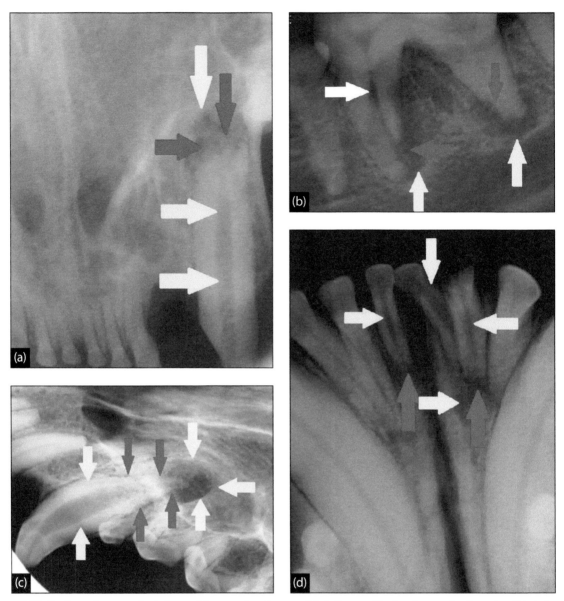

Fig. D8.11 In these images of a left maxillary canine in a cat (a), left mandibular first molar in a dog (b), left maxillary canine in a dog (c) and mandibular incisors in a dog (d) there are areas of external resorption, which is indicative of endodontic infection (red arrows). In addition, all involved teeth demonstrate periapical rarefaction (blue arrows). The affected canines as well as the incisors in (a), (b), and (d) also demonstrate a wider endodontic system (yellow arrows). The first molar in (b) has an area of internal resorption in the mesial root (white arrow). All of these are signs of endodontic disease.

complete resolution of a periapical lucency. However, many veterinary dentists consider a reduction of a periapical lucency as successful.[26] Finally, it is possible that the lucency will remain static due to apical 'scar' formation, even with successful treatment. It is also important to ensure that the endodontic filling material is stable.

Monitoring of surgical endodontic therapy is directed mostly at the treated apex. With successful therapy, the bone should fill in the area of the removed apex. The retrofill should also be examined to ensure it is still intact (**Figure D8.15**).

In cases of treatment failure, further therapy is required. For failed vital pulp therapy, standard

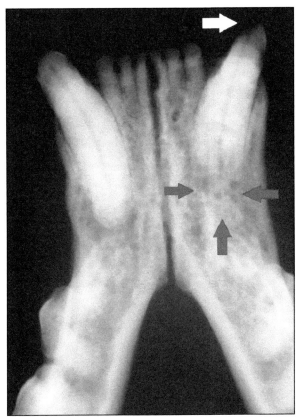

Fig. D8.12 **Intraoral dental radiograph of a chronically fractured (white arrow) left mandibular canine in a cat. Note the advanced external resorption (red arrows).**

endodontics should be performed, provided that the canal is mature (i.e. has completed apexogenesis). If the canal is immature, treatment options include surgical endodontics, apexification, or extraction. For standard endodontic therapy failures, the best option depends on the quality of the initial treatment. If the obturation was poor, reinstrumentation (débridement and shaping) and obturation is recommended. If the fill was complete, this procedure could still be attempted, but will not have as good a prognosis. In these cases, surgical endodontics (or extraction) should be performed. Surgical endodontics is a technique that involves removing the apical portion of the root and then removing a small amount of the now exposed apical endodontic obturation material, and then placing a retrograde filling (**Figure D8.15a**). One limitation for endodontic treatment/monitoring of standard endodontic therapy is that endodontic systems are not perfect cylinders. This is especially true of canine teeth in dogs (**Figure D8.9**). Consequently, a fill that appears adequate on an image obtained with a straight over the nose projection (i.e. more parallel and in line with the long axis of the nose) may actually have a poor fill in the ventrodorsal (VD) direction, which can only be appreciated on a more lateral view (**Figure D8.16**). For this reason, it is recommended that two images of the endodontic fill are obtained for the canine teeth.

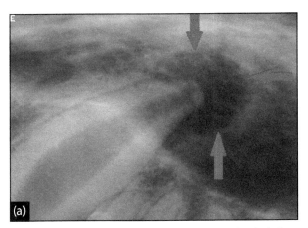

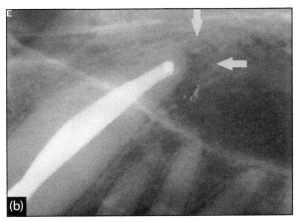

Fig. D8.13 **(a) This preoperative radiograph of a left maxillary canine reveals a widened endodontic system and periapical rarefaction (arrows), which demonstrates endodontic infection. (b) Nine-month recheck dental radiograph of the same patient demonstrating the regrowth of the periapical bone (arrows). This indicates successful therapy.** *(Continued)*

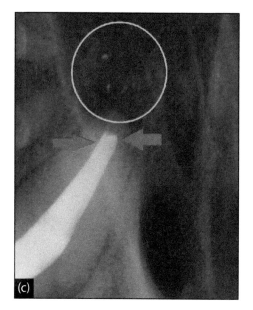

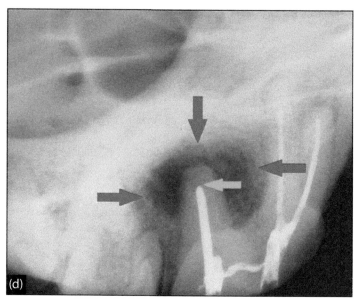

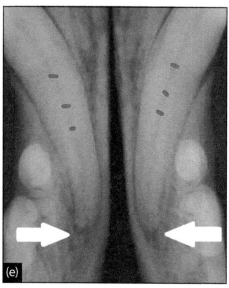

Fig. D8.13 *(Continued)* (c) This recheck image of the right maxillary canine (104) in a dog reveals periapical rarefaction associated with the tooth (circle), which indicates a failed endodontic treatment, despite apparently adequate obturation (arrows). (d) This recheck image of the right maxillary fourth premolar (108) in a dog reveals periapical rarefaction associated with the distal root (red arrows), which indicates a failed endodontic treatment, likely caused by a slightly short fill (blue arrow). (e) Seven-year recheck radiograph of a vital pulp therapy performed when the dog was 6 months of age. In this image, the endodontic systems are of similar diameter (red lines). This, along with the lack of periapical rarefaction (white arrows), indicates a vital tooth and successful therapy.

Finally, in cases of failed surgical endodontic therapy, extraction is generally the treatment of choice. An exception may be those cases where there is an obvious reason for prior failure, in which case surgical retreatment many be considered.

Questionable teeth

There are numerous teeth that require regular radiographic follow-up. This is because the teeth may be nonvital at the time of treatment but the lesion is not yet radiographically evident. Although radiographs are a critically important tool, it is important to keep in mind that they have been shown to be an inaccurate means of determining *true* success or failure.[27] There are several factors that contribute to the limitation of dental radiographs. Firstly, 40–60% of the mineralization of bone must be lost before it is evident radiographically. Next, dental radiographs are a 2D image of a 3D structure. Finally, the degree of change in the width of the endodontic system decreases very *slowly* in older animals, which means that a noticeable radiographic change may take years to occur.[4,28,29] Despite these limitations, radiographs are a valuable tool, and they can

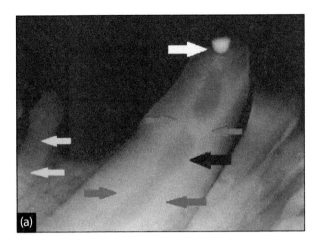

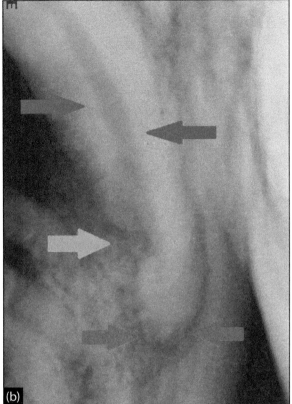

Fig. D8.14 In these 6-year recheck images of the right mandibular canine (104) in a dog, the restoration is intact (a, yellow arrow) and there is an apparently adequate dentinal bridge (although possibly a little short) (a, red arrows). However, the tooth is nonvital and infected as evidenced by (1) the widened endodontic system (a, blue arrows) as opposed to the surrounding premolars (a, green arrows); (2) the periapical rarefaction (b, purple arrows); (3) the internal resorption (a, black arrow); and (4) the external resorption (b, orange arrow).

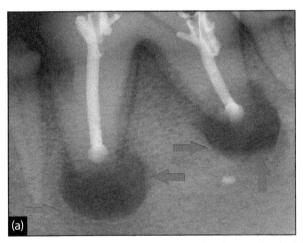

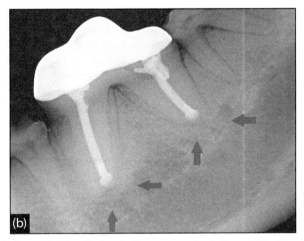

Fig. D8.15 (a) Postoperative intraoral radiograph of a failed standard endodontic therapy on the left mandibular first molar of a dog (arrows). (b) Nine-month dental recheck of the same tooth. The bone has regrown in the area (arrows), which is indicative of successful therapy. Note that the pulp chamber was not filled in this case, which in some dentists' opinion improves the success rate of endodontic therapy.

be used and interpreted more wisely when this information is kept in mind. There are several indications for utilizing strict radiographic monitoring. The most common scenario for this involves radiographic monitoring of uncomplicated crown fractures. These teeth can be radiographically normal at the initial diagnosis and treatment (typically bonded sealant), yet found to be nonvital on the 6–9 month recheck.[30]

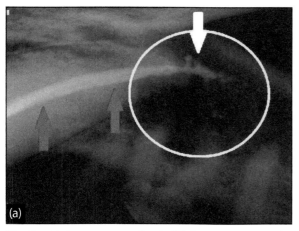
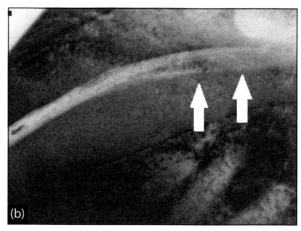

Fig. D8.16 **Importance of a 3D fill for successful endodontic therapy. (a) One-year recheck of a dog treated with standard root canal therapy. There is significant periapical rarefaction (circle), indicating failed therapy. This is despite there appearing to be adequate obturation (red arrows). However, there is significant overfill (white arrow). (b) When the same tooth is imaged more laterally, the very poor fill is evident (arrows).**

Another indication for strict monitoring are teeth with discoloration at the cusp *tip*, but which appear otherwise normal. It is very important for these teeth to be radiographically monitored. Finally, teeth with any type of pathology (periodontal disease, caries, enamel hypocalcification, attrition/abrasion) should also be regularly monitored.

KEY POINTS

- Dental radiography is crucial in the diagnosis and treatment of endodontic disease.
- Wider root canals and periapical rarefaction are the two main indicators of endodontic disease/inflammation.
- Occasionally the diseased canal will be *narrower*.
- Carnassials and canines may have widened periapical PDL spaces (chevron effect), which is a normal phenomenon.
- Resorption (internal and external) is a potential sign of inflammation.
- Radiographic monitoring is critical for treated as well as potentially diseased teeth.
- Dental radiographs do have limitations, and these should be kept in mind when interpreting and utilizing radiographic images in the overall treatment and management plan.

REFERENCES

1 Niemiec BA (2005) Dental radiographic interpretation. *J Vet Dent* **22(1):**53–9.
2 Niemiec BA (2010) Veterinary dental radiology. In: *Small Animal Dental, Oral and Maxillofacial Disease: A Color Handbook*. (ed. BA Niemiec) Manson Publishing, London, pp. 63–87.
3 Dupont G (2010) Pathologies of the dental hard tissues In: *Small Animal Dental, Oral and Maxillofacial Disease: A Color Handbook*. (ed. BA Niemiec) Manson Publishing, London, pp. 127–157.
4 Startup S (2011) Tooth response to injury. In: *Veterinary Endodontics*. (ed. BA Niemiec) Practical Veterinary Publishing, Tustin, pp. 16–36.
5 Niemiec BA (2011) Surgical endodontics. In: *Veterinary Endodontics*. (ed. BA Niemiec) Practical Veterinary Publishing, Tustin, pp. 161–174.
6 Niemiec BA (2005) Endodontics. *Vet Clin North Am Small Anim Pract* **35(4):**837–868.
7 Niemiec BA (2008) Oral pathology. *Top Companion Anim Med* **23(2):**59–71.
8 Niemiec BA (2008) Case based dental radiology. *Top Companion Anim Med* **24(1):**4–19.
9 Niemiec BA (2011) The importance of dental radiology. *Eur J Comp Anim Pract* **20(3):**219–229.
10 Anthony JMG, Marretta SM, Okuda A (2000) Feline endodontics. In. *An Atlas of Veterinary Dental Radiology*. (eds. DH DeForge, BH Colmery. Iowa State University Press, Ames, pp. 149–158.

11 Marretta SM, Anthony JMG (2000) Canine endodontics. In. *An Atlas of Veterinary Dental Radiology.* (eds. DH DeForge, BH Colmery. Iowa State University Press, Ames, pp. 35–58.

12 Bellows J (2008) Dental radiography. In: *Small Animal Dental Equipment, Materials, and Techniques: A Primer.* Wiley-Blackwell, Ames, pp. 63–104.

13 Mulligan TW, Aller MS, Williams CA (1998) Interpretation of endodontic disease. In: *Atlas of Canine and Feline Dental Radiography.* Veterinary Learning Systems, Trenton, pp. 124–152.

14 Bellows J (2010) Radiology. In: *Feline Dentistry: Oral Assessment, Treatment, and Preventative Care.* Wiley-Blackwell, Ames, pp. 39–83.

15 Strepaniuk K, Hinrichs JE (2013) The structure and function of the periodontium. In: *Veterinary Periodontology.* (ed. BA Niemiec) Wiley-Blackwell, Ames, pp. 3–17.

16 Matsuo M, Takahashi K (2002) Scanning electron microscopic observation of microvasculature in periodontium. *Microsc Res Tech* **56(1):**3–14.

17 Rochette J (1996) Identification of the endodontic system in carnassial and canine teeth in the dog. *J Vet Dent* **13(1):**35–37.

18 Moore JI (2011) Vital pulp therapy. In: *Veterinary Endodontics.* (ed. BA Niemiec) Practical Veterinary Publishing, Tustin, pp. 78–92.

19 Niemiec BA, Mulligan TW (2001) Vital pulp therapy. *J Vet Dent* **18(3):**154–156.

20 Wiggs R, Lobprise H (19970 Advanced endodontic therapies. In: *Oral Surgery in Veterinary Dentistry: Principles and Practice.* (eds. R Wiggs, H Lobprise) Lippincott-Raven, Philadelphia, pp. 325–345.

21 Kuntsi-Vaattovaara H, Verstraete FJ, Kass PH (2002) Results of root canal treatment in dogs: 127 cases (1995–2000). *J Am Vet Med Assoc* **220(6):**775–780.

22 Niemiec BA (2001) Assessment of vital pulp therapy for nine complicated crown fractures and fifty-four crown reductions in dogs and cats. *J Vet Dent* **18(3):**122–125.

23 Trope M, Blanco L, Chivian N *et al.* (2006) The role of endodontics after dental traumatic injuries. In: *Pathways of the Pulp*, 9th edn. (eds. S Cohen, K Hargreaves) Mosby, St. Louis, pp. 610–645.

24 Clarke D (2001) Vital pulp therapy for complicated crown fracture of permanent canine teeth in dogs: a three-year retrospective study. *J Vet Dent* **18(3):** 117–121.

25 Trowbridge H, Kim S, Suda H (2002) Structure and function of the dentin and pulp complex. In: *Pathways of the Pulp*, 8th edn. (eds. S Cohen, RC Burns) Mosby, St. Louis, pp. 411–456.

26 Ng YL, Mann V, Rahbaran S *et al.* (2007) Outcome of primary root canal treatment: systematic review of the literature - part 1. Effects of study characteristics on probability of success. *Int Endod J* **40(12):** 921–939.

27 Wu MK, Shemesh H, Wesselink PR (2009) Limitations of previously published systematic reviews evaluating the outcome of endodontic treatment. *Int Endod J* **42(8):**656–666.

28 Luukko K, Kettunen P, Fristad I *et al.* (2011) Structure and function of the dentin-pulp complex. In: *Pathways of the Pulp*, 9th edn. (eds. S Cohen, K Hargreaves) Mosby, St. Louis, pp. 452–495.

29 Andreasen JO, Lovschall H (2007) Response of oral tissue to trauma. In: *Textbook and Color Atlas of Traumatic Injuries to the Teeth*, 4th edn. (eds. JO Andreasen, FM Andreasen, L Andreasen) Blackwell, Victoria, Australia, pp. 62–113.

30 Theuns P, Niemiec BA (2001) Bonded sealants for uncomplicated crown fractures. *J Vet Dent* **(28)2:**130–133.

PART E

TOOTH HARD TISSUE DISEASES

Jerzy Gawor

INTRODUCTION

The dental hard tissues include enamel, dentin, and cementum, which are the major structures of the crown and root of the teeth. Diseases or defects of the dental hard tissues may have various origins and etiologies. However, traumatic, congenital, inflammatory, neoplastic, and idiopathic etiologies are the most common. This chapter will discuss the following pathologies that create radiographically visible lesions of the hard dental substances: tooth resorption, caries, enamel hypoplasia, enamel hypocalcification, dentinal dysplasia, and a selection of abnormalities in tooth shape and structure.

When tooth structure is weakened by one of the above conditions, fracture of or defects in the tooth can occur even during normal use. In addition, traumatic defects to enamel and/or dentin, luxation, or attrition/abrasion can cause significant changes in hard dental tissue. The nature of these pathologies is complex and almost always multifactorial. Radiography shows only the consequences of pathology; however, by properly interpreting the radiograph, the etiology can occasionally be determined.

TOOTH RESORPTION

Physiologically, tooth resorption (TR) occurs during the changing of dentition from deciduous to permanent teeth. The eruption of permanent teeth is normally preceded by resorption of the root of the deciduous tooth.[1] Persistent deciduous teeth very often undergo resorption even without permanent tooth eruption, therefore the lifespan and duration of functionality of these teeth is often limited (**Figures E8.1–8.4**).[2]

In general, TR is subdivided into external and internal types. External resorption originates in the

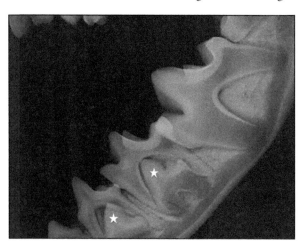

Fig. E8.1 **Six-month-old Yorkshire terrier just prior to eruption of the mandibular cheek teeth. The left mandibular third and fourth premolars (307 and 308) (stars) are very close to their deciduous predecessors (707, 708) but have not yet begun starting progression towards their structures.**

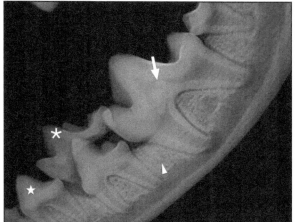

Fig. E8.2 **A 7.5-month-old Yorkshire terrier in the process of changing dentition. The left mandibular third premolar (307) (star) has already erupted and 707 has exfoliated. The fourth premolar (708) (asterisk) is undergoing physiologic resorption and this tooth is close to being exfoliated; however, its distal root (arrowhead) is still present. Note the radiopacity in the pulp chamber of the left mandibular first molar (309) (arrow), which is possibly a pulp stone.**

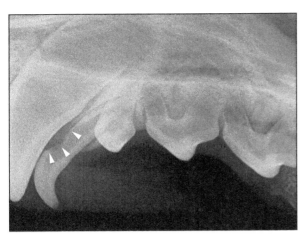

Fig. E8.3 **Resorption in a deciduous left maxillary canine tooth (604) (arrowheads) likely caused by pressure from the erupting permanent successor (204). This will result in a high likelihood of fracture during an extraction attempt.**

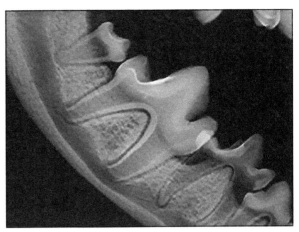

Fig. E8.4 **Resorption in a deciduous right mandibular fourth premolar (808) without any influence from the eruption process.**

periodontal ligament (PDL) or tissues surrounding the teeth, and internal resorption is initiated within the endodontic system.[3] External root resorption, which has a known mechanism in man, includes surface resorption, replacement resorption associated with ankylosis, and inflammatory resorption. Finally, inflammatory resorption refers to an apical root resorption and two other additional forms: peripheral inflammatory root resorption (PIRR) and external inflammatory root resorption (EIRR). If the etiology is unknown, it is termed idiopathic.[4]

The radiographic appearance of different types of resorption does not always relate to the type of disease; however, replacement resorption has some typical features. In addition, the location of the lesion can also be linked to the specific type. For example, PIRR is often located at the cervical area of the tooth as a consequence of damaged cervical root surface and therefore was previously called a 'neck lesion'.[4]

Feline tooth resorption

Feline TRs are the result of odontoclastic destruction of teeth and, based on their radiographic appearance, are classified as either type (stage) 1, 2, or 3 (**Figures E8.5–8.7**). In Type 1 there is no replacement by bone, whereas in type 2 there is replacement of the resorbed root structure by bone. Type 3 represents the combined presence of types 1 and 2 in the same tooth.

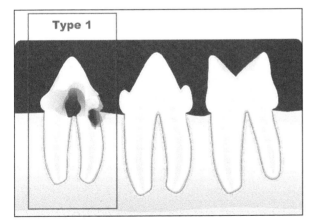

Fig. E8.5 **Type 1 tooth resorption. (Copyright© AVDC®, used with permission.)**

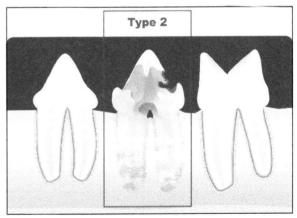

Fig. E8.6 **Type 2 tooth resorption. (Copyright© AVDC®, used with permission.)**

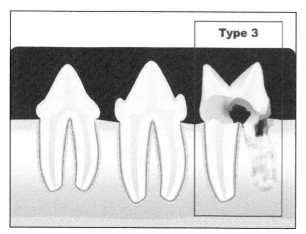

Fig. E8.7 **Type 3 tooth resorption. (Copyright©
AVDC®, used with permission.)**

TRs are very common in felines. The prevalence
of TRs in a cat population of 109 cats, based on
clinical and radiologic assessment, was reported to
be 30%.[5] The etiology of TR in cats is inflammatory for type 1 and unknown for type 2. TRs are
not bacterial in nature, although in some cases the
periodontal inflammation (which is caused by plaque
bacteria) may have activated the odontoclasts. There
are numerous theories; however, none have been
proven at this time. Odontoclastic resorption generally begins at the cervical area of the tooth and
progresses at varying rates until in some cases no
identifiable tooth remains (**Figure E8.8**).

- **Type 1 TRs** are typically associated with
  inflammation such as stomatitis, gingivitis, or
  periodontal disease. Thus, they are often seen
  with alveolar bone loss on dental radiographs.
  In these cases, it is believed that the soft tissue
  inflammation activated the odontoclasts. The
  teeth will have normal root density in some areas
  and a well-defined PDL space (**Figure E8.9**). In
  addition, there is often a definable root canal in
  the intact part of the tooth. This type will have
  significant resorption of the teeth and tooth roots,
  which is *not* replaced by bone.

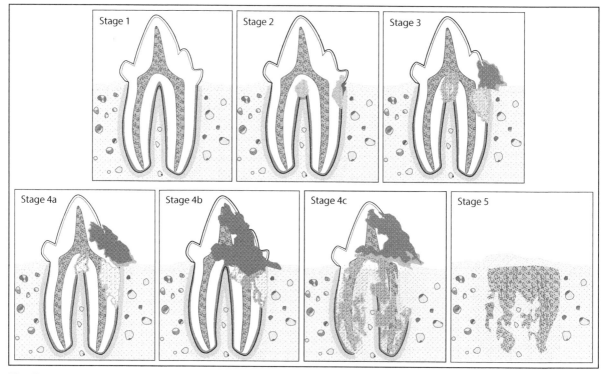

Fig. E8.8 **Stages of tooth resorption. (Copyright© AVDC®, used with permission.)**

- **Type 2 TRs** are usually associated with only localized gingivitis and/or gingival enlargement on oral examination, in contrast to the more severe inflammation seen with type 1 TRs. In these cases, the gingival inflammation is usually a result of the TR. The radiographic appearance is that of teeth that have a different radiographic density compared with normal teeth, as they have undergone significant replacement resorption (**Figure E8.10**). Findings will include areas with no discernable PDL space (dentoalveolar

ankylosis) or root canal. The ankylosis and osteoid remodeling that are characteristic of type 2 TRs result from the degradation and modification of dentin and cementum into osteoid repair tissue.[6] In the late stages, there will be little to no discernable root structure (ghost roots). In these cases, the lost root structure is replaced by bone.

- **Type 3 TRs** are 'simply' a combination of the first two types affecting different areas of the same tooth at the same time (**Figures E8.11, E8.12**).

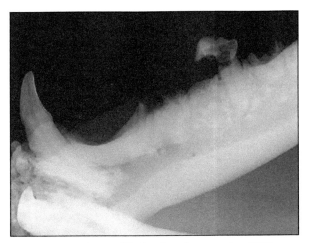

Fig. E8.9 This right mandibular first molar (409) is affected by a type 1 TR, stage 4c.

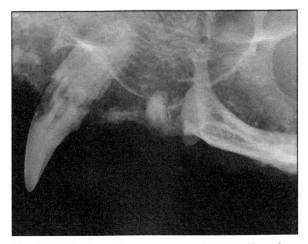

Fig. E8.10 Left maxillary canine tooth (204) affected by a type 2 TR, stage 4c. Note the presence of root remnants of 206, 207, and 208 distal to the canine tooth.

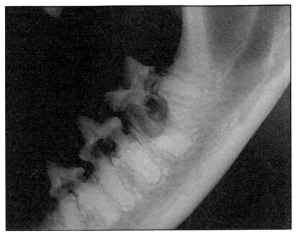

Fig. E8.11 Left mandibular fourth premolar (308) affected by a type 3 TR, stage 4b. Root remnants of the left mandibular third premolar and first molar (307 and 309) indicate possible previous type 1 TRs affecting them and causing their fracture.

Fig. E8.12 In this cat, the left mandibular third premolar (307) has features of a type 2 TR whereas the fourth premolar and first molar (308 and 309) are affected by type 1 TRs. Obviously it is possible that the same cat may have representation of all 3 types of TR.

Type 1 TRs are typically associated with periodontal bone loss, while type 2 TRs are poorly linked to periodontal variables.[7] Periodontitis in cats may result in TRs that do not have root replacement as the component of the disease (**Figures E8.13–8.18**).[8] There is also an association between tooth extrusion (particularly maxillary canines) and teeth resorption.[9]

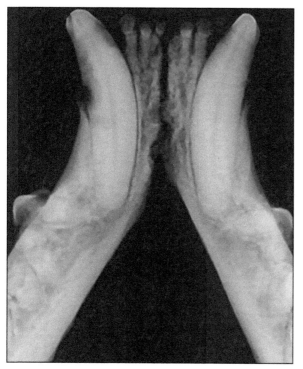

Fig. E8.13 **Type 1 TR, stage 2. Moderate dental hard tissue loss (cementum or cementum and enamel with loss of dentin that does not extend into the pulp cavity). In this case, the right mandibular canine tooth (404) is affected.**

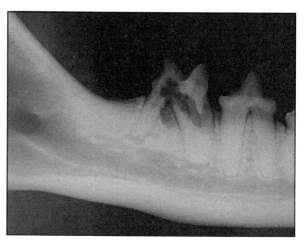

Fig. E8.14 **Type 1 TR, stage 3. Deep dental hard tissue loss (cementum or cementum and enamel with loss of dentin that extends to the pulp cavity); most of the tooth retains its integrity. In this case, the right mandibular first molar (409) is affected.**

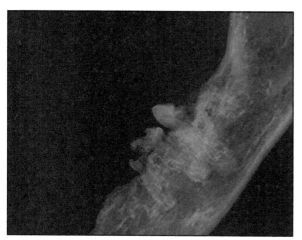

Fig. E8.15 **Type 2 TR. Extensive dental hard tissue loss (cementum or cementum and enamel with loss of dentin that extends to the pulp cavity); most of the tooth has lost its integrity. Stage 4a TR: the crown and root are equally affected. The left mandibular fourth premolar and first molar teeth (308, 309) are affected. The surrounding bone has a changed structure. Based on biopsy osteomyelitis was diagnosed.**

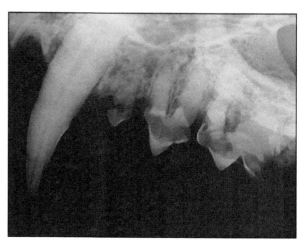

Fig. E8.16 **Stage 4b TR. The crown is more severely affected than the root. Type 1 TRs are present in the left maxillary second, third, and fourth premolars (206, 207, 208). Note the radiographic features of periodontitis in all affected teeth.**

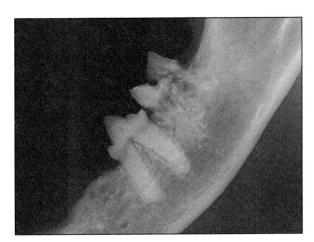

Fig. E8.17 **Type 2 TR, stage 4c. The root is** more severely affected than the crown in this left mandibular first molar tooth (309). Note the missing left mandibular third premolar (307).

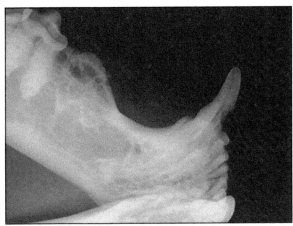

Fig. E8.18 **Type 2 TR, stage 5. Remnants of dental** hard tissue are visible only as irregular radiopacities, and gingival covering is complete. The stage 5 refers to the right mandibular third premolar (407), while the right mandibular canine tooth (404) has stage 4c TR.

The importance of dental radiography in TR cases cannot be overstated. Type 1 lesions typically retain a viable root canal system, and will result in pain and probable endodontic infection if the roots are not completely extracted. However, the concurrent presence of a normal PDL often makes these extractions less complicated.[10] With type 2 lesions, there are areas lacking a normal PDL (ankylosis), which also demonstrate varying degrees of root resorption, making extraction by conventional elevation difficult to impossible. Alterations in the PDL have been proposed by some authors as a preclinical stage of TR.[8] The fact that resorption will generally continue and progress is the basis for crown amputation therapy in teeth affected by advanced type 2 lesions. Teeth with an identifiable root canal on dental radiographs MUST be extracted completely, while teeth with no discernable root canal may be treated with crown amputation. As a standard of care it is important to look at the exposed root after crown amputation to check for the presence of an intact PDL or root canal. If these structures are present, further root removal is necessary.

Teeth resorption can also be associated with neoplastic and traumatic conditions, which are discussed in Chapter 8, Part G.

Canine tooth resorption

The American Veterinary Dental College (AVDC) classification of TR was the subject of a survey in dogs, which found that 90.2% of dogs affected with TR met the radiographic characteristics of 1 of the 5 types of TR.[11] The types of TR in dogs that were examined included: external surface resorption, external replacement resorption, external inflammatory resorption, external cervical root surface resorption, and internal resorption (**Figures E8.19–8.23**).[12]

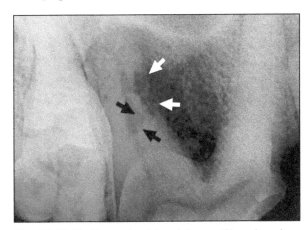

Fig. E8.19 **Radiograph of the right maxillary fourth** premolar (208) in a dog. External surface resorption (white arrows) and internal resorption (black arrows) can occur in the same root.

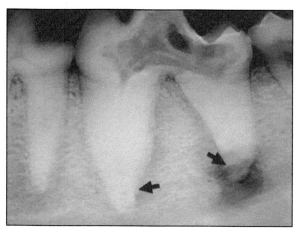

Fig. E8.20 **Idiopathic resorption in the coronal part of the left mandibular first molar (309), with external inflammatory resorption in both roots (arrows). Note the periapical lesion in the distal root.**

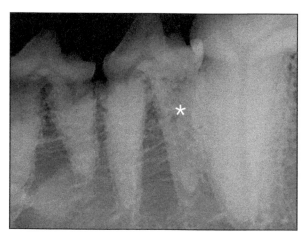

Fig. E8.21 **External replacement resorption in the distal root (asterisk) of a left mandibular fourth premolar (308).**

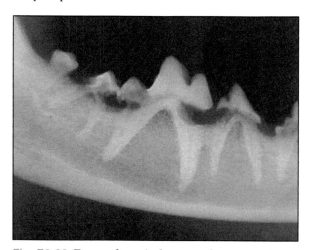

Fig. E8.22 **External cervical root surface resorption of the right mandibular fourth premolar (408) and first and second molar teeth (409, 410) in a 12-year-old dachshund. All the radiographed roots have no visible periodontal ligament space.**

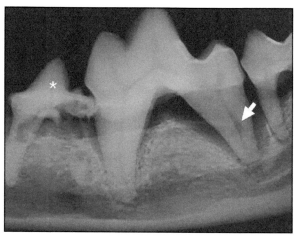

Fig. E8.23 **Idiopathic resorption of the left mandibular fourth premolar (308) (asterisk) and internal resorption in the distal root of the left mandibular first molar (309) (arrow). All the radiographed teeth are also affected by periodontal disease.**

CARIES

Carious lesions are the result of acidic degradation of the calcified dental tissues (enamel, dentin, and cementum).[3] They appear radiographically as areas of decreased radiodensity in the crown and/or root of the tooth (*Table E8.1*). In the vast majority of cases, there will be an obvious lesion noted on oral examination. The extent of lost tooth structure will be clinically evident to a certain extent and thus help with

treatment planning. As in periodontal disease, remember that approximately 30–60% of the mineral in the tooth must be lost before radiographic changes will be noticeable. Therefore, radiographs always underestimate carious loss. Radiography is essential to rule out endodontic disease in teeth with carious lesions. Endodontic involvement must be evaluated prior to initiation of cavity preparation, since the owner may elect extraction as opposed to root canal therapy on an endodontically diseased tooth.[13] The prevalence

Table E8.1 **Crown defects according to the GV Black modified classification.**[15,16]

Class I	Incisors, premolars, molars	Structural defects: pits and fissures on occlusal surface
Class II	Premolars, molars	Defect on interproximal surface does not involve incisal surface
Class III	Incisors canines	Interproximal surface does not involve incisional surface
Class IV	Incisors canines	Proximal surface involves incisional surface
Class V	Incisors, canines, premolars, molars	Facial, palatal or lingual gingival third
Class VI	Incisors, canines, premolars, molars	Incisal edge of rostral teeth or a cusp in caudal teeth

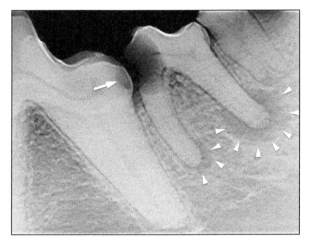

Fig. E8.24 **Class VI crown defect caused by caries in a left mandibular second molar (310). The defect reaches the pulp chamber and has caused pulp disease with periapical complications (arrowheads). In addition, there is an early stage of caries creating a class II defect visible at the distal interproximal surface of the left mandibular first molar (309) (arrow).**

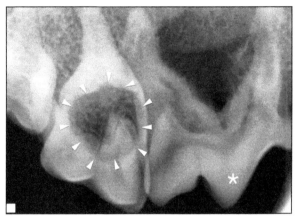

Fig. E8.25 **Caries (class I defect) affecting a right maxillary first molar (109), resulting in significant destruction of a large portion of the crown (arrowheads). Note the resorption affecting the right maxillary fourth premolar (108) (asterisk).**

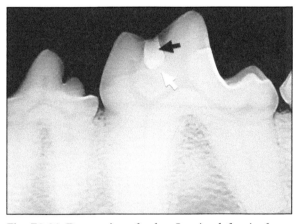

Fig. E8.26 **Restoration of a class I caries defect in the left mandibular first molar (309), where the mesial defect wall wall was close to the pulp horn. This case required using a glass ionomer liner (white arrow) prior to composite restoration (black arrow). Prior to restoration the apical portions of both roots were radiographed and assessed to rule out endodontic involvement.**

of caries in dogs was found to be 5.3% in one referral dental practice (**Figures E8.24, E8.25**).[14]

Radiolucent areas of demineralized dentin are not always obvious, therefore the extent of necessary débridement should be based on clinical evaluation during removal of the softened dentin, rather than on radiographic appearance. Radiography is important for evaluating the distance to the pulp chamber, the selection of restorative material, as well as the lining cement (**Figure E8.26**).

DEVELOPMENTAL DENTAL ABNORMALITIES OF HARD TISSUE

Dentinal dysplasia

Dentinal dysplasia is characterized by abnormal dentin formation following the initial deposition of mantle dentin, which results in abnormally short or absent roots and a narrow pulp chamber. Clinical and radiographic findings are consistent with descriptions of odontodysplasia in humans, and (as in humans) it typically affects the entire dentition. The teeth have abnormal structure, with very thin dentin due to defective mineralization. In human dentistry, two types of dentin dysplasia are described:

- Type 1: teeth have normal crowns (shape and color) but short roots (**Figure E8.27**).[17]
- Type II: the color of the deciduous dentition is opalescent but the color of the permanent dentition is normal.[18]

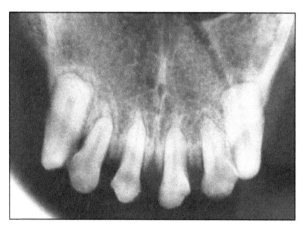

Fig. E8.27 **Type I dentin dysplasia. The crowns of all the maxillary incisors are normal size but the roots are short.**

Regional odontodysplasia (also described as 'ghost teeth') affects both dentin and enamel in one or several teeth in a localized area (**Figure E8.28**).[19]

Abnormalities of enamel formation

Amelogenesis imperfecta includes genetic and/or developmental enamel formation and maturation abnormalities such as enamel hypoplasia and enamel hypomineralization.[20]

Enamel hypoplasia refers to a disturbance in the formation of a tooth leading to visible defects in the enamel (**Figure E8.29**).[21] Enamel hypomineralization may be caused by local, systemic, or hereditary factors, which disturb the mineralization of matrix during enamel development (**Figure E8.30**).[22–24] The process of enamel formation consists of two phases: enamel matrix formation and its subsequent maturation. The consequences of abnormal enamel formation are:

- Hypoplasia (an incomplete formation that has a quantitative character).
- Hypomineralization (lack of quality of the enamel).

The qualitative problem affecting the enamel has a tendency to worsen during mastication, as the soft, brittle enamel breaks off. The circumscribed hypoplasia (deficiency in thickness of external enamel layer) is defined early and does not enlarge as the

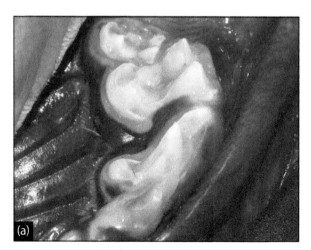
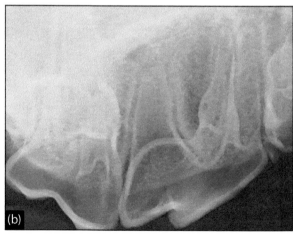

Fig. E8.28 **Regional odontodysplasia. Clinical appearance (a) and radiograph (b).**

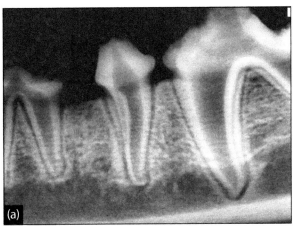

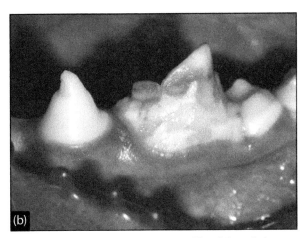

Fig. E8.29 **Enamel hypoplasia. (a) The rough surface of the crown and uneven radiopacity of hard dental tissues are radiographically visible on the crown of both imaged teeth – left mandibular fourth premolar and first molar (308, 309). With 308 only a small area at the tip of the crown is affected, but it is additionally deformed (peg tooth). (b) Radiographic assessment is mandatory to confirm or rule out endodontic complications.**

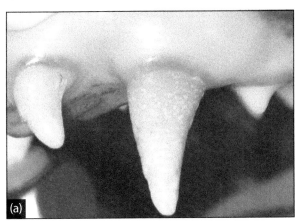

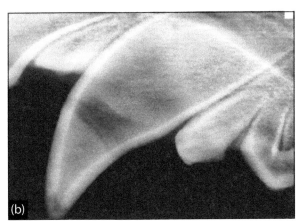

Fig. E8.30 **(a) Enamel hypomineralization. (b) This radiograph reveals a thin wall of the crown without the presence of radiopaque enamel.**

surrounding tissues are normal. Systemic and hereditary factors usually affect the whole dentition, but occasionally only a few teeth are affected. Local factors such as inflammation, injury, or infection (e.g. abscess) cause local defects to one or a few teeth in the same area.

The minerals contained in saliva *may* eventually obliterate the dentinal tubules if there is connection with the dentin.[16] However, this type of defect may also enable transfer of bacteria from the oral cavity through the dentinal tubules into the pulp chamber, resulting in endodontic infection.[25] In addition, dentinal exposure is known to cause tooth sensitivity. The currently accepted fluid dynamic theory of tooth sensitivity is summarized as follows:

- 'Dentin exposure will change the fluid dynamics within the dentinal tubules, especially in response to stimuli such as heat, cold, or desiccation. The change in fluid velocity within the tubules is translated into electrical signals by the sensory fibers located within the tubules or subjacent odontoblast layer. These signals result in the sensation of pain within the tooth.[26]

Treatment is necessary to eliminate sensitivity, protect against pulp infection, and control plaque accumulation from the rough surface of the crown.[2] The radiographic appearance of enamel hypoplasia is one of a missing radiopaque line of enamel, provided that the x-ray beam is tangential to the area of hypoplasia (**Figure E8.31**).

Intrinsically stained (discolored) teeth

These teeth can appear pink, purple, yellow, brown, or gray. The most common intrinsic stain seen in dogs is caused by pulp hemorrhage due to trauma. Endodontic disease can be also manifested by intrinsic staining. A study by Hale (2001) showed that only 40% of intrinsically stained teeth had radiographic signs of endodontic disease; however, 92.7% are nonvital.[27] Therefore, in AVDC nomenclature, discolored teeth are defined as nonvital.[20]

Discolored teeth affected by pulpitis may show a narrowed root canal and pulp chamber compared with unaffected teeth, but, conversely, some nonvital teeth have terminated dentin deposition and their endodontic system can appear wider (**Figures E8.32, E8.33**).[28]

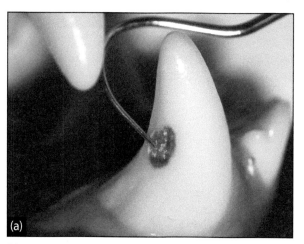
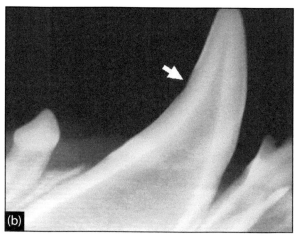

Fig. E8.31 (a) Localized enamel hypoplasia. (b) This is visible radiographically in this right mandibular canine tooth (404) as it is missing the radiopaque line of enamel (arrow). The x-ray beam must be tangential to the area of hypoplasia otherwise the defect will not be visible.

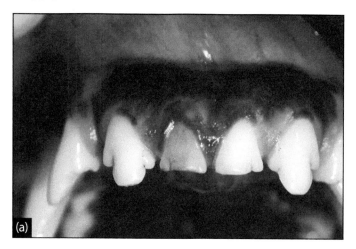
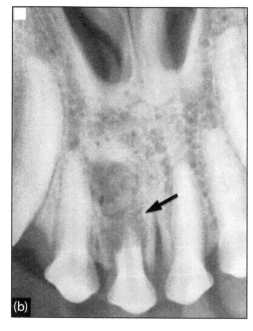

Fig. E8.32 Intrinsically stained right maxillary first incisor (101) (a) with obvious pulp necrosis (wider pulp chamber than adjacent teeth) and root resorption present on the radiograph (b) (arrow).

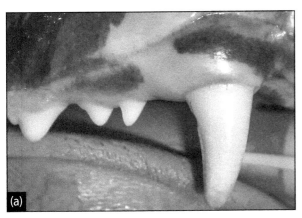

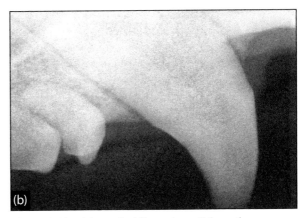

Fig. E8.33 **Intrinsically stained right maxillary canine tooth (104) (a) with total obliteration of the pulp chamber (b). Note the supernumerary right maxillary first premolar (105).**

ANATOMIC ANOMALIES OF DENTAL HARD TISSUE

Many of the conditions listed below refer to abnormal shape, structure, or orientation of teeth, which are detectable only with the use of radiography. Most of them have an impact on treatment plans (e.g. dilacerated teeth in extraction or pulp stones in endodontic treatment) or require action (e.g. endodontic treatment or extraction of an invaginated tooth). Regardless of their origin or etiology, it is important to be aware of the anomaly before performing any procedure on an affected tooth, therefore preoperative radiography is invaluable.

- Supernumerary roots: most commonly found in maxillary third premolars (**Figures E8.34, E8.35**).[29]

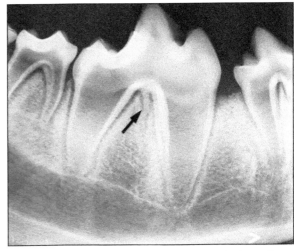

Fig. E8.34 **Supernumerary root present in furcation area of the right mandibular first molar (409) in a dog (arrow).**

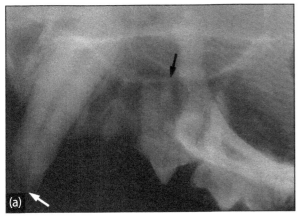

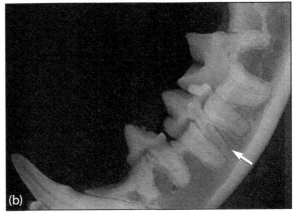

Fig. E8.35 **Supernumerary roots of the left maxillary third premolar 207 (a, black arrow) and left mandibular fourth premolar (308) (b, arrow) in a cat. Note the fractured left maxillary canine tooth (204) in (a) (white arrow).**

- Gemination: single tooth bud splits, but not always completely (**Figure E8.36**).
- Twinning: complete splitting of the geminated tooth. Causes appearance of supernumerary teeth (**Figure E8.37**).
- Concrescense: fusion of the cementum of adjacent teeth roots (**Figure E8.38**).
- Fusion: two separate teeth joined at the crown by enamel and dentin, creating a reduction in number of teeth. This may be seen in deciduous or permanent dentition (**Figure E8.39**).

- Root and crown dilaceration: abnormal, curved shape of either the apical part of the root or the crown. These conditions can be caused by trauma (**Figures E8.40, E8.41**).
- Convergent roots: usually occur in mandibular first and second molar teeth in small breed dogs or in premolars (**Figure E8.42**).
- Fused roots: very common in small breed dogs and typically affect the second molars and premolars (**Figure E8.43**).

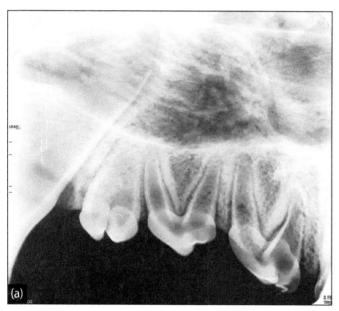
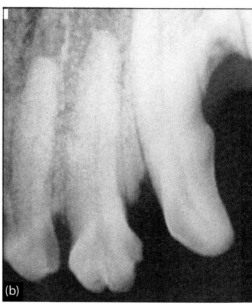

Fig. E8.36 **Gemination of the left maxillary first premolar (205) (a) and second incisor (202) (b) in a dog.**

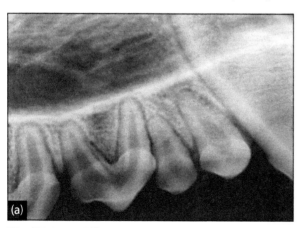
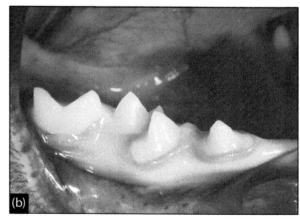

Fig. E8.37 **(a) The twinning of the right maxillary first premolar (105) in this dog creates the appearance of supernumerary teeth, but as there is room for a supernumerary tooth, it is not causing crowding. (b, c) The twinning of the right mandibular fourth premolar (408) in this cat has created crowding and will require interceptive extraction.**

(Continued)

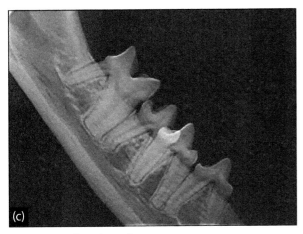

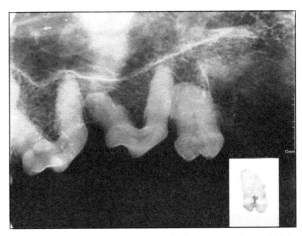

Fig. E8.37 *(Continued)*

Fig. E8.38 **Radiograph exposed after extraction of 104. Note the fusion of the cementum and dentin of the adjacent supernumerary 105 after extraction (insert).**

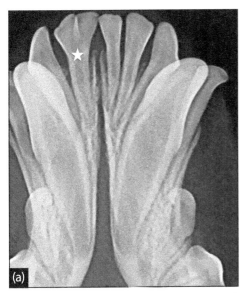

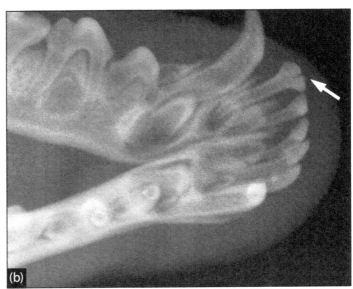

Fig. E8.39 (a) **Fusion of the right mandibular first and second incisors (401, 402) (star) resulting in a reduction of the number of mandibular incisors. (b) The same situation can apply to deciduous dentition. Fusion of the right mandibular second and third incisors (802, 803) (arrow).**

- Taurodontia: crown and pulp chamber are relatively larger than the root and root canal (**Figure E8.44**).
- Microdontia: the crown is shaped normally but is smaller in relation to size of the dog or adjacent teeth (**Figure E8.45**).
- Invagination: infolding of the tooth wall causing presence of additional layers of enamel and dentin. This condition can be confirmed either clinically, when the folding and entry to the pulp chamber is visible or can be felt with an explorer, or histologically (**Figure E8.46**).

- Peg tooth: small conical or cone-shaped teeth with a single cusp (**Figure E8.47**).
- Shell teeth: teeth with a crown but underdeveloped root(s) (**Figure E8.48**).
- Pulp stones: presence of radiopaque mineralized structures within the endodontic system. Large pulp stones that are located in the central portion of the canal and either bulging or constricting it are the features of a subcategory of dentin dysplasia (**Figure E8.49**).[17]

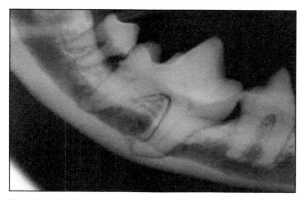

Fig. E8.40 Root dilacerations. Abnormal, curved shape of the apical part of the roots of the right mandibular first molar (409).

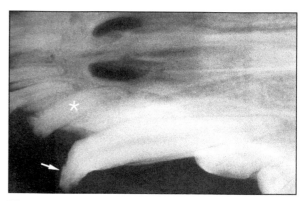

Fig. E8.41 Crown dilaceration in the right maxillary canine (204) (arrow). The most likely origin of this deformation is trauma. Note the fractured crown of the right maxillary third incisor (203) (asterisk).

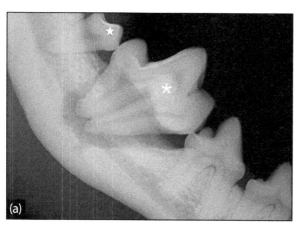

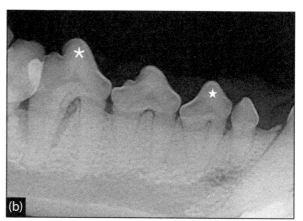

Fig. E8.42 Convergent roots occur most commonly in the mandibular first molar teeth (a) or premolars (b) of small breed dogs. In (a) note the presence of the radiopaque structure in the coronal part of the right mandibular first molar (409) (asterisk), which appears as an invaginated tooth, as well as the fused roots of the right mandibular second molar (410) (star) and the missing right mandibular third molar (411). In (b) note that the right mandibular second premolar (406) (star) has convergent roots and the distal root of the right mandibular fourth premolar (408) (asterisk) has vertical bone loss.

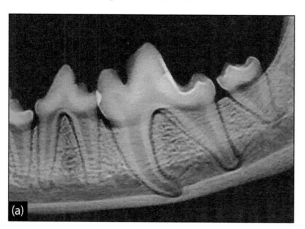

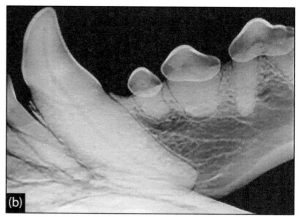

Fig. E8.43 Fused roots. (a) Mandibular second molar (310); (b) left mandibular second premolar (306).

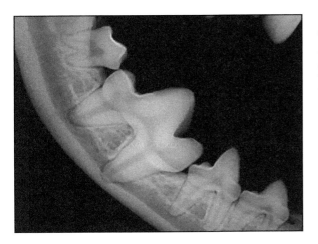

Fig. E8.44 Taurodontia in a Yorkshire terrier. The crown and pulp chamber of the right mandibular first and second molar teeth (409, 410) are relatively larger than the roots and root canal. Note the missing mandibular third molar (411).

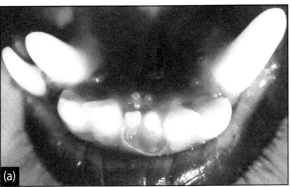

Fig. E8.45 (a) Microdontia of the right and left mandibular first incisors (401, 301). The affected teeth are relatively smaller than the adjacent incisors. (b) The radiographic appearance of the teeth confirms that they are not deciduous. Note the presence of a persistent right mandibular canine tooth (804).

Fig. E8.46 Invagination. In this case the right mandibular first molar (409) is afffected. Note the presence of a radiopaque structure in 409, its wider root canals, and periapical radiolucency. The latter two findings indicate endodontic infection following pulp necrosis. After extraction of the affected tooth, the presence of folding and entry to the pulp chamber was confirmed.

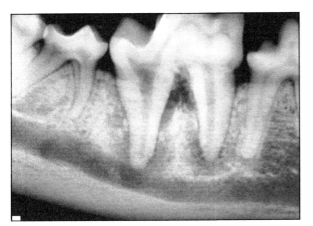

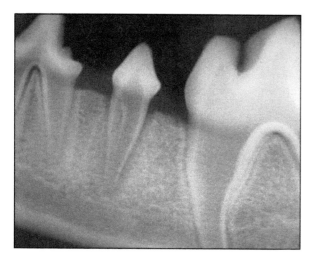

Fig. E8.47 Peg tooth. The left mandibular fourth premolar (308) appears as a small conical or cone-shaped tooth with a single cusp.

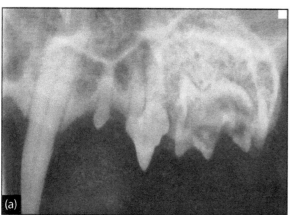

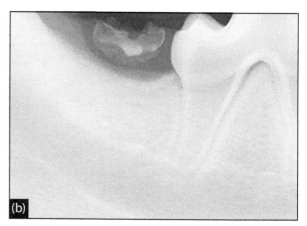

Fig. E8.48 Shell teeth. (a) The left maxillary fourth premolar (208) in a cat with a crown but with underdeveloped roots. (b) Right mandibular second molar (410) in a dog.

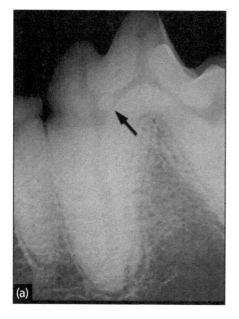

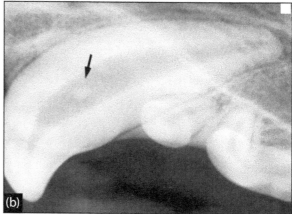

Fig. E8.49 Pulp stones (arrows) in a left mandibular first molar (309) (a) and a left maxillary canine (204) (b).

REFERENCES

1 Gracis M (2007) Orodental anatomy and physiology. In: *BSAVA Manual of Canine and Feline Dentistry*, 3rd edn. (eds. C Tutt, J Deeprose, DA Crossley) British Small Animal Veterinary Association, Gloucester, pp. 13–21.

2 Niemiec BA (2010) Pathology in the pediatric patient. In: *Small Animal Dental, Oral and Maxillofacial Disease: A Color Handbook*. (ed. BA Niemiec) Manson Publishing, London, pp. 89–126.

3 DuPont GA (2010) Pathologies of the dental hard tissue. In: *Small Animal Dental, Oral and Maxillofacial Disease: A Color Handbook*. (ed. BA Niemiec) Manson Publishing, London, pp. 127–157.

4 Gorrel C (2008) Root resorption: an introduction. In: *Saunders Solutions in Veterinary Practice: Small Animal Dentistry*. (series ed. F Nind) Saunders Elsevier, Edinburgh, pp. 105–107.

5 Girard N, Servet E, Hennet P *et al*. (2010) Tooth resorption and vitamin D3 status in cats fed premium dry diets. *J Vet Dent* **27(3)**:142–147.

6 Mihaljevic SY, Kernmaier A, Mertens-Jentsch S (2012) Radiographic changes associated with tooth resorption type 2 in cats. *J Vet Dent* **29(1)**:20–26.

7 Girard N, Servet E, Bourse V *et al*. (2008) Feline tooth resorption in a colony of 109 cats. *J Vet Dent* **25(3)**:166–174.

8 DuPont G, DeBowes L (2002) Comparison of periodontitis and root replacement in cat teeth with resorptive lesions. *J Vet Dent* **19(2)**:71–75.

9 Lewis J, Eked A, Shofer F *et al*. (2008) Significant association between tooth extrusion and tooth resorption in domestic cats. *J Vet Dent* **25(2)**:86–95.

10 Niemiec BA (2011) The importance of dental radiology. *Eur J Comp Anim Pract* **20(3)**:219–229.

11 Nomenclature Committee of the American Veterinary Dental College. Veterinary dental nomenclature – classification of tooth resorption. Available at: www.avdc.org/Nomenclature.html#resorption.

12 Peralta S, Verstraete FJ, Kass PH (2010) Radiographic evaluation of the classification of the extent of tooth resorption in dogs. *Am J Vet Res* **71(7)**:794–798.

13 Verstraete FJ (1999) *Self-Assesment Colour Review of Veterinary Dentistry*. Manson Publishing, London, p. 194.

14 Hale FA (1998) Dental caries in the dog. *J Vet Dent* **15(2)**:79–83.

15 Mulligan TW (1998) Acquired defects: caries and regressive changes. In: *Atlas of Canine and Feline Dental Radiography*. Veterinary Learning Systems, Trenton, pp. 153–169.

16 Wiggs RB, Lobprise HB (1997) Operative and restorative dentistry. In: *Veterinary Dentistry: Principless and Practice*. Lippincott-Raven, Philadelphia, pp. 351–394.

17 Smithson CW, Smith MM, Gamble DA (2010) Multifocal odontoblastic dysplasia in a dog. *J Vet Dent* **27(4)**:242–247.

18 Hoffman S (2008) Abnormal tooth eruption in a cat. *J Vet Dent* **25(2)**:118–122.

19 Schwamberger G, Maretta SM, Dubielzig R *et al*. (2010) Regional odontodysplasia in a juvenile dog. *J Vet Dent* **27(2)**:98–103.

20 www.avdc.org. Recommendation from AVDC Nomenclature.

21 Arzi B, Fiani N (2009) Diagnostic imaging in veterinary dental practice. *J Am Vet Med Assoc* **235(10)**:1149–1151.

22 Neville BW, Damm DD, Allen CM *et al*. (2002) Abnormalities of teeth. In: *Oral and Maxillofacial Pathology*, 2nd edn. Saunders, Philadelphia, pp. 49–106.

23 Harvey CE, Emily PP (1993) Restorative dentistry. In: *Small Animal Dentistry*. Mosby, St. Louis, pp. 213–265.

24 Colyer JF (1990) Enamel hypoplasia. In: *Colyer's Variations and Diseases of the Teeth of Animals*. (eds. AEW Miles, C Grigson) Cambridge University Press, Cambridge, pp. 437–454.

25 Nair R (2002) Pathobiology of the periapex. In: *Pathways of the Pulp*, 8th edn. (eds. A Cohen, RC Burns) Mosby, St. Louis, pp. 457–500.

26 Trowbridge HO, Syngcuk K, Hideaki S (2002) Structure and functions of the dentin-pulp complex. In: *Pathways of the Pulp*, 8th edn. (eds. A Cohen, RC Burns) Mosby, St. Louis, pp. 411–456.

27 Hale FA (2001) Localized intrinsic staining of teeth due to pulpitis and pulp necrosis in dogs. *J Vet Dent* **18(1)**:14–20.

28 DuPont GA, DeBowes LJ (2009) Intraoral radiographic anatomy of the dog. In: *Atlas of Dental Radiography in Dogs and Cats*. Saunders, Philadelphia, pp. 5–80.

29 Verheart L (2007) Developmental oral and dental conditions. In: *BSAVA Manual of Canine and Feline Dentistry*, 3rd edn. (eds. C Tutt, J Deeprose, DA Crossley) British Small Animal Veterinary Association, Gloucester, pp. 77–95.

PART F

TRAUMA

Jerzy Gawor

INTRODUCTION

Maxillofacial diagnostic imaging in trauma patients is never the first part of the management. The first goal of therapy is to stabilize the patient and perform a thorough clinical assessment. However, without a diagnosis and identification of all injured structures, it is impossible to create an appropriate treatment plan.

A thorough clinical examination of the orofacial structures will provide a list of injuries and, based on this, a treatment plan with specified priorities can be created.

In post-traumatic situations, computed tomography (CT) is superior to traditional radiography.[1] Additionally, 3D imaging is more beneficial in the diagnosis of temporomandibular joint (TMJ) injuries and allows for the formulation of a precise treatment plan.[2] As access to 3D imaging technology is still not universal, routine extraoral and intraoral imaging should be performed first.

DENTAL TRAUMA

Fractured teeth are a relatively common finding in dogs and cats.[3] The teeth most frequently involved are the canines, carnassials, and incisors.[4] Tooth fractures result from trauma such as biting on hard objects or being hit accidentally. Many fractures remain unnoticed by the owners until complications occur or they are found during a thorough oral examination. All fractured teeth need an accurate diagnostic approach, as almost all fractures require some form of treatment. Neglecting fractures often leads to infections and painful complications.

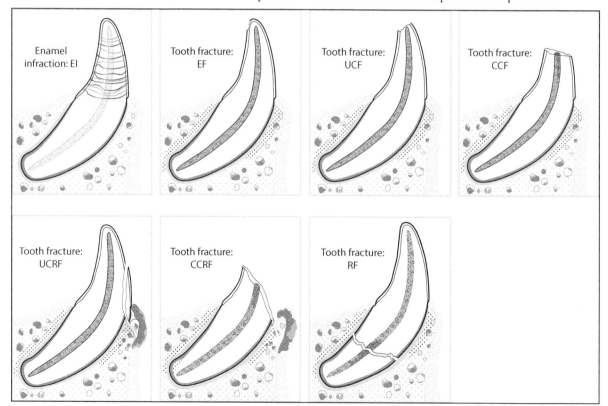

Fig. F8.1 **Tooth fracture classification. (Adapted from the American Veterinary Dental College website.)**

The American Veterinary Dental College (AVDC) classification of tooth fractures is illustrated in **Figures F8.1–8.9**.[5] Radiographic evaluation is required to assess the entire tooth structure, particularly the part that cannot be assessed clinically (the roots). In addition, it is important to evaluate surrounding tissues. Finally, it is important to have preoperative images for comparison at the time of follow-up. However, infractions are nondetectable radiographically and occasionally vertical root fractures cannot be seen even at the best resolution.

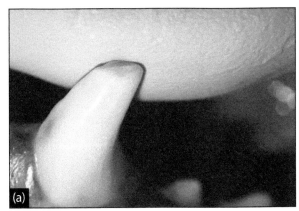

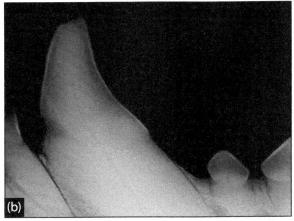

Fig. F8.4 Uncomplicated crown fracture (UCF). A fracture of the crown that does not directly expose the pulp chamber. Fractured tip of the crown of the left mandibular canine tooth (304) in clinical appearance (a) and radiograph (b).

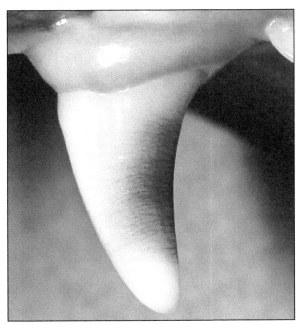

Fig. F8.2 Enamel infraction (EI).

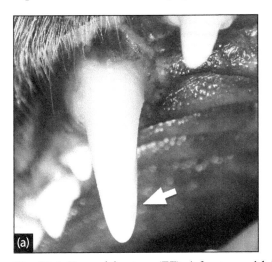

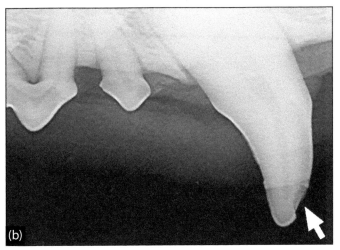

Fig. F8.3 Enamel fracture (EF). A fracture with loss of crown substance that is confined to the enamel. Clinical appearance of EF in right maxillary canine tooth (104) (a, arrow) and radiograph (b, arrow)

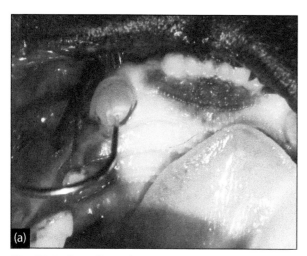
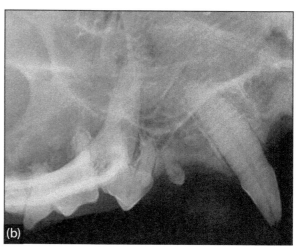

Fig. F8.5 Complicated crown fracture (CCF). A fracture of the crown that directly exposes the pulp chamber. Dental explorer entering exposed pulp chamber of the fractured right maxillary canine tooth (104) in a cat (a) and radiograph of the fractured tooth (b).

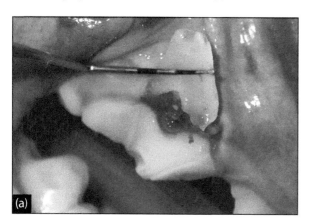
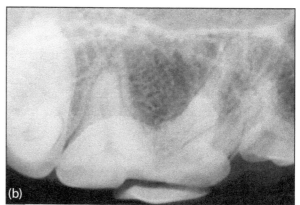

Fig. F8.6 Uncomplicated crown-root fracture (UCRF). A fracture of the crown and root that does not expose the pulp canal. Clinical (a) and radiographic (b) evaluation of a right maxillary fourth premolar tooth (108) fracture.

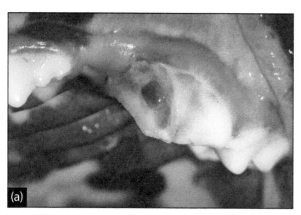
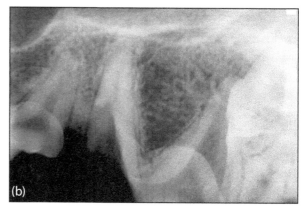

Fig. F8.7 Complicated crown-root fracture (CCRF). A fracture of the crown and root that exposes the pulp canal. Clinical appearance of a fractured left maxillary fourth premolar tooth (208) with visible exposed pulp (a) and radiographic evaluation of the tooth (b).

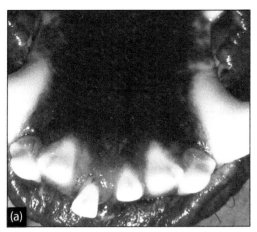
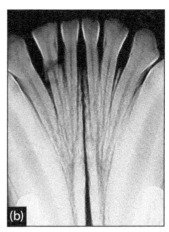

Fig. F8.8 **Root fracture (RF). A fracture involving only the root, in this case a horizontal fracture (a). Radiograph of a fractured right mandibular second incisor (402) (b).**

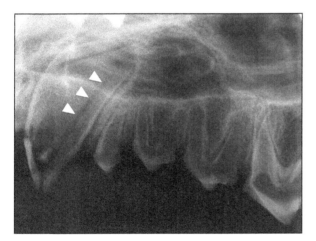

Fig. F8.9 **Root fracture (RF). In this case the fracture involves the crown and root of the left maxillary canine tooth (204). Note the vertical fracture of the root (arrowheads).**

An accurate diagnosis of fracture type has an important prognostic value. Treatment options depend on the extent of the injury, any additional complications, the periodontal status of the injured tooth, the age and condition of the patient, the decision of the owner and, finally, the competence of the veterinarian. Extraction, endodontic treatment, splinting, and restorations, including prosthetics (crowns), are the most common options for management of fractured teeth.

Apart from the above traumatic injuries, dentition can also undergo chronic trauma. Attrition is the process whereby the crowns are worn due to tooth on tooth trauma.[6] This is most commonly the case in class III malocclusions. When chewing is more intensive, for example as the consequence of skin disease and pruritus or habit (bruxism), teeth are worn quickly, even to the extent of pulp exposure (**Figure F8.10**).

When the loss of tooth structure happens through wear against material other than opposing dentition it is termed abrasion.[7] Abrasion results from biting hard objects (cage biter syndrome), retrieving, or excessive playing with abrasive toys (e.g. a tennis ball on the beach). Radiographs are necessary to determine the thickness of the reparative dentin that protects the pulp chamber, and to reveal possible endodontic complications (**Figures F8.11–8.13**).

TOOTH LUXATION

This condition can be divided into one of six categories: concussion, subluxation, lateral luxation, extrusive luxation, intrusive luxation, and avulsion.[8] The most common presenting signs of luxation are change in tooth position and increased mobility. Only radiographic evaluation can differentiate luxation from tooth fracture. Replacement resorption, inflammatory root resorption, ankylosis, and periapical changes are potential complications.[9] Subluxation can be seen radiographically as a widened periodontal ligament space (**Figure F8.14**). Lateral luxation is always accompanied by fracture of the buccal and possibly palatal/lingual wall of the alveolus (**Figure F8.15**). Intrusion appears as an

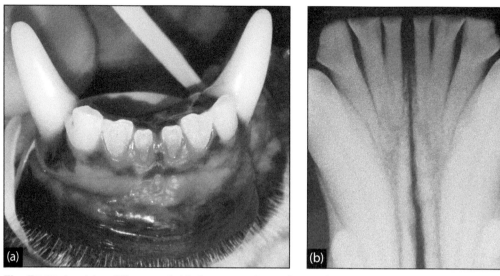

Fig. F8.10 Attrition. Worn teeth (a) always require radiographic evaluation (b).

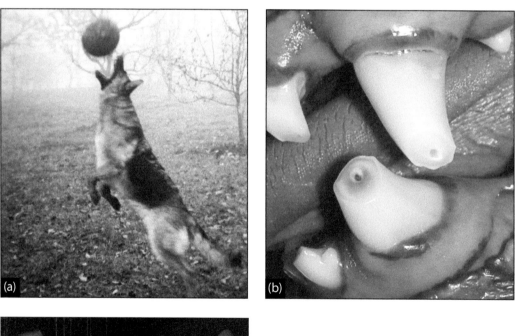

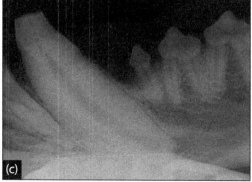

Fig. F8.11 Abrasion. (a) This can result from excessive playing with an abrasive toy and may lead to destruction of the hard dental tissue, including exposure of the pulp chamber (b). Dental radiographs are mandatory to rule out or confirm periapical pathology (c).

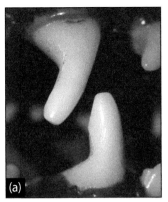
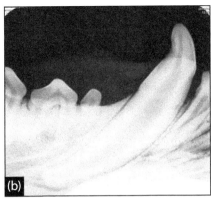
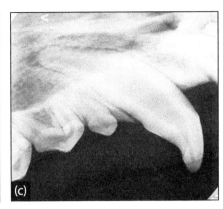

Fig. F8.12 Abrasion. (a) In cage biter syndrome, the typical location of the defect is the distal surface of the canine teeth. (b, c) Dental radiographs may allow the practitioner to determine how close the damage is to the pulp.

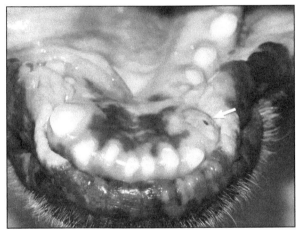

Fig. F8.13 Typical abrasion caused by retrieving stones. Quite often, damaged teeth have pulp exposure and require management appropriate for the endodontic problems. Note the direct root canal exposure in the left mandibular canine tooth (304) associated with this tooth discoloration (arrow).

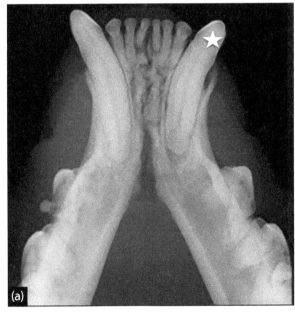

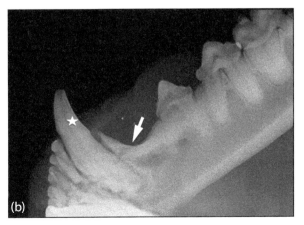

Fig. F8.14 A left mandibular canine tooth (star) (304) with subluxation: occlusal view (a) and lateral oblique view (b). Note that the luxated tooth has an uncomplicated crown fracture and there is also a fracture of the surrounding alveolar bone (b, arrow). In addition, there is a fracture of 407 (a).

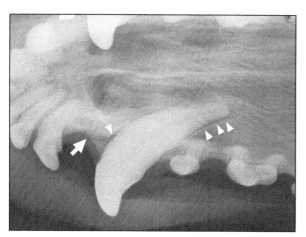

Fig. F8.15 **Lateral luxation accompanied by fracture of the buccal (arrow) and possibly palatal wall of the alveolar bone. Note the widened periodontal ligament space (arrowheads).**

apical shift of the tooth, which always causes fracture of the apical part of the alveolus and vascular/nerve bundle at the apical delta (**Figure F8.16**). Avulsion and extrusion are not typically associated with alveolar bone fracture (**Figure F8.17**).

All of the above injuries can cause intrinsic staining of the tooth, usually due to pulpal hemorrhage, followed by pulpits and ultimately pulp necrosis and infection (**Figure F8.18, F8.19**).

FOREIGN BODIES

The presence of foreign bodies in the oral cavity, even if they are not traumatic in origin, have an influence on the therapy of traumatic injuries. Bone chips present between teeth, needles in the tongue or palate, and rings around the tongue are difficult to diagnose because most patients do not allow a thorough oral examination without anesthesia. Therefore, it is not until the outward clinical signs of drooling, abscess, or malodor are present will the issue be detected and the foreign object removed. The long-term presence of these foreign bodies in the oral cavity often causes irreversible damage to the surrounding tissue (**Figures F8.20, F8.21**).

Another type of foreign object is a pellet or bullet, which occasionally creates hard tissue trauma in the oral cavity. Unfortunately, it is

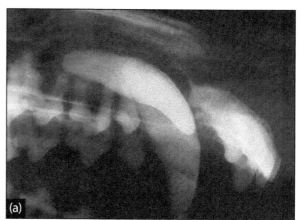

(a)

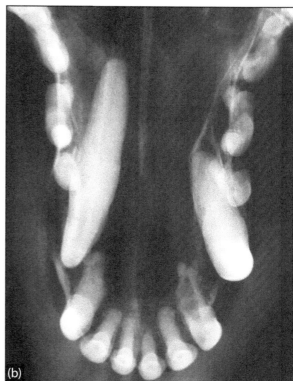

(b)

Fig. F8.16 **Lateral (a) and ventrodorsal (b) radiographic views of an intruded right maxillary canine tooth (104) that required extraction.**

not uncommon for people to shoot cats or dogs and many of these cases are diagnosed spuriously (**Figure F8.22**). Whenever the practitioner suspects breakage of an instrument, a dental radiograph should be exposed. A radiopaque piece of broken curette or other instrument can be easily detected radiographically (**Figure F8.23**).

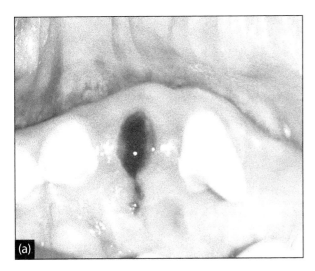

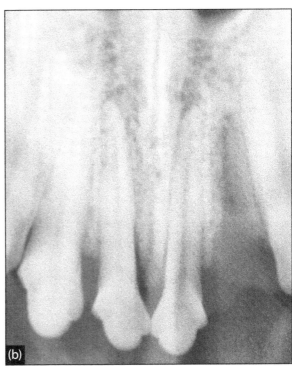

Fig. F8.17 **Avulsion and/or extrusion. All areas with missing teeth after injury (a) should be radiographed. An empty alveolus without any fractures indicates likelihood of avulsion (b).**

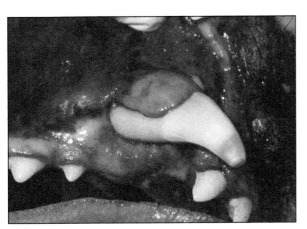

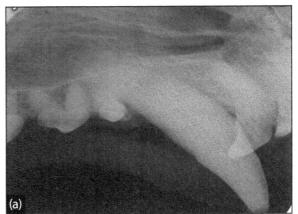

Fig. F8.18 **Intrinsic staining of the tooth due to pulpal hemorrhage caused by a luxation. This tooth required endodontic therapy following replacement and fixation.**

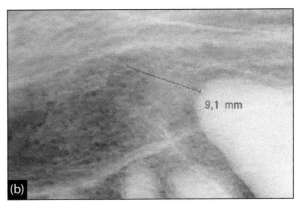

Fig. F8.19 **(a) This radiograph shows dislocation of the tooth in Fig. F8.18 (right maxillary canine 104) in relation to the alveolar socket. (b) Intraoperative radiograph showing the remaining distance to complete reduction of the luxated tooth. The distance is measured to the site of the alveolus that the contralateral canine tooth apex occupies.**

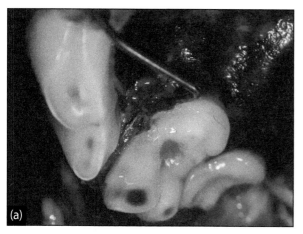

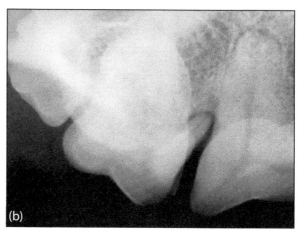

Fig. F8.20 (a) Foreign body in oral tissues causing irreversible damage to the surrounding tissue. (b) Note the worn hard dental tissue of the right maxillary fourth premolar and first molar (108, 109), with the presence of brown colored reparative dentin in worn areas.

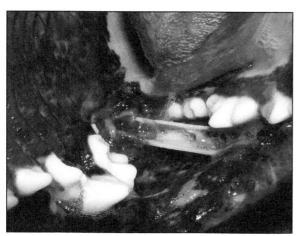

Fig. F8.21 Gross appearance of a radiopaque foreign body in the mouth of a dog. Remember that postoperative radiographs are required.

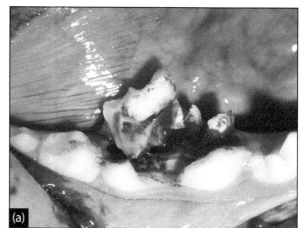

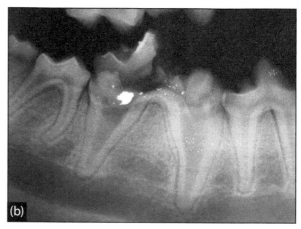

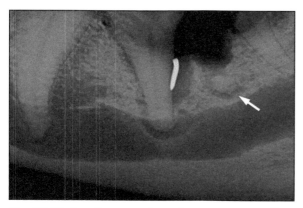

Fig. F8.23 A radiopaque piece of a curette can easily be seen in this radiograph. Note also the retained mesial root tip of 310 (arrow)

Fig. F8.22 (a) The comminuted fracture of this right mandibular molar tooth (409) was caused by a gun shot. (b) Radiopaque remnants of the pellet are visible on the radiograph.

JAW FRACTURES

Accurate examination after head trauma typically cannot be performed until sedation or anesthesia can be safely administered. Localization of jaw fractures has been studied, with the most common fracture location in the dog involving the molar region (47.1% of fractures), followed by the symphyseal area (30.6%) and finally the maxilla (10%).[10]

Different types of jaw fractures may occur: simple, multiple, comminuted, pathologic, compound stable or nonstable (**Figures F8.24–8.29**).

Currently, instead of 'favorable' and 'unfavorable' the terms used to describe fractures are stable and nonstable. For mandibular fractures, the proposed classification is determined by location (*Table F8.1*).

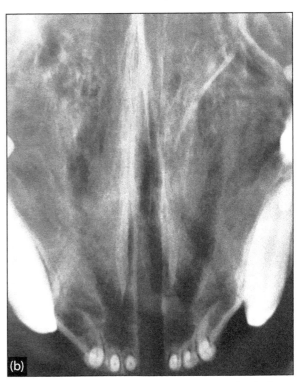

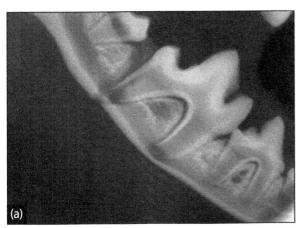

Fig. F8.24 **Simple fracture of the right mandible between 409 and 410 in a dog (a) and the incisive and palatine bones in a cat, with separation of the palatine process of the maxilla (b).**

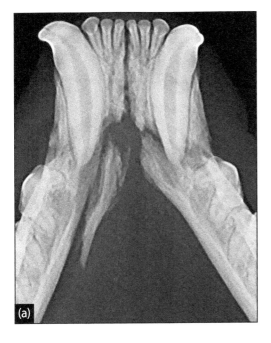

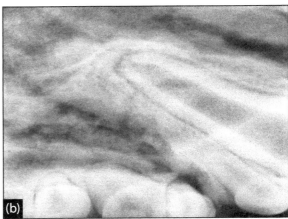

Fig. F8.25 **Multiple fractures of the rostral mandible in a cat (a) and the right maxilla in a dog (b).**

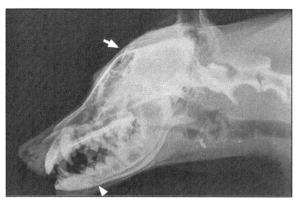

Fig. F8.26 Comminuted fracture of the frontal bone (arrow) and multiple fractures of the rostral mandible (arrowheads) in a dog. To obtain diagnostic radiographs of the mandibular fractures, a series of intraoral images was performed.

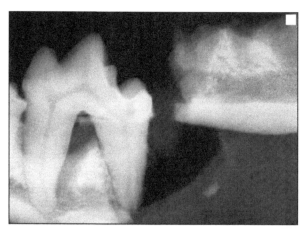

Fig. F8.27 Fracture of the mandible at the site of a periodontally affected molar tooth. There was no history of injury in this dog. Rather, the fracture occurred during normal play. Note the periodontal disease affecting the left mandibular first molar (309), which weakened the mandible and predisposed it to pathologic fracture. Note also the absence of the left mandibular second molar (310), which was lost during manipulation due to its severe attachment loss.

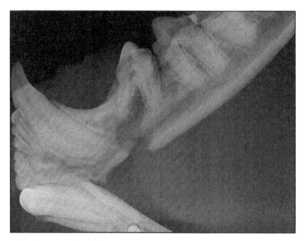

Fig. F8.28 Stable type of mandibular fracture. Note the rostroventral–caudodorsal oblique direction of the fracture line.

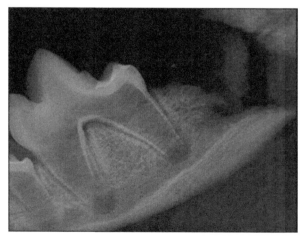

Fig. F8.29 Nonstable type of mandible fracture. Note the rostrodorsal–ventrocaudal oblique direction of the fracture line.

Table F8.1 **Mandibular fractures types.**[11]

TYPE	AREA OF MANDIBLE AFFECTED
A	Symphyseal area to canine tooth (**Figures F8.30a, b**)
B	Canine to second premolar (**Figure F8.30c**)
C	Second premolar to first molar (**Figure F8.30d**)
D	First molar to angle of mandible (**Figure F8.30e**)
E	Angle of mandible (**Figure F8.30f**)
F	Coronoid process (**Figure F8.30g**)
G	Condylar process (**Figure F8.30h**)

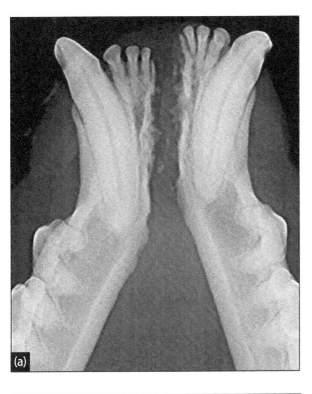

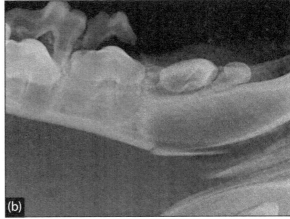

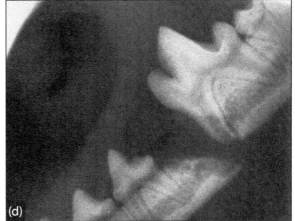

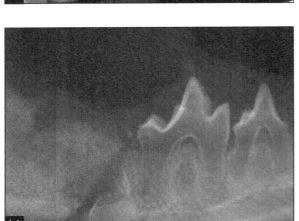

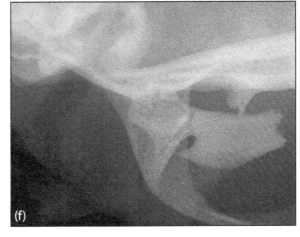

Fig. F8.30 Mandibular fractures in relation to the part of the mandible affected. (a) Symphysis separation; (b) symphyseal area; (c) mandibular canine area to second mandibular premolar; (d) second premolar to first molar tooth; (e) first molar tooth to mandibular angle; (f) mandibular angle area.

(Continued)

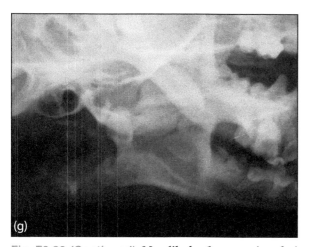
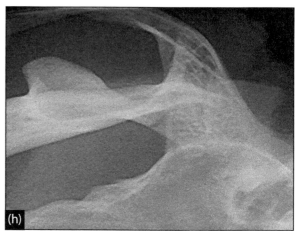

Fig. F8.30 *(Continued)* **Mandibular fractures in relation to the part of the mandible affected. (g) Coronoid process; (h) condylar process fracture.**

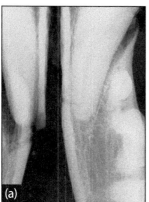
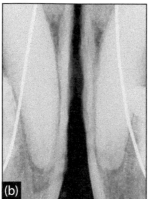
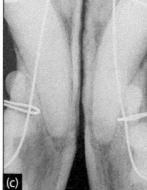
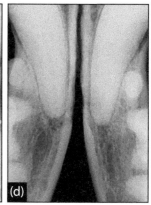

Fig. F8.31 **(a) Multiple fractures of the rostral mandible at the site of the canine teeth apicies; (b) reduction of the fractures and preliminary stabilization; (c) recheck after 6 weeks just prior to removal of the wire reinforced splint; (d) after removal of the splint.**

Proper radiographic diagnosis is critical for selecting the best option for treatment and controlling the results of reduction and stabilization as well as monitoring treatment (**Figure F8.31**). Treatment of teeth present in the fracture line is also based on radiographic evaluation. Depending on the fracture type, its location, and teeth involvement, the optimal treatment method can be selected.

HIGH-RISE SYNDROME

High-rise syndrome is the term used to describe cases where cats fall from balconies or windows of high-rise buildings. The minimal height of the fall is the second story.[12] Orofacial findings include epistaxis, abrasions, jaw fractures, symphyseal separation, hard palate fractures, tooth fracture, and TMJ luxation.[13] Studies show that most maxillofacial and oral injuries are not diagnosed when the examination is not performed by a dental specialist.[13] Even with a very careful examination followed by standard radiographic 2D imaging, some important pathologies can be missed. Diagnostic imaging performed in cats after maxillofacial trauma using CT demonstrates twice the number of injuries compared with using conventional radiography.[1] As previously mentioned, until 3D methods are widely accessible, patients suffering from head injuries have to undergo a thorough clinical and radiographic examination, which will allow for the diagnosis and treatment of the majority of issues (**Figure F8.32**).

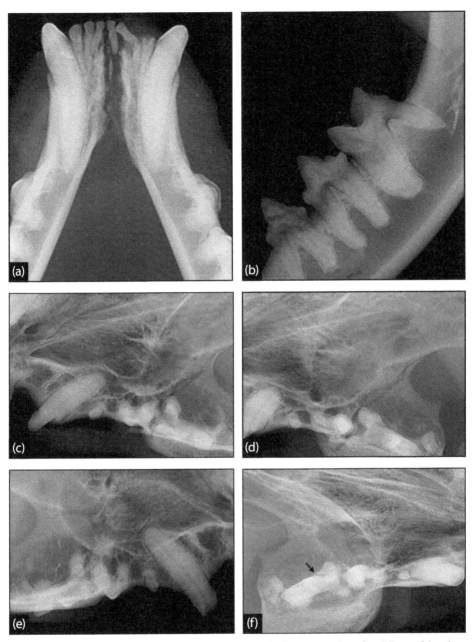

Fig. F8.32 This cat with high-rise syndrome was referred with the suggestion that "Something is not normal with its mandible". Oral examination followed by a full-mouth dental as well as temporomandibular joint radiographs revealed numerous dental injuries including: (a) symphyseal separation with fracture of the left rostral part of parasymphyseal area, avulsion of the left mandibular first incisor (301), horizontal root fracture of the left mandibular second incisor (302), and a complicated crown-root fracture of the left mandibular third incisor (303); (b) a complicated crown fracture of the left mandibular third premolar (307); (c) a complicated crown-root fracture of the left maxillary canine (204) and a fracture of the palatine process of the maxillary bone; (d) better visibility of the maxillary bone fracture and a complicated crown-root fracture of the left maxillary fourth premolar (arrow); (e) a complicated crown fracture of the right maxillary canine (104); (f) a complicated crown-root fracture of the right maxillary fourth premolar (108) (arrow).

TEMPOROMANDIBULAR JOINT AND SYMPHYSEAL INJURIES

These are discussed in Chapter 10.

OTHER TRAUMATIC ISSUES

Iatrogenic trauma, unfortunately, is the main issue among possible complications during extractions. Extractions are the most common oral surgical procedure, for which all standard requirements have been thoroughly listed elsewhere. Despite this, due to improper technique, lack of appropriate equipment, or underestimation of existing conditions, iatrogenic complications such as incomplete extraction (retained roots), fracture of the alveolar bone, and iatrogenic jaw fracture are often diagnosed and require further treatment (**Figures F8.33–8.35**). The only way to avoid these complications is to follow the standards listed in appropriate references.[14,15]

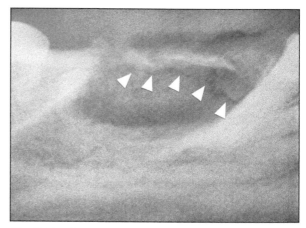

Fig. F8.34 **Iatrogenic fracture of the alveolar process (arrowheads) that occurred during extraction of the right mandibular canine (404).**

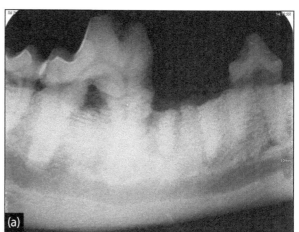

(a)

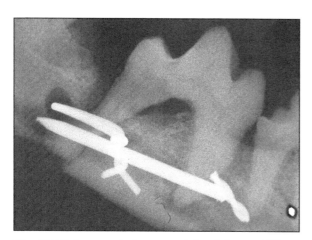

Fig. F8.33 **Iatrogenic fracture of the right mandible in a Yorkshire terrier, which occurred during extraction of the compromised right mandibular first molar (409). The referring veterinarian made an attempt to reduce and stabilize this fracture. A periodontally compromised 409 is present at the fracture line. This, combined with a single interosseous suture, lack of additional splint, and presence of wire within the mandibular canal, makes a poor prognosis for healing of this fracture.**

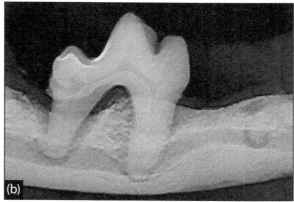

(b)

Fig. F8.35 **(a, b) Retained roots (two visible in [a]) with periapical radiolucency as a result of improperly performed extraction of the fourth right mandibular premolar (408). Note the periodontal disease affecting the right mandibular first molar (409).**

HEALING, REMODELING OF THE FRACTURE LINE AND SCAR TISSUE

The process of fracture healing should be monitored radiographically. Good monitoring can influence the timing of fixation removal as well as aid in the early detection of complications (**Figure F8.36**). Possible complications that may occur during the fracture treatment process include sequesterum formation, nonunion, and osteomyelitis (**Figure F8.37**). The radiographic appearance of osteomyelitis is presented in Chapter 8, Part G. The most important goal of fracture management is achievement of functional nontraumatic occlusion and optimal masticatory functions. Fractures or injuries that affect the TMJ area or change the length or shape of the jaw carry potentially higher risks of long-term problems. In these cases, because of bone remodeling or scar formation, malocclusion or limitations in TMJ mobility may occur. Both problems require additional surgical procedures such as interceptive orthodontics or condylectomy.

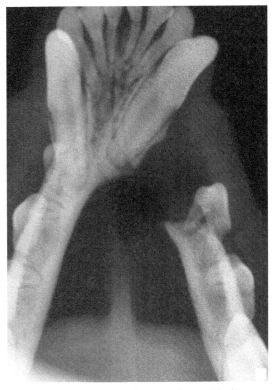

Fig. F8.37 **Nonunion of a rostral mandibular fracture due to a sequestrum of small bony fragment between the left mandibular canine (304) and the third premolar (307). Note the mesial root of 307 has no attachment and requires extraction. It is likely that 304 will require endodontic treatment.**

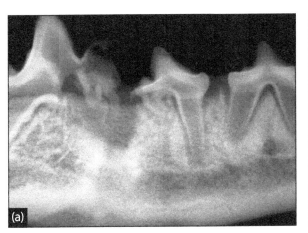
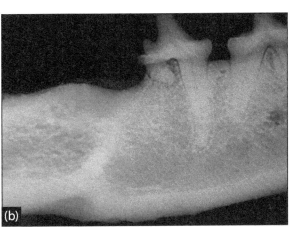

Fig. F8.36 **(a) Mandibular fracture in the area of the right mandibular first molar (409) in a puppy treated conservatively with the use of a muzzle. 409 was severely damaged and required extraction. The right mandibular fourth premolar (408) had dilacerations of the distal root, but was otherwise healthy. Therefore, the tooth was not extracted and was radiographically monitored. (b) Recheck radiograph after 4 years showing further development of 408.**

COMPLICATIONS AND CONSEQUENCES OF TRAUMATIC INJURIES

Traumatic injury is mentioned as the causative factor in multiple oral pathologies. Some problems require immediate action because the affected patients cannot function properly (e.g. jaw fractures, TMJ luxation). Some complications occur a long time after the injury happened and pathologies can be predictable and management of post-traumatic conditions should be performed with respect to anatomy and functionality. For example, endodontic treatment of a fractured or luxated tooth prevents periapical inflammation and proper anatomic reduction of fracture prevents traumatic malocclusion. In some instances prevention of such complications is not possible, therefore monitoring helps in the management of complications before they become painful and cause decreased quality of life (**Figures F8.38, 8.39**).

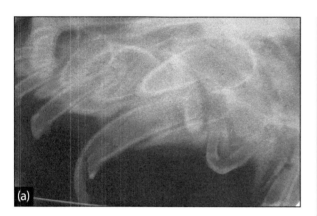

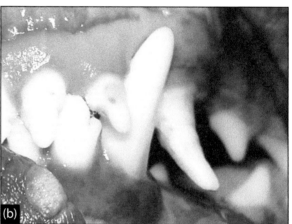

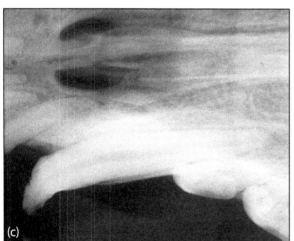

Fig. F8.38 (a) Complicated fracture of a deciduous left maxillary canine (604) consulted via the internet. (b) The patient underwent extraction of 604 by the referring veterinarian. The same dog was presented after 5 years with a dilacerated crown of the left maxillary canine (204) and enamel hypoplasia of the left maxillary third incisor (203); (c) neither affected tooth showed radiographic evidence of endodontic disease.

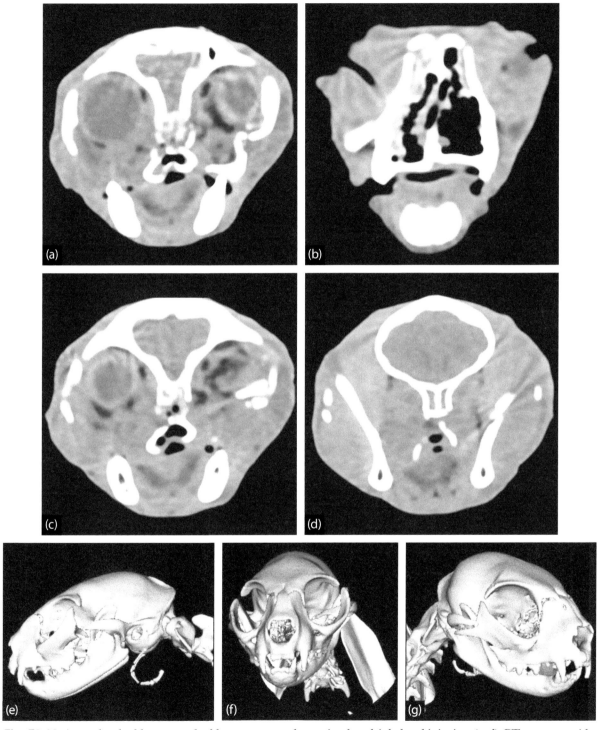

Fig. F8.39 A cat that had been attacked by a coyote and sustained multiple head injuries. (a–d) CT scans provide details; (e–g 3D reconstruction allows for easier analysis and discussion of the treatment plan. (Courtesy Dr Seth Wallack)

REFERENCES

1 Bar-Am Y, Pollard RE, Kass PH *et al.* (2008) The diagnostic yield of conventional radiographs and CT in dogs and cats with MFT (maxillofacial trauma). *Vet Surg* **37(3):**294–299.

2 Soukup J, Snyder C, Gengler W (2009) Computed tomography and partial coronoidectomy for open mouth jaw locking in two cats. *J Vet Dent* **26(4):**226–233.

3 Harvey CE Emily P (1993) Restorative dentistry. In: *Small Animal Dentistry.* Mosby, St. Louis, pp. 213–265.

4 Schreyer J (2010) Management of tooth fracture. *Eur J Companion Anim Pract* **20(3):**230–235.

5 Nomenclature Committee of the American Veterinary Dental College. *Veterinary Dental Nomenclature: Dental Fracture Classification.* Available at: www.avdc.org/Nomenclature. html#dental fracture.

6 Wiggs RB (1997) Glossary of terms. In: *Veterinary Dentistry: Principles and Practice.* (eds. RB Wiggs, HB Lobprise) Lippincott-Raven, Philadelphia, pp. 628–676.

7 DuPont GA (2010) Pathologies of the dental hard tissue. In: *Small Animal Dental, Oral and Maxillofacial Disease: A Color Handbook.* (ed. BA Niemiec) Manson Publishing, London, pp. 127–157.

8 Startup S (2010) Wire-composite splint for luxation of the maxillary canine tooth. *J Vet Dent* **27(3):**198–202.

9 Ulbricht RD, Manfra Maretta S, Klippert LS (2004) Mandibular canine tooth luxation injury in a dog. *J Vet Dent* **21(2):**77–83.

10 Lopes FM, Gioso MA, Ferro D *et al.* (2005) Oral fractures in dogs of Brazil - a retrospective study. *J Vet Dent* **22(2):**86–90.

11 Wiggs RB (1997) Oral fracture repair. In: *Veterinary Dentistry: Principles and Practice.* (eds. RB Wiggs, HB Lobprise) Lippincott-Raven, Philadelphia, pp. 259–279.

12 Vnuk D, Pirkic B, Maticic D *et al.* (2004) Feline high-rise syndrome: 119 cases (1998–2001). *J Feline Med Surg* **6(5):**305–312.

13 Bonner SE, Reiter AM, Lewis JR (2012) Orofacial manifestations of high-rise syndrome in cats: a retrospective study of 84 cases. *J Vet Dent* **29(1):**10–18.

14 Colmery B (2005) The gold standard of veterinary oral health care. *Vet Clin North Am Small Anim Pract* **35(4):**781–787.

15 DeBowes L (2005) Simple and surgical exodontia. *Vet Clin North Am Small Anim Pract* **35(4):**963–984.

PART G

PROLIFERATIVE LESIONS

Jerzy Gawor

INTRODUCTION

Any deformities or defects in the oral/maxillofacial area should be evaluated and radiographed. The causes of swellings are varied and different pathologies (sometimes coexisting) have to be confirmed or ruled out when dealing with proliferative lesions. Imaging is necessary to evaluate the affected tissues and surrounding anatomy as well as to select the optimal management or further diagnostic efforts. It is important to remember that radiography is a complementary diagnostic tool, which must be followed by biopsy submission and histopathologic evaluation. Many cases of osteomyelitis (particularly in cats) can mimic neoplasia radiographically (**Figures G8.1–8.3**).

The non-neoplastic lesions that can deform the face or oral cavity include:

- Abscess with endodontic and/or periodontal origin as well as those caused by foreign bodies or injuries (see Chapter 8, Parts C, E, and G).
- Inflammatory lesions with an immunologic or traumatic cause.
- Trauma.
- Developmental disorders.

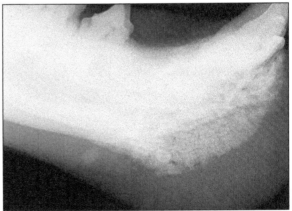

Fig. G8.2 **Osteomyelitis of the rostral mandible of a cat with severe periosteal reaction.**

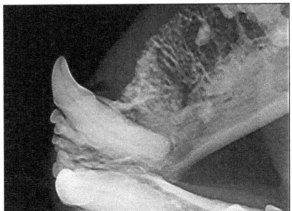

Fig. G8.3 **Osteomyelitis of the left mandible in a cat with proliferation of alveolar bone.**

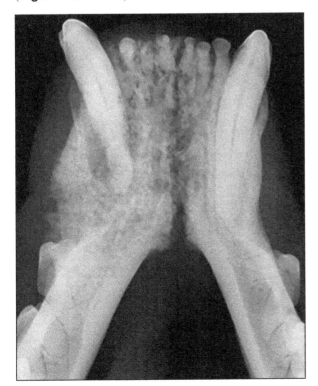

Fig. G8.1 **Osteomyelitis in a cat surrounding the right mandibular canine (404) and incisors.**

Definitive diagnosis is possible only after receiving the histopathologic evaluation. Each proliferative or ulcerative lesion should be considered a potential tumor. Radiography is a part of the TMN (Tumor/Node/Metastasis) clinical evaluation adopted by the World Health Organization – Collaborating Center for Comparative Oncology and described in many textbooks.[1]

Radiographic evaluation is necessary to determine underlying bony reaction, the size of the affected area, and the characteristics of the lesion. In the TNM staging system, radiography is required to determine a Ta or Tb tumor. The first type (Ta) has no underlying bony reaction, whereas Tb does have underlying bony reaction (**Figures G8.4, G8.5**).

Radiographic evaluation of maxillofacial tumors is currently considered insufficient. 3D imaging methods are more informative. Firstly, CT is more sensitive and accurate in the evaluation of lesions (in particular the radiodensity of the lesion is better assessed). Secondly, superimposition of structures in the head complicates diagnostic attempts using conventional radiography. In animals with oral tumors, radiography of the entire head is also important for revealing accompanying pathologies (e.g. teeth resorption).[2]

Diagnostic imaging of suspected neoplastic lesions does not provide a definitive diagnosis. The first impression created during radiographic interpretation may be helpful in making a tentative diagnosis.

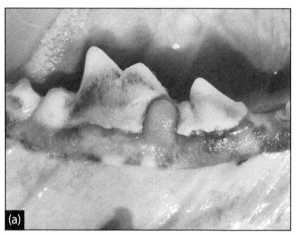 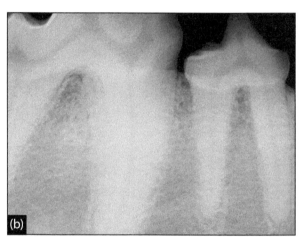

Fig. G8.4 (a) Oral mass (peripheral odontogenic fibroma) with T1 characteristic in TNM classification. (b) Radiograph showing that this tumor has no bony reaction and so is classified as T1a.

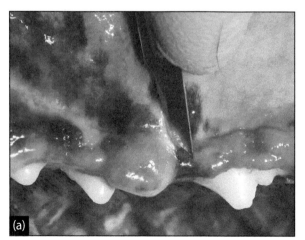 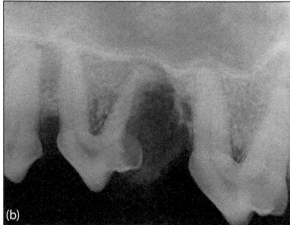

Fig. G8.5 (a) Oral mass (fibrosarcoma) with T1 characteristic in TNM classification. (b) Radiograph showing that this tumor has caused bony reaction and so is classified as T1b.

However, even though it may adequately characterize the lesion, it does not define it.

The radiographic description of proliferative lesions takes into account the type, shape, borders, density, tooth involvement, and adjacent structures.[3] All of the characteristics have their own radiographic description (**Figures G8.6–8.9**):

- Type: solitary, multiple, generalized.
- Shape: unilocular, multilocular, nonlocular.
- Borders: well defined, poorly defined.
- Density: radiolucent/radiopaque, mixed.
- Tooth involvement: no involvement, active involvement: resorption, displacement.
- Adjacent structures: displaced, eroded, no effect.

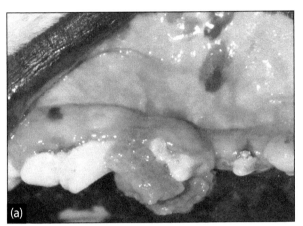
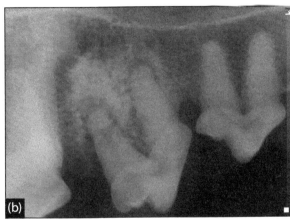

Fig. G8.6 (a) Clinical appearance of a canine oral tumor (ameloblastoma). (b) Radiographic description: solitary unilocular, well-defined, radiopaque, involving and displacing affected tooth with erosion of surrounding alveolar bone.

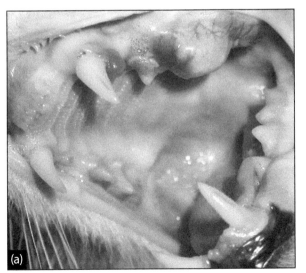
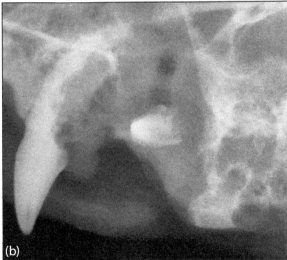

Fig. G8.7 (a) Inductive odontogenic tumor affecting the left maxilla of a cat. (b) Radiographic description: multiple, multilocular, poorly defined borders, mixed pattern, involving tooth and causing resorption of affected teeth.

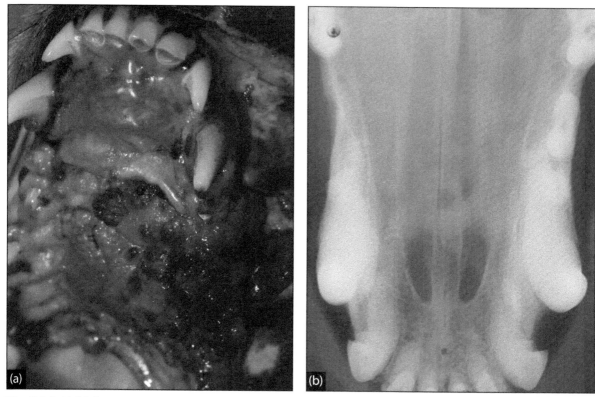

Fig. G8.8 (a) Melanoma malignum affecting the palate and nasal cavity of a dog. (b) Radiographic description: generalized, poorly defined, radiopaque, surrounding teeth with no effect on dentition.

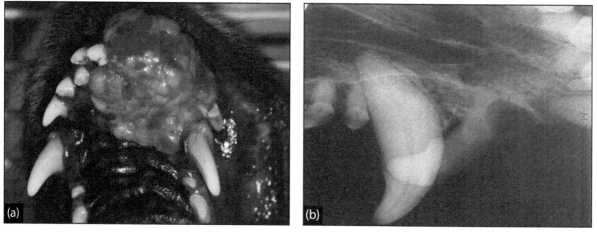

Fig. G8.9 (a) Amelanotic melanoma of the rostral maxilla of a dog. (b) Radiographic description: solitary, unilocular, poorly defined, radiolucent, involving and displacing incisor tooth.

Another categorization is based on of the radiographic appearance of the lesion and includes: geographic, moth-eaten, and permeative bone loss (**Figures G8.10–8.12**):

- The geographic type is a destructive osseous lesion that is uniform in appearance and generally well-circumscribed. These 'holes' in bone can be further subclassified by the

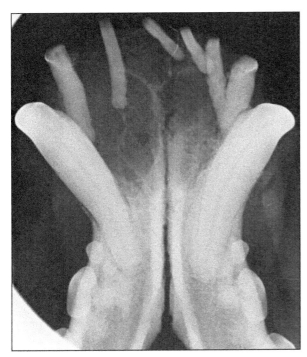

Fig. G8.10 **This geographic type radiographic appearance indicates a destructive osseous lesion (fibrosarcoma, which is uniform in appearance and generally well-circumscribed).**

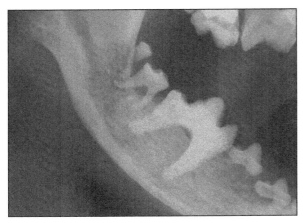

Fig. G8.12 **The permeative processes of bone loss preserve the outline of the bone but reveal numerous small, diffuse lytic lesions (osteosarcoma).**

appearance of the border as sclerotic, well defined, or poorly defined.[4]

- Moth-eaten lesions represent a confluence of multiple small lytic areas in the bone.
- Permeative processes of bone preserve the outline of the bone but reveal numerous small, diffuse lytic lesions.[5]

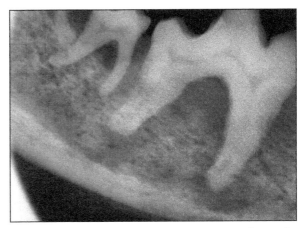

Fig. G8.11 **The moth-eaten lesions in this radiograph represent multiple small lytic areas in the bone (osteosarcoma).**

Apart from destruction of bone surrounding the lesion, it is important to note the involvement of adjacent or distant dentition. Tumor-associated dental structure disruption is reported to develop in 60% of dogs with malignant tumors.[6] In tumor sites, the most common types of resorption are: external inflammatory resorption, external replacement resorption, and external surface resorption (**Figures G8.13–8.15**).[2]

Based on the radiographic appearance and length of time the growth has been present (if known), the aggressiveness of the lesion can be estimated.[1] Benign lesions are usually discrete, slow growing, homogeneous, regular shaped, sclerotic, or smooth with distinct margins and a narrow distance between margins and normal tissue. Teeth involved in benign lesions are displaced and the bone cortex either thinned or expanded. Aggressive lesions grow rapidly and have disseminated margins that are ragged with a wide transition zone from lesion to normal area. The bone cortex undergoes lysis and the involved teeth often stay in their natural position, but have increased mobility (**Figures G8.16, G8.17**).[3]

When a neoplasm is suspected, a complex diagnostic imaging approach is required. This is typically performed using the intraoral techniques described in Chapter 2. It is important to assess the whole region (head) utilizing the extraoral techniques discussed in Chapter 5. Finally, ruling out potential metastases requires CT scans or chest radiographs and ultrasonic evaluation of the abdomen.

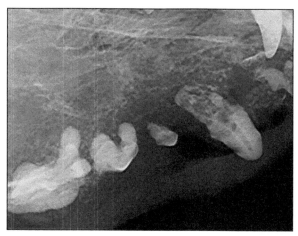

Fig. G8.13 This radiograph shows external inflammatory resorption affecting the right maxillary canine tooth (104) surrounded by squamous cell carcinoma in a cat.

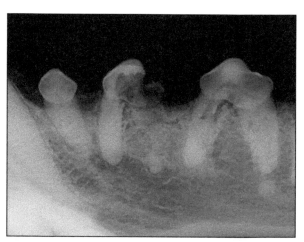

Fig. G8.14 This radiograph shows external replacement resorption of the mandibular left second and third premolars (306 307) associated with malignant melanoma in a dog.

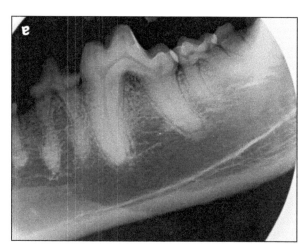

Fig. G8.15 External surface resorption of the left mandibular fourth premolar (308) of a dog with fibrosarcoma.

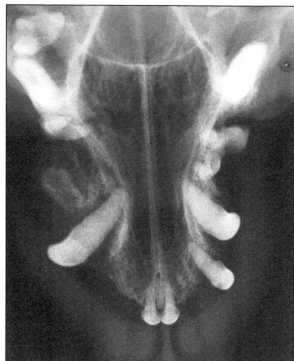

Fig. G8.16 In this radiograph the right maxillary canine (104) is displaced and the bone cortex expanded (histopathology revealed hemangioma capillare).

Fig. G8.17 This CT scan shows a rapidly growing mandibular tumor (squamous cell carcinoma) in a cat, with mandibular teeth present in their natural position. (Courtesy Dr Lisa Mestrinho.)

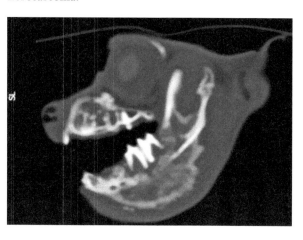

ODONTOGENIC CYSTS

Many odontogenic cysts are diagnosed in cats and dogs including dentigerous, lateral radicular, eruption, and follicular cysts. Again, the definitive diagnosis can only be made histologically, as radiographic appearance is not diagnostic but may limit the range of differential diagnoses (**Figures G8.18–8.23**).

The radiographic appearance provides important diagnostic information; however, it is not definitive as other lesions (e.g. ameloblastoma) can appear radiographically similar to odontogenic cysts. Commonly, clinical assessment underestimates tumor size compared with the radiographic appearance (**Figure G8.24**). In addition, 2D conventional radiography underestimates the extent of bony invasion compared with 3D imaging.[7]

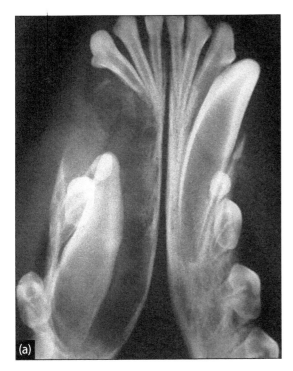

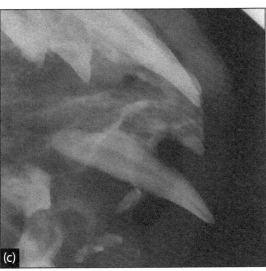

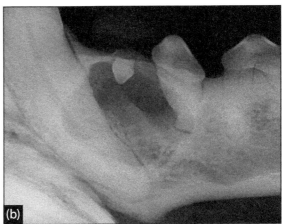

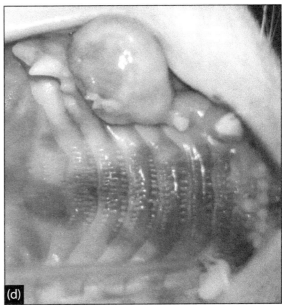

Fig. G8.18 Dentigerous cyst in a dog caused by an impacted right mandibular canine tooth (404) (a) and left mandibular first premolar (205) (b) This type of cyst may also occur in cats (c, d). (Courtesy Dr Kadri Kaaramees.)

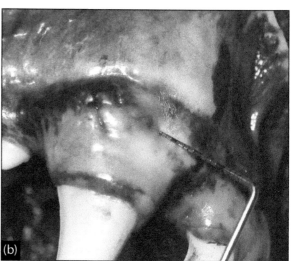

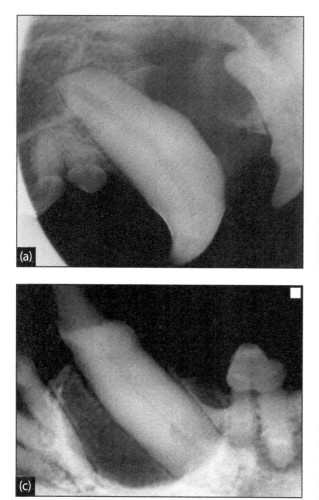

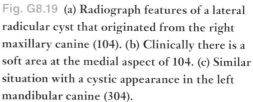

Fig. G8.19 (a) Radiograph features of a lateral radicular cyst that originated from the right maxillary canine (104). (b) Clinically there is a soft area at the medial aspect of 104. (c) Similar situation with a cystic appearance in the left mandibular canine (304).

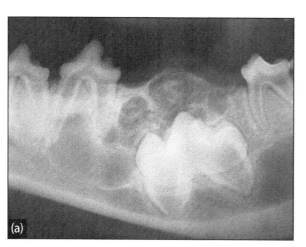

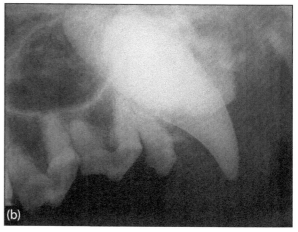

Fig. G8.20 (a) Keratocyst surrounding an impacted left mandibular first molar (309) in a dog. (b) Keratocyst surrounding a partially retained right maxillary canine (104).

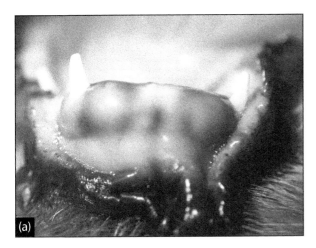

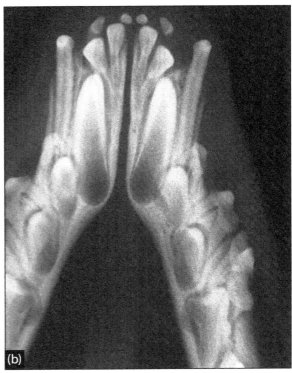

Fig. G8.21 (a) Eruption cyst in a Tibetan terrier puppy that had no erupted deciduous incisors at the age of 10 weeks. (b) Radiograph revealing a reduced number of unerupted deciduous as well as permanent incisor teeth.

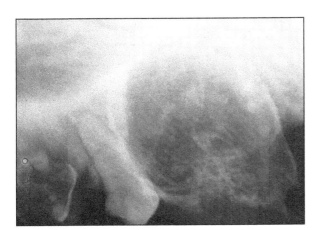

Fig. G8.22 Follicular cyst at the area where the right maxillary canine (104) should be present. (Courtesy Dr M. Stasiowska.)

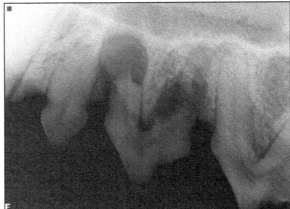

Fig. G8.23 Radicular periapical cyst in the mesial root of 206. Both roots are undergoing tooth resorption. (Courtesy Dr Brook Niemiec.)

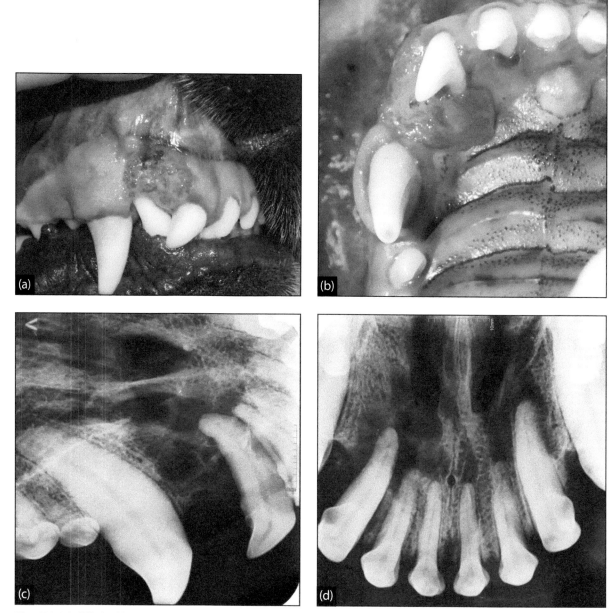

Fig. G8.24 Clinical lateral (a) and palatal (b) views of a central ameloblastoma in a dog. Lateral (c) and palatal (d) radiographs reveal larger affected areas than are clinically apparent.

NONODONTOGENIC TUMORS

Feline tumors

Seven point four per cent of all feline tumors occur in the oropharynx[8] with 89% of them being malignant.[9] The most prevalent feline oral tumor is squamous cell carcinoma. The radiographic appearance of malignant feline tumors consists of bone lysis and, in some areas, new bone formation. The radiographic extent of tumors always exceeds that found on clinical examination (**Figures G8.25–8.30**).

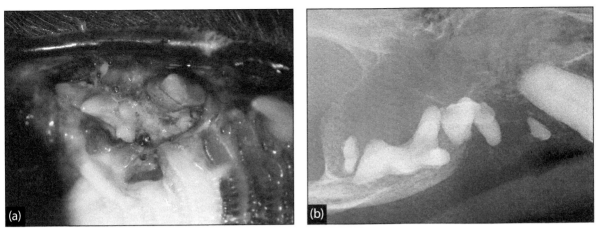

Fig. G8.25 Feline maxillary squamous cell carcinoma: (a) clinical and (b) radiographic appearance.

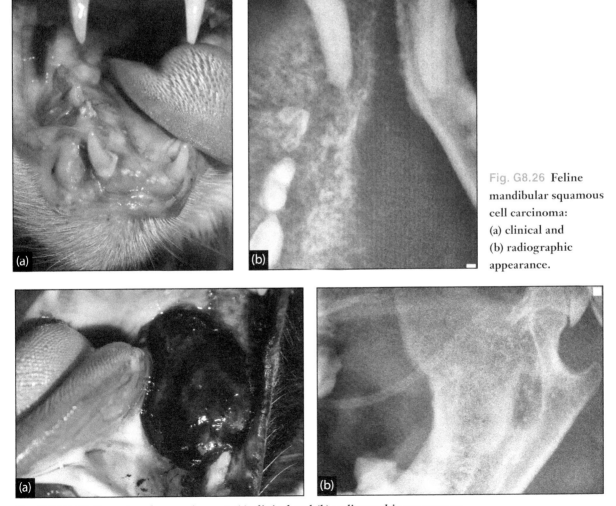

Fig. G8.26 Feline mandibular squamous cell carcinoma: (a) clinical and (b) radiographic appearance.

Fig. G8.27 Malignant melanoma in a cat: (a) clinical and (b) radiographic appearance.

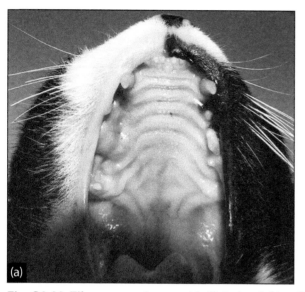
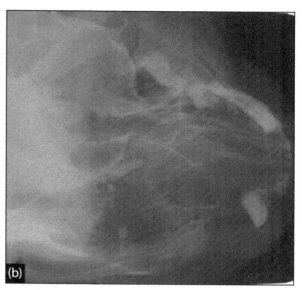

Fig. G8.28 **Fibrosarcoma in a cat: (a) clinical and (b) radiographic appearance in an extraoral lateral oblique projection.**

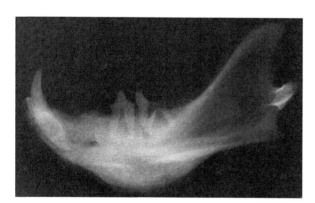

Fig. G8.29 Osteosarcoma: radiograph of affected mandible after mandibulectomy.

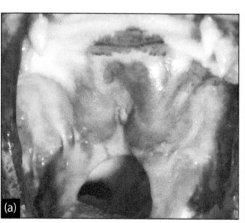
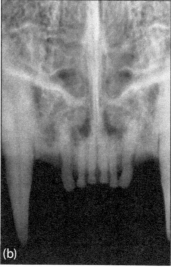
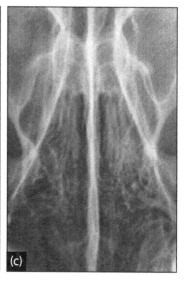

Fig. G8.30 Oral lymphoma in a cat: (a) clinical and (b, c) radiographic appearance. The radiographs show no bone involvement.

Canine tumors

The prevalence of oropharyngeal tumors in dogs was 5.4% of all canine tumors in one report.[8] Canine tumors have various radiographic appearances, and therefore none of the presented radiographs is pathognomic for a specific neoplasm (**Figures G8.31–8.39**).

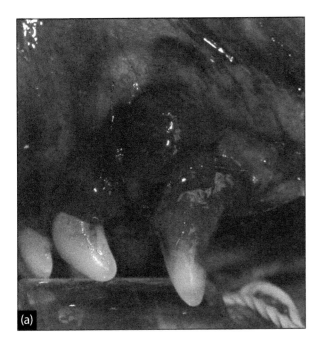

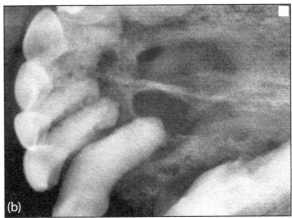

Fig. G8.31 Oral malignant melanoma in a dog: (a) clinical and (b) radiographic appearance.

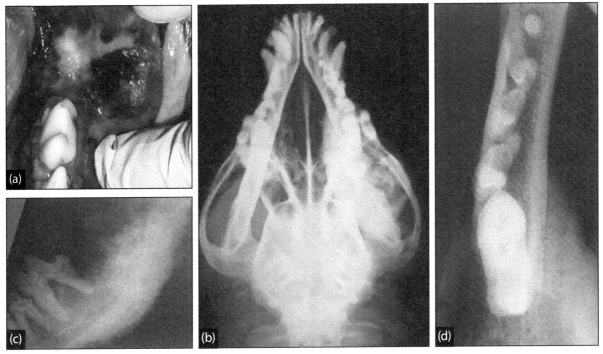

Fig. G8.32 Canine squamous cell carcinoma in mandible. (a) Clinical appearance. Radiographic appearance: (b) extraoral VD view; (c) intraoral lateral view; (d) intraoral VD view.

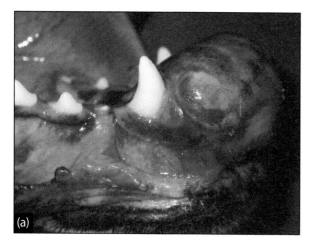

Fig. G8.33 Oral fibrosarcoma in a dog: (a) clinical and (b) radiographic appearance.

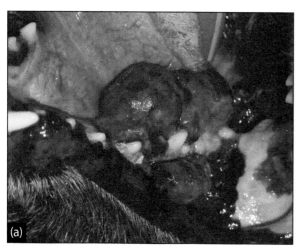

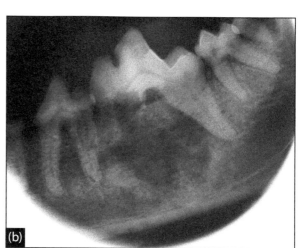

Fig. G8.34 Mandibular osteosarcoma in a dog: (a) clinical and (b) radiographic appearance.

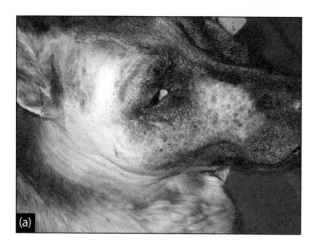

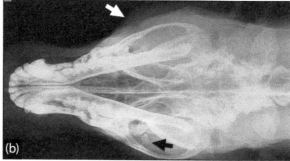

Fig. G8.35 Hemangiosarcoma of the masseter muscle in a dog. (a) Clinical appearance, (b) radiograph showing only greater thickness of the soft tissues (white arrow) (note the radiopaque mass on the unaffected side [black arrow]).   *(Continued)*

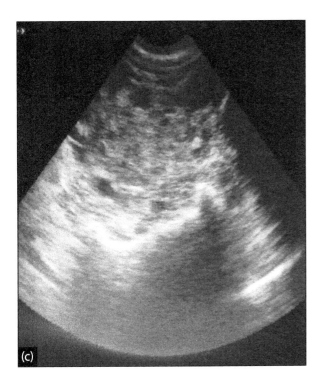

Fig. G8.35 *(Continued)*
Hemangiosarcoma of the masseter
muscle in a dog. (c) Ultrasonic
image providing assessment of the
character of the mass.

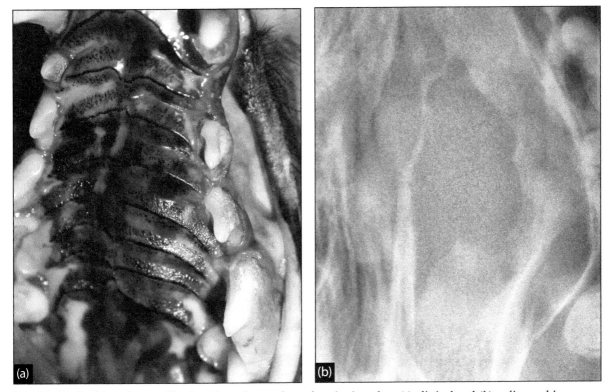

Fig. G8.36 Oral lymphoma affecting the palate and nasal cavity in a dog: (a) clinical and (b) radiographic
appearance.

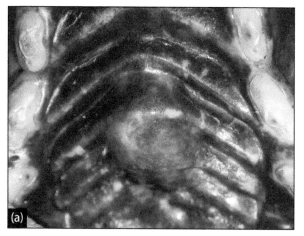

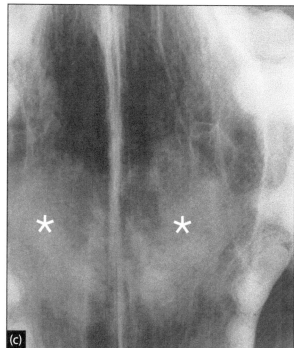

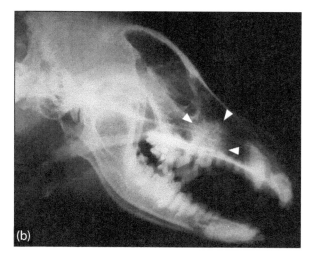

Fig. G8.37 Multilobular tumor of bone typically affects the flat bones of the cranium. (a) Clinically visible deformation of hard palate, (b) extraoral lateral radiograph reveals radiodense mass dorsally from the third maxillary premolars (arrowheads), (c) intraoral radiograph shows two symmetric radiopaque lesions (asterisks).

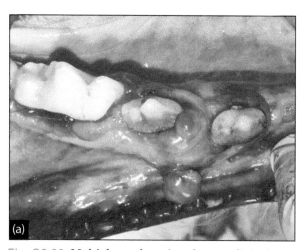

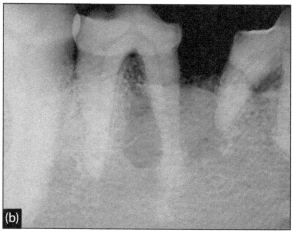

Fig. G8.38 Multiple myeloma in a dog: (a) clinical and (b) radiographic appearance.

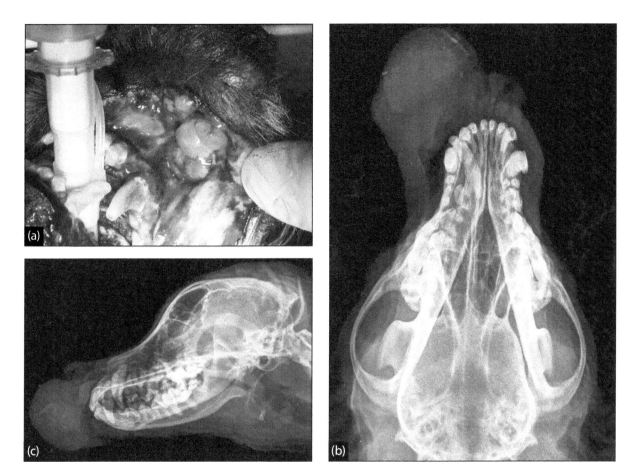

Fig. G8.39 **Mast cell tumor normally does not affect the surrounding bone regardless of its size. (a) Clinical appearance. Radiographic appearance: (b) extraoral DV view; (c) extraoral lateral view.**

ODONTOGENIC TUMORS

Odontogenic tumors (OTs) arise from remnants of odontogenic epithelium located in the periodontal ligament space (rests of Malassesz) and gingiva (rests of Serres) (**Figure G8.40**). Some typical radiographic findings for OT are described below. Central ameloblastoma (CA) most often appears as an osteolytic unilocular or multilocular cystic lesion with well-defined sclerotic margins (**Figure G8.41**).

Canine acanthomatous ameloblastoma is infiltrative and expansive in growth, which distinguishes this tumor from CA (**Figure G8.42**). Odontomas or non-neoplastic hamartomas have two major types: compound odontoma is comprised of tooth-like structures (**Figure G8.43**), whereas complex odontoma has more of a conglomerate appearance, which does not look like teeth particles (**Figure G8.44**).[10] Another rare type of odontogenic tumor is the odontogenic myxoma (**Figure G8.45**).[11]

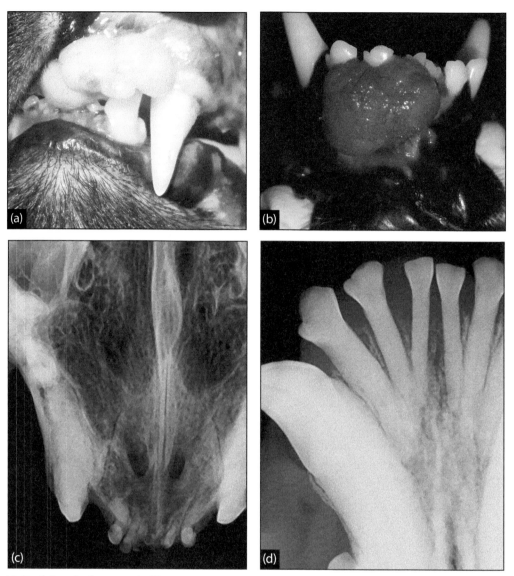

Fig. G8.40 Peripheral odontogenic fibroma in a cat (a) and a dog (b) affecting the gingiva. However, it does not create significant bony reaction in the cat (c) or in the dog (d).

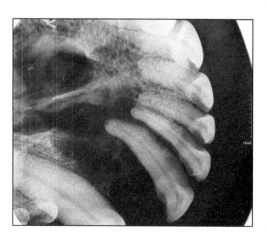

Fig. G8.41 Central ameloblastoma most often appears as an osteolytic unilocular or multilocular cystic lesion with well-defined sclerotic margins.

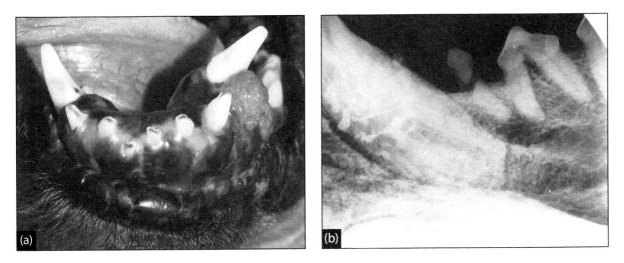

Fig. G8.42 Canine acanthomatous ameloblastoma is infiltrative in behavior: (a) clinical and (b) radiographic appearance.

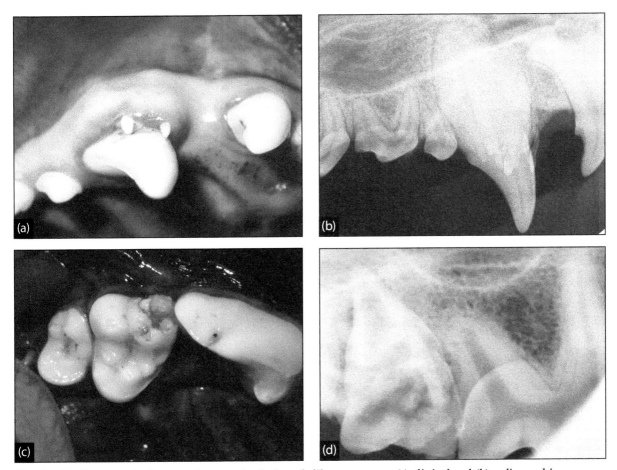

Fig. G8.43 Compound odontoma is comprised of tooth-like structures: (a) clinical and (b) radiographic appearance. (c, d) Occasionally, an odontoma can be attached to an otherwise normal tooth.

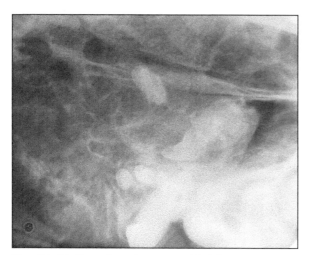

Fig. G8.44 **Complex odontoma, which has a more conglomerated appearance radiographically.**

COMPLICATIONS OF NEOPLASTIC DISEASE

Treatment of most tumors begins with surgery, and 12-month tumor-free survival is necessary before full remission can be pronounced. During this period, the most common complications are recurrence and metastases. The former is typically observed at the surgical margins or in the surgical area, and the latter normally in the predictive sites for each specific tumor (**Figures G8.46, G8.47**).

In certain tumors an additional radiographic assessment (three-view thoracic radiographs) are used to reveal/rule out metastases in lungs , bronchi, ribs, or lymph nodes located in the chest.

Another possible complication of maxillofacial bone tumors is pathologic (spontaneous) fracture. Statistically this occurs more often with mandibular tumors, which weaken the mandibular body, and fracture occurs even with normal force applied to the jaws (**Figure G8.48**).

OSSEOUS LESIONS

Non-neoplastic lesions occurring in the maxillofacial bones cannot be diagnosed exclusively by imaging techniques. It is always necessary to submit a biopsy for histopathologic evaluation and treat the lesion as potentially neoplastic until the biopsy is returned.

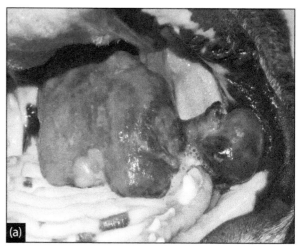

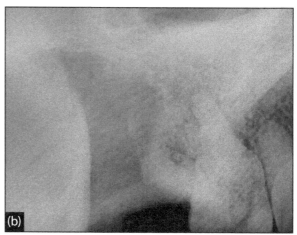

Fig. G8.45 **Odontogenic myxoma in a dog: (a) clinical and (b) radiographic appearance.**

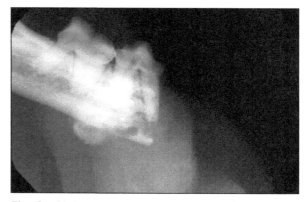

Fig. G8.46 **Reoccurrence of squamous cell carcinoma at the surgical margin.**

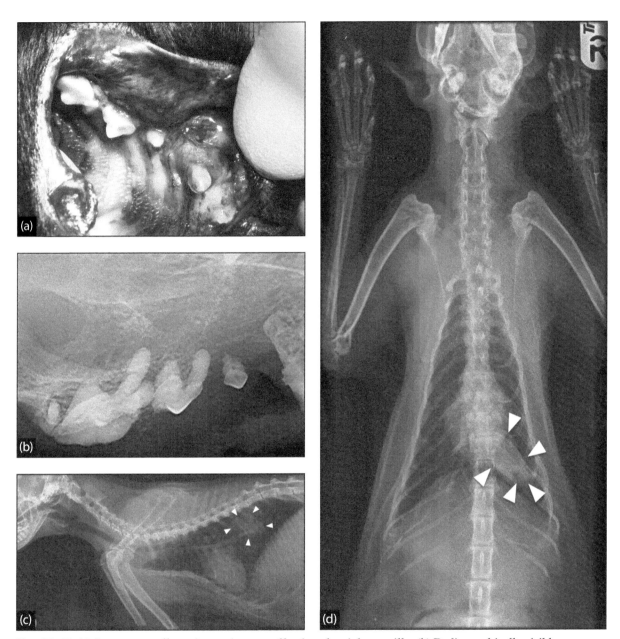

Fig. G8.47 (a) Squamous cell carcinoma in a cat affecting the right maxilla. (b) Radiographically visible severe destruction of the surrounding bone. Chest radiographs reveal the presence of radiopaque lesions in the lungs (arrowheads): (c) lateral right view; (d) VD view.

Secondary hyperparathyroidism

Secondary hyperparathyroidism results in low blood calcium concentration and secondary stimulation of parathyroid hormone (PTH) production. The normal range of PTH is 2–13 pmol/l; in this condition the PTH level is 84 pmol/l or more.

Hyperostotic osteodystrophy is more common in the jaws of young dogs, whereas generalized osteodystrophy resulting in rubber jaw is more common in old dogs.[12] Radiographically, it appears as decalcification and loss of density of the head bones (**Figure G8.49**).

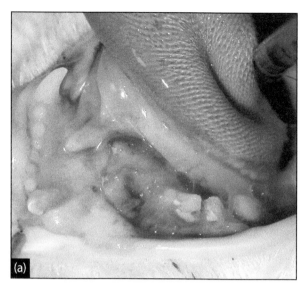

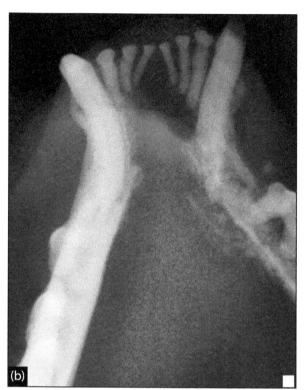

Fig. G8.48 **Pathologic fracture of a left mandible affected by squamous cell carcinoma: (a) clinical and (b) radiographic appearance. The fracture is located between the mandibular canine and premolar teeth. Note the lack of mandibular symphysis structures due to tumor expansion.**

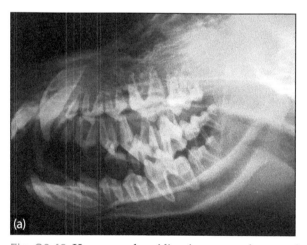

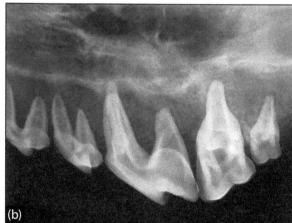

Fig. G8.49 **Hyperparathyroidism in a young dog associated with renal insufficiency. (a) Decalcification and loss of density of the alveolar bone visible in the entire head. (b) Better visualization of the problem is possible with an intraoral projection of the maxilla.**

Osteonecrosis

Radiographically, necrotic bone is more radiopaque and is distinct from vital bone, with the possible presence of the sequestrum surrounded by a radiolucent margin (**Figure G8.50**).[13]

Craniomandibular osteopathy

Craniomandibular osteopathy (CMO) is a non-neoplastic, proliferative bony disease of the dog, affecting primarily the mandible, tympanic bullae and, occasionally, other bones of the head. Scottish terriers, West Highland white terriers and Cairn terriers

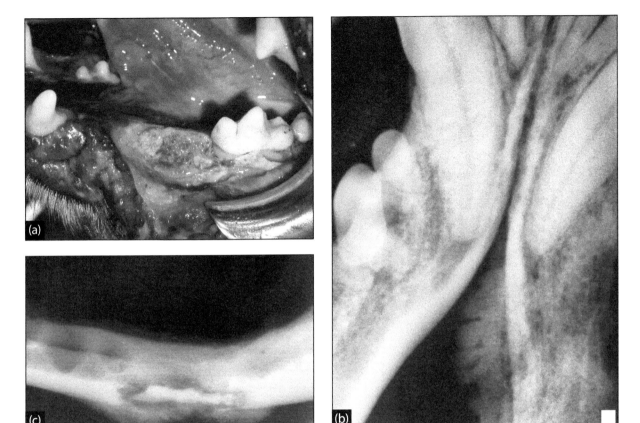

Fig. G8.50 **Osteonecrosis (a) is distinct from the vital bone (b) with the possible presence of sequestra surrounded by a radiolucent margin (c).**

are overrepresented. In West Highland white terriers, the condition is an autosomal recessive trait.[14] Radiographically, there is enlargement of the mandibles and a cortical periosteal reaction. It is important to rule out or confirm involvement of the tympanic bullae and temporomandibular joint area because it worsens the prognosis (**Figure G8.51**).[15]

Osteomyelitis

The radiographic signs of acute osteomyelitis include decreased radiodensity of the affected area with scattered regions of radiolucency. In contrast, in chronic osteomyelitis the bone is more radiodense and sclerotic with possible periosteal new bone formation (**Figures G8.1–8.3**).[13,16]

Periostitis ossificans

Periostitis ossificans (PO) appears clinically as jaw swelling in immature, large breed dogs.

The differential diagnoses include bone fracture, callus formation, cellulitis, soft tissue abscess, tooth root abscess, dentigerous cyst, CMO, developmental abnormalities, fibrous osteodystrophy, odontoma, and neoplasia. Fine needle aspirates are an excellent way to noninvasively obtain diagnostic samples, although cytology does not provide information about tissue architecture. In non-oral tumors the accuracy of cytology after fine needle aspiration for determining malignancy is over 90%.[17]

The typical radiographic finding is a 'double cortex formation', usually from the ventral or lingual aspect of the mandible. Mandibular PO in large breed dog puppies results from an inflamed or infected dental follicle, developing unerupted tooth, (most likely the mandibular first molar), and/or secondary to pericoronitis (**Figure G8.52**).[18]

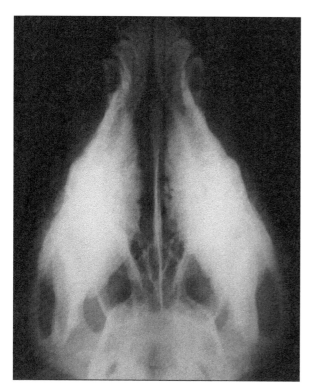

Fig. G8.51 **Radiographic appearance of craniomandibular osteopathy in a dog. Note the enlargement of the mandibles and a cortical periosteal reaction.**

Hyperostosis

Hyperostosis is bone enlargement that appears as a large, irregular, thickened bony mass surrounding the normally present bone. Histologically, hyperostosis has no signs of malignancy; however, due to the change of shape of the bone it may cause either malocclusion or malfunctions of the jaws (**Figure G8.53**).[19] Infantile calvarial hyperostosis presents as cortical thickening of the calvarium in young male mastiffs. It is self-resolving and has no known causes other than a possible familiar predisposition.[20]

Fibrous dysplasia

Fibrous dysplasia is a non-neoplastic lesion thought to be developmental in origin. Fibrous dysplasia has a major component of fibrovascular stroma. It may be an inherited trait in the Doberman pinscher and Old English sheepdog. It shows morphologic similarity with osteoma and ossifying fibroma.[21] Radiographically, there is no clear pattern to the lesion nor its margins (**Figure G8.54**).

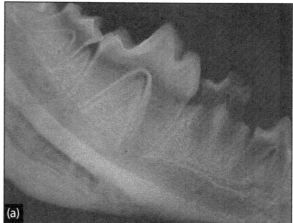

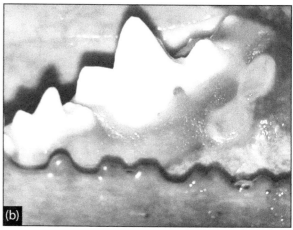

Fig. G8.52 **(a) The typical radiographic finding in periostitis ossificans is a 'double cortex formation', usually from the ventral or lingual aspect of the mandible. (b) It is typically associated with pericoronitis of the first mandibular molar tooth.**

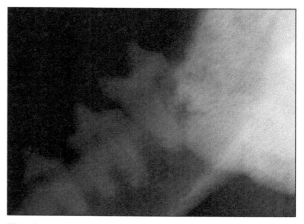

Fig. G8.53 **Hyperostosis in a cat affecting unilaterally the caudal part of the mandible.**

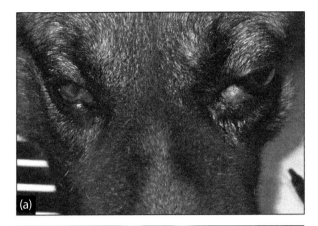

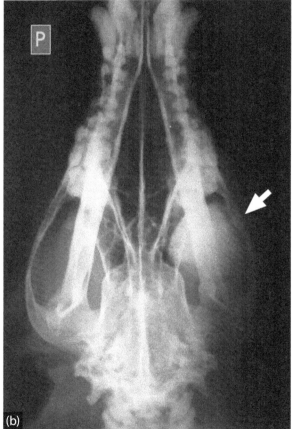

Osteosclerosis

Osteosclerosis is a benign lesion, found mostly in mandibular bone, with distinct margins and a significantly radiopaque character. There are no obvious causative factors such as nonvital teeth or injury (**Figure G8.55**).

Hypercementosis

Hypercementosis (cemental dysplasia) is an excessive production of cementum formed on the root surface (**Figure G8.56**).

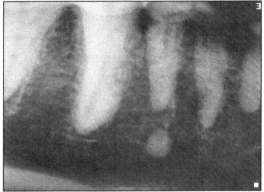

Fig. G8.55 This osteosclerosis lesion is located ventrally from the distal root of the right mandibular fourth premolar (408). Note the features of teeth resorption in 408.

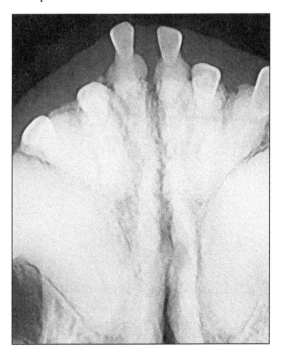

Fig. G8.54 (a) German shepherd dog with unilateral (left) exophthalmos. (b) Radiograph showing the presence of a radiopaque lesion (arrow) affecting the caudal part of the left mandible. The histopathologic diagnosis of the mass was fibrous osteodystrophy.

Fig. G8.56 Hypercementosis is present in all the mandibular incisors of this boxer. The increased cementum enlarges the roots of affected teeth.

3D RECONSTRUCTION

3D reconstruction is one of the advantages available when performing CT scans. This tool is particularly useful in treatment planning of neoplastic conditions. Currently it is also possible to produce 3D models with the use of a 3D printer and plan the operative technique prior to the real procedure (**Figures G8.57, G8.58**).

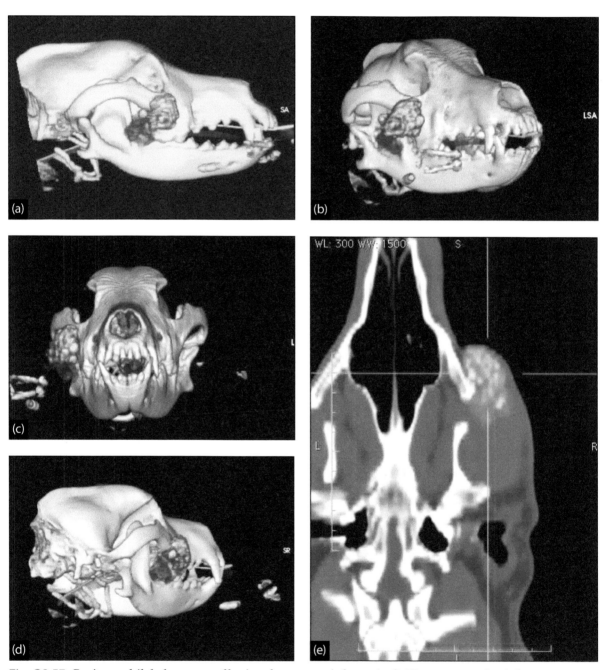

Fig. G8.57 **Canine multilobular tumor affecting the zygomatic bone. (a–d) 3D reconstruction helps define the external margins of the tumor; (e) CT scan showing the depth of tumor infiltration. (Courtesy Dr Lisa Mestrinho.)**

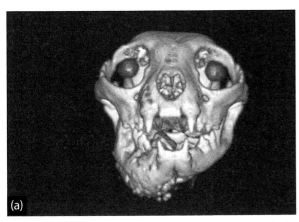
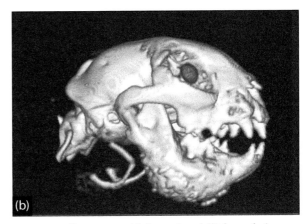

Fig. G8.58 **3D reconstruction in a cat with mandibular squamous cell sarcoma: (a) frontal and (b) lateral views. (Courtesy Dr Lisa Mestrinho.)**

REFERENCES

1 Arzi B, Verstraete FJ (2012) Clinical staging and biopsy of maxillofacial tumors. In: *Oral and Maxilloafacial Surgery in Dogs and Cats*. (eds. FJM Verstraete, MJ Lommer) Saunders/Elsevier, Edinburgh, pp. 373–380.

2 Nemec A, Arzi B, Murphy B *et al.* (2012) Prevalence and types of tooth resorption in dogs with oral tumors. *Am J Vet Res* **73:**1057–1066.

3 Mulligan TW (1998) Osseous lesions. In: *Atlas of Canine and Feline Dental Radiography*. Veterinary Learning Systems, Trenton, pp. 184–203.

4 Sanders TG, Parsons TW III (2001) Radiographic imaging of musculoskeletal neoplasia. *Cancer Control* **8(3):**221–231.

5 Lodwick GS, Wilson AJ, Farrel C *et al.* (1980) Determining growth rates of focal lesions of bone from radiographs. *Radiology* **134:**577–583.

6 Frew DG, Dobson JM (1992) Radiological assessment of 50 cases of incisive or maxillary neoplasia in the dog. *J Small Anim Pract* **33:**11–18.

7 Ghirelli O, Vilamizar L, Carolina A *et al.* (2013) Comparison of standard radiography and CT in 21 dogs with maxillary masses. *J Vet Dent* **30(2):**72–76.

8 McEntee CM (2012) Clinical behaviour of nonodontogenic tumors. In: *Oral and Maxilloafacial Surgery in Dogs and Cats*. (eds. FJM Verstraete, MJ Lommer) Saunders/Elsevier, Edinburgh, pp. 387–402.

9 Stebbins KE, Morse CC, Goldschmidt HM (1989) Feline oral neoplasia: a ten year survey. *Vet Pathol* **26:**121–128.

10 Chamberlain TP, Lommer M (2012) Clinical behavior of odontogenic tumors. In: *Oral and Maxilloafacial Surgery in Dogs and Cats*. (eds. FJM Verstraete, MJ Lommer) Saunders/Elsevier, Edinburgh, pp. 403–410.

11 Meyers B, Boy S, Steenkamp G (2007) Diagnosis and management of odontogenic myxoma in a dog. *J Vet Dent* **24(3):**166–171.

12 Sarkiala E, Harvey CE (1994) Jaw lesions resulting from renal hyperparathyroidism in a young dog – a case report. *J Vet Dent* **11(4):**121–124.

13 Maretta SM Lommer JM (2012) Management of maxillofacial osteonecrosis. In: *Oral and Maxilloafacial Surgery in Dogs and Cats*. (eds. FJM Verstraete, MJ Lommer) Saunders/Elsevier, Edinburgh, pp. 519–524.

14 Padgett GA, Mostosky UV (1986) The mode of inheritance of craniomandibular osteopathy in West Highland White terrier dogs. *Am J Med Genet* **25(1):**9–13.

15 Gawor J (2004) Case reports of four cases of craniomandibular osteopathy. *Eur J Companion Anim Pract* **14(2):**209–213.

16 Boutoille F, Hennet P (2011) Maxillary osteomyelitis in two Scottish terrier dogs with chronic ulcerative parental stomatitis. *J Vet Dent* **28(2):**96–100.

17 Ghisleni G, Roccabianca P, Ceruti R *et al*. (2006) Correlation between fine-needle aspiration cytology and histopathology in the evaluation of cutaneous and subcutaneous masses from dogs and cats. *Vet Clin Pathol* **35(1):**24–30.

18 Blazejewski SW, Lewis JR, Gracis M *et al*. (2010) Mandibular periostitis ossificans in immature large breed dogs: 5 cases (1999–2006). *J Vet Dent* **27(3):**148–159.

19 Gawor J, Niemiec B (2011) Unilateral mandibular hyperostosis in a cat. *J Vet Dent* **28(4):**250–252.

20 McConnell JF, Hayes A, Platt SR *et al*. (2006) Calvarial hyperostosis syndrome in two bullmastiffs. *Vet Radiol Ultrasound* **47(1):**72–77.

21 Fitzgerald W, Slocombe R, Caiafa A (2001) Fibrous dysplasia of mandibular bone in a dog. *J Vet Dent* **19(2):**77–81.

INTRODUCTION

The relationship between nasal and oral cavity pathologies is based on their anatomic proximity and common structures (palatal bone, vomeronasal organ), as well as the close position of the maxillary teeth root apices to the lateral and/or rostral walls of the nasal cavity. More commonly, oral pathologies influence the health and functionality of the nose (cleft palate, periapical abscesses, oral tumors) but the opposite situation also happens. Mouth breathing caused by brachycephalic breed syndrome, nasal tumors, or idiopathic rhinitis is a predisposing factor for periodontal disease due to overdrying of the oral mucosa (xerostomia). Chronic rhinitis can lead to destruction or significant weakness of the palatine bone and compromise its function. In fungal infections of the sinuses and the nasal and oral cavities, the organism very often enters through the nose (sniffing infectious material) and affects the function of the entire area.[1]

Nasal discharge is a common indication for oral radiographic diagnostics. Ideally, the causative factor is diagnosed on the first attempt. However, a full diagnostic plan and differential diagnosis protocol is always required so that coincidental pathologies are not missed. For example, a nasal discharge (**Figure 9.1a**) was seen in a dog with an odontogenic cyst that originated from the left maxillary second premolar (206) (**Figure 9.1b**), an oral mass at the area of left maxillary canine and first and second premolars (**Figure 9.1c**), and a foreign body in the left nasal cavity. In all likelihood, the main cause of the nasal discharge was the presence of a foreign body, which was revealed and removed during the final part of the management procedure: rhinoscopy (**Figure 9.1d**).

The nasal cavity is a 3D space, therefore interpretation with 2D imaging has certain limitations. Diagnostic imaging with CT or MRI is superior to conventional radiography; however, the initial evaluation should still be performed with 2D methods.

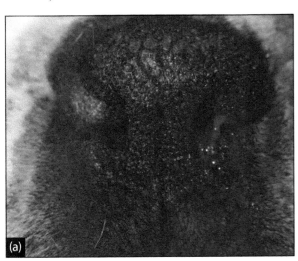

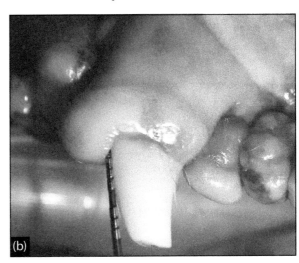

Fig 9.1 (a) The unilateral nasal discharge resulted in the decision to sedate this patient and perform diagnostic imaging and endoscopy. (b) After sedation an oral mass was discovered in the area of the left maxillary canine and first and second premolars.

(Continued)

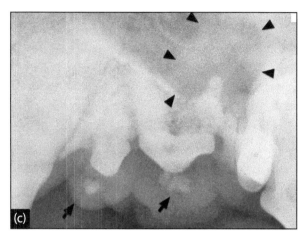

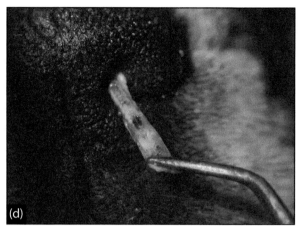

Figs 9.1 *(Continued)* **(c) Intraoral radiograph of the left maxillary first and second premolars showing calcifications within gingival growth (arrows) and the presence of a cystic lesion (arrowheads). (d) Endoscopy revealed the presence of a foreign body.**

The major clinical signs of nasal pathology are sneezing and nasal discharge, therefore these are the most common indications for obtaining a series of diagnostic radiographs of the nose. Neither the fact that the discharge is unilateral or bilateral nor the character of discharge is pathognomic. Among identified problems causing epistaxis in 115 dogs, 78% were caused by local diseases and included tumors (30%), trauma (29%), idiopathic rhinitis (17%), and periapical abscess (2%).[2] Bleeding and a purulent, mucous, or mucopurulent character of the nasal discharge appears with all nasal problems regardless of the causative factor (**Figures 9.1–9.5**).

PROJECTIONS

There are four main projections used for evaluation of the nasal cavity, with the dorsoventral (DV) projection being the most commonly used. DV projections of the nasal cavity are performed intraorally and ventrodorsal (VD) projections extraorally. The other two projections are the lateral and frontal projections.

In cats, a size 2 sensor allows for evaluation of the nasal cavity in two intraoral images (**Figures 9.6a, b**). Size 4 plates may be too large to fit in the caudal part of the nose in a cat if inserted along its axis. However, if the corner of the plate

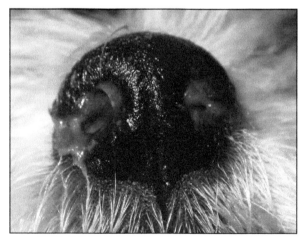

Fig. 9.2 Bleeding from the nose associated with *Aspergillus* infection of the frontal sinus.

Fig. 9.3 A purulent discharge may indicate a foreign body.

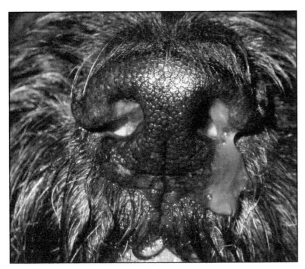

Fig. 9.4 **Nasal discharge with blood associated with adenocarcinoma.**

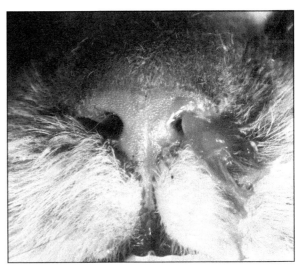

Fig. 9.5 **Solid mucopurulent discharge in a cat with nasal lymphoma.**

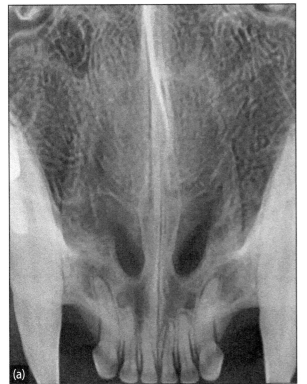

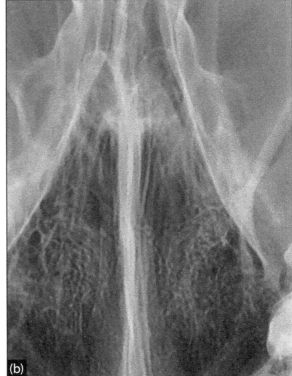

Fig. 9.6 **Intraoral exposure of the rostral (a) and caudal (b) parts of the nasal cavity in a cat using a size 2 sensor.**
(Continued)

is placed into the pharynx, perfect views can be obtained (**Figure 9.6c**). It is also possible to image the nasal cavity of a cat with an extraoral projection (**Figure 9.7**). This requires maximal opening

of the jaws and therefore must be performed as quickly as possible because such wide opening will cause pressure on the maxillary artery, which in turn can compromise the blood supply

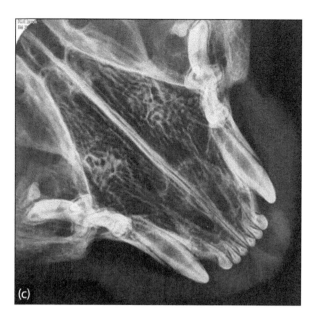

Fig. 9.6 *(Continued)* **(c) The corner of a size 4 plate has been placed into the pharynx to obtain a perfect view.**

and increase the risk of neurologic complications such as blindness.[3] In dogs, depending on the breed, a size 4 plate is easy to use for the intraoral DV projection (**Figure 9.8**). The VD projection can be performed in dogs with ease because the mouth can be opened wider. Care must be taken not to have superimposition of mandibular structures on the nasal passages, choanae, or pharynx (**Figure 9.9**).

Lateral projections are complementary to DV and VD projections. It is very difficult to locate any pathology within the nasal cavity based on one radiograph (**Figure 9.10**), therefore at least two projections (and ideally all three possible planes) are recommended (**Figure 9.11**).

To visualize the left and right nasal cavity separately, a frontal projection is exposed, which makes evaluation of the nasal cavities and frontal sinuses possible (**Figure 9.12**). To obtain a frontal projection, the position of the body must be stable in sternal recumbency and the central beam should be pointing at the nose. It is not easy to create a perfectly symmetric projection, therefore exposing a series of radiographs is often necessary.

A partial frontal projection can also be obtained with an open-mouth projection, when the central beam is directed at the pharynx. Such an exposure enables evaluation of the nasal cavity and tympanic bullae at the same time (**Figure 9.13**).

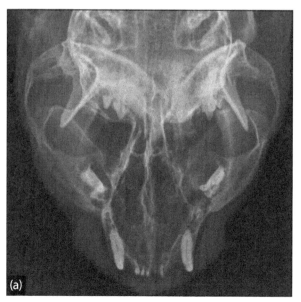

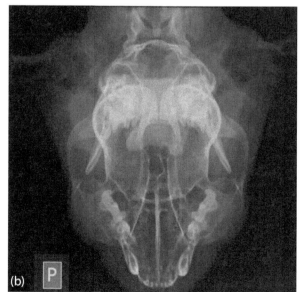

Fig. 9.7 **(a, b) Radiographs showing that it is possible to expose the feline nasal cavity with only an extraoral projection.**

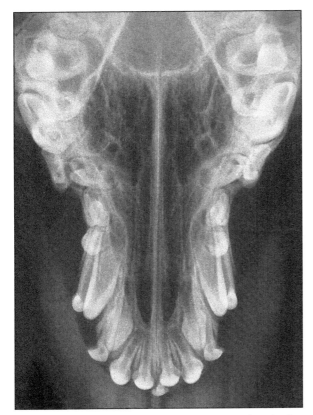

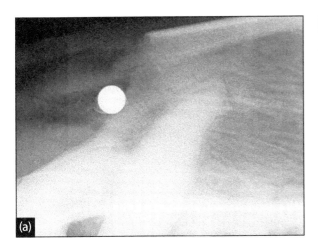

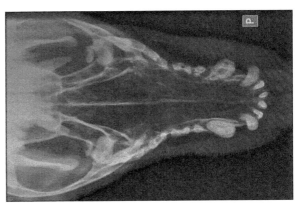

Fig. 9.9 Extraoral VD projection of the nasal cavity in a dog with a large format film in a cassette.

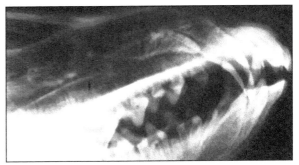

Fig. 9.8 Intraoral DV projection of the nasal cavity in a dog using a size 4 dental film. Note the numerous persistent deciduous teeth and open apices of canines and incisors, indicating the young age of the dog.

Fig. 9.10 Lateral projection of the nasal cavity in a dog revealing the presence of an impacted canine tooth. Based on this radiograph it is not possible to determine which side is affected.

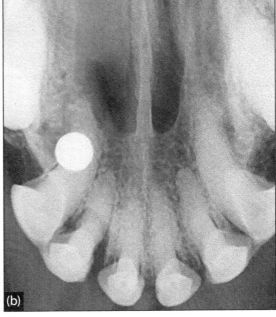

Fig. 9.11 Foreign body in the rostral part of the nose (metal ball). Two projections (lateral [a] and DV [b]) enable accurate location of the object.

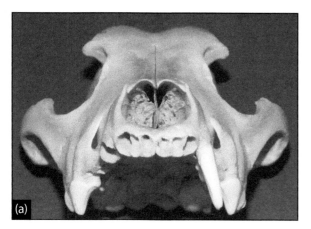

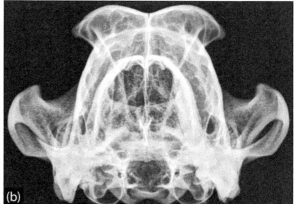

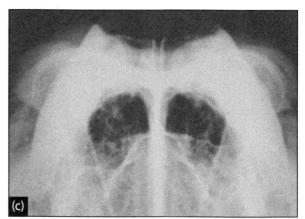

Fig. 9.12 **Frontal projection of the nasal cavity. Anatomic orientation (a), skull radiograph (b), and clinical appearance (c).**

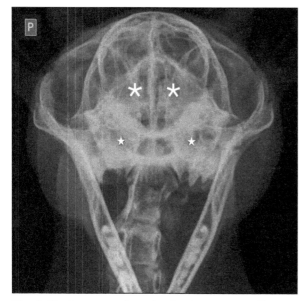

Fig. 9.13 **Open-mouth projection in a cat revealing part of the nasal cavity (asterisks) and tympanic bullae (stars).**

NASAL PATHOLOGY

The nasal cavity, due to its topography and location, is commonly affected by pathology present in the oral cavity. Some oral/dental pathology creates signs from the nasal cavity, such as nasal discharge, bleeding, sneezing, breathing problems, snoring, panting, and deformations of the face, palate, or muzzle. The problems discussed in this chapter are categorized into four groups according to their etiology: infectious, inflammatory, proliferative, and other.

Radiographically, nasal structures should be comparable and symmetrical on both sides of the nose. The structures visible on radiographs are mostly turbinates and ethmoidal bone. Additionally, anatomic structures (i.e. palatine fissures, vomer, and incisive foramen) are visible (**Figure 9.14**). The sagittal portion of the vomer, the perpendicular plate of the ethmoid, and the septal processes of the frontal and nasal bones divide the nasal cavity into

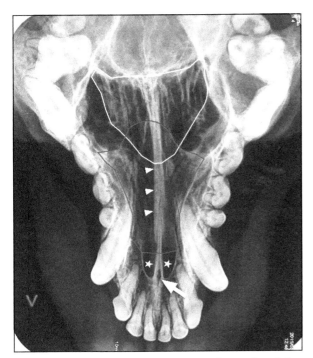

Fig. 9.14 **The structures visible on radiographs of the nasal cavity are mostly endoturbinates (red line) and ethmoidal bone with ethmoturbinates (white line). Additionally, the following anatomic structures are visible: palatine fissures (stars), nasal septum with vomer (arrowheads), and interincisive canal (arrow).**

two equal parts.[4] The 2D radiographic evaluation is based on comparing the left and right cavities, or by comparing them with the anatomically normal structure of a healthy patient. It seems that these structures are unique for individual patients; however, it has not been studied in animals. In human forensic medicine the importance of dental sinus radiography was appreciated in the identification of unidentified humans through the comparison of antemortem and postmortem 2D imaging.[5]

Among possible radiographic signs in feline patients affected by nasal diseases are the following: soft tissue opacity, loss of turbinate detail, destruction of nasal bones, and lysis of midline nasal structures.[6]

CT scanning provides more accurate assessment because the extent of the lesions can be evaluated in all three dimensions. This has a particularly high value in neoplastic lesions (**Figure 9.15**).

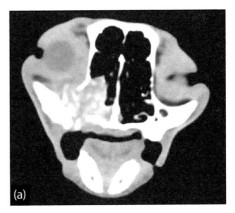
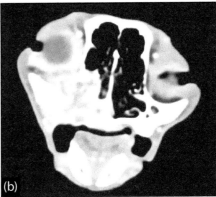
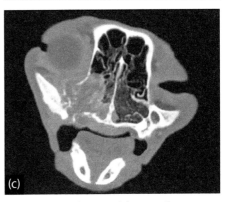

Fig. 9.15 **CT scan of a cat with a nasal tumor destroying the palatal bone and affecting the caudal part of the oral cavity. Three different filters show different aspects of pathology. The first one (a) demonstrates a soft tissue window, which provides optimal conditions to diagnose soft tissue tumors and/ or hematomas. The second (b) is typical for the brain window; however, there is no brain at this image. The third (c) is a bone window used for assessment of hard tissues of the face and cranium. This window is optimal for nasal cavity evaluation. (Courtesy Dr Seth Wallack.)**

Infectious

Foreign bodies

Nasal foreign bodies are the cause of 1.3–8% of nasal disease in dogs.[7] Commonly diagnosed radiopaque foreign bodies include teeth, bones, small stones, and other objects (**Figures 9.16, 9.17**). Radiolucent foreign bodies are not visible nor easy to diagnose until their long-term presence creates chronic inflammation and destruction of nasal structures (**Figure 9.18**). The use of contrast can be helpful in visualizing radiolucent objects.[8]

Odontogenic problems

- Pulpal pathology and periapical complications. The apices of the maxillary dentition are separated from the nasal cavity by a relatively thin plate of bone. Periapical inflammation and abscesses may destroy this bone and create a communication into the nasal cavity. Such a communication may with time become a fistula, which may drain directly into nasal cavity, or it may appear as a sinus tract on the oral mucosa or facial skin. (**Figures 9.19–9.21**).[9]
- Periodontal disease. Combined perio-endo (type II) and endo-perio (type 1) lesions have the same destructive result on the alveolar bone as a periapical abscess. Breed predilection to periodontal disease on the palatal aspect of the maxillary canines and subsequent oronasal fistulas is common in dolichocephalic breeds such as dachshunds, Shetland sheepdogs, and greyhounds.[10] Sneezing, epistaxis, or nasal discharge in such dogs requires an accurate oral assessment concentrating on a specific area (**Figures 9.22–9.24**).

- Retention of maxillary teeth. Partially impacted maxillary teeth (especially canines) create a periodontal pocket where foreign material is easily packed (**Figures 9.25, 9.26**). Fully embedded/impacted teeth predispose to dentigerous cyst formation and may affect the nasal respiratory passage when these develop in the maxilla (see Chapter 8, Part G).[11]

Fungal infection

The most common fungal infection of the nose in canine veterinary patients is aspergillosis.[12] This infection particularly affects sinuses and ethmoidal bones.[13] Chronic nasal discharge is unfortunately routinely and symptomatically treated by antibiotics prior to final diagnosis, therefore the clinical situation worsens. Because of chronic overuse of antibiotics, there is currently widespread antibiotic resistance. Nasal discharge is very irritating to the soft tissues and dogs with significant discharge often have erosions and ulceration on the nasal mucosa and skin (**Figure 9.27**). Definitive diagnosis is based on mycologic culture, but a rhinoscopy and cytologic evaluation of an impression smear of the exudate can also provide useful information and support suspicion of fungal infection (**Figures 9.28, 9.29**).

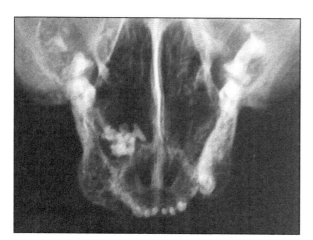

Fig. 9.16 **Radiopaque foreign body in the right nasal cavity of a cat.**

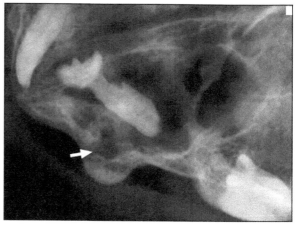

Fig. 9.17 **Canine tooth intruded into the nasal cavity causing chronic rhinitis and oronasal fistula (arrow).**

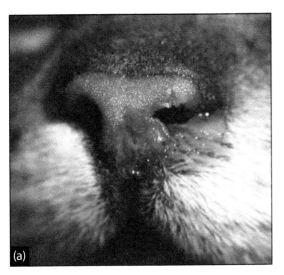

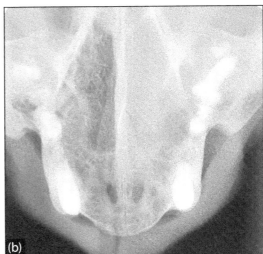

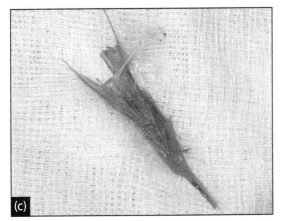

Fig. 9.18 Unilateral purulent nasal discharge (a) associated with significant unilateral generalized loss of turbinate detail in the left nasal cavity (b) caused by a foxtail present for at least 3 months (c).

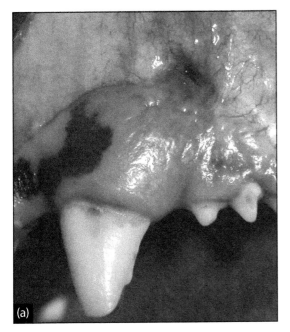

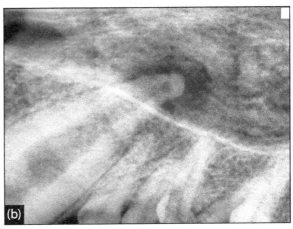

Fig. 9.19 (a) Unilateral (left) nasal discharge in a dog with a fractured left maxillary canine (204) and a sinus tract entering the oral cavity. (b) Radiographically visible periapical lucency. The drainage to the nasal cavity was confirmed by rhinoscopy.

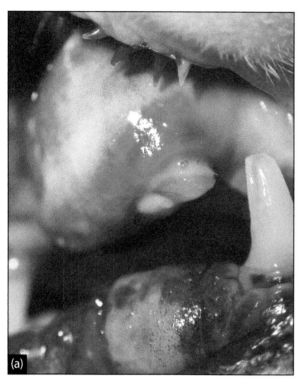

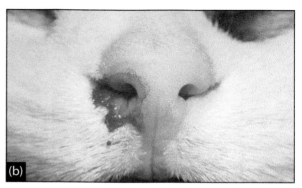

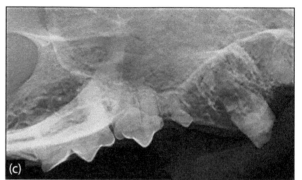

Fig. 9.20 Fractured right maxillary canine tooth (104) (a) in a cat with frequent bleeding from the right nasal cavity (b). Radiograph shows root resorption with radiolucent area surrounding the affected root (c).

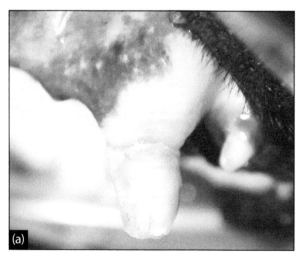

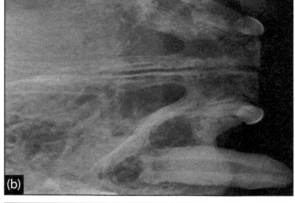

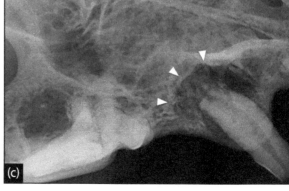

Fig. 9.21 Sneezing cat with a fractured canine tooth (a). Radiographs of the fractured tooth reveal periapical radiolucency (b, c) that breaks the radiopaque line (junction of the palatal process of maxilla and vertical body of the maxilla, arrowheads). Note the open apex of the affected canine tooth and its wide root canal as well as the missing incisors (b).

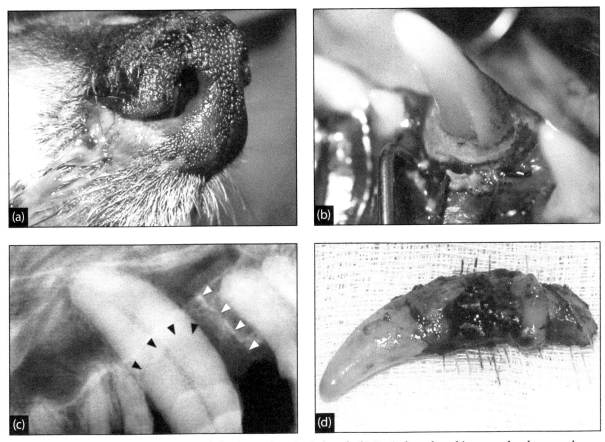

Fig. 9.22 (a) Chronic right-sided nasal discharge in a dachshund. (b) Periodontal probing to a depth more than 17 mm from the distopalatal aspect of 104. (c) Radiograph confirming the periodontal disease: alveolar bone loss (black arrowheads), widening of the periodontal ligament space around canine tooth (white arrowheads). (d) Extracted tooth with granulation tissue and subgingival calculus on the palatal surface.

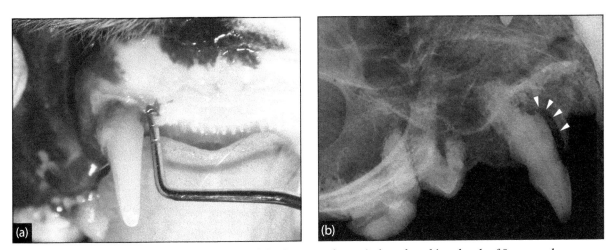

Fig. 9.23 (a) Sneezing cat with unilateral nasal discharge and a periodontal probing depth of 8 mm at the mesiopalatal aspect. (b) Radiograph revealing that the canine tooth is affected by TR type 3 with a periodontal pocket (arrowheads).

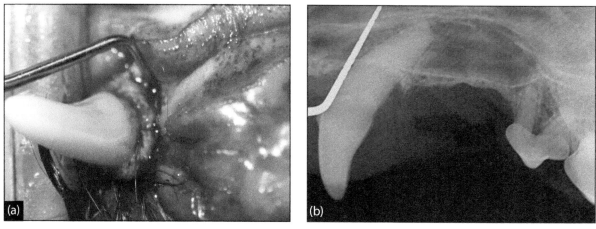

Fig. 9.24 Ten-year-old dachshund with a nasal discharge. The periodontal probe enters the nasal cavity from the palatal aspect. (a) Probing reveals periodontal pockets. (b) The depth of the periodontal pocket is recorded.

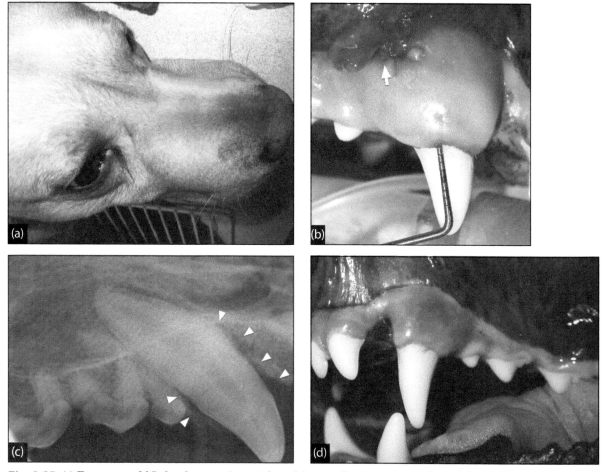

Fig. 9.25 (a) Four-year-old Labrador retreiver with no history of trauma presenting with a swelling of the right muzzle and purulent nasal discharge. (b) Sinus tract present at the mucogingival junction of 104 (arrow). Periodontal probing depth of 12 mm on the lateral aspect. (c) Radiograph confirming partial retention of 104 with a periodontal pocket from the mesial and distal aspect (arrowheads). (d) For comparison the contralateral canine tooth is shown fully erupted.

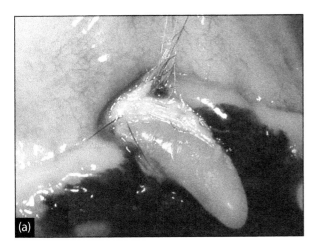

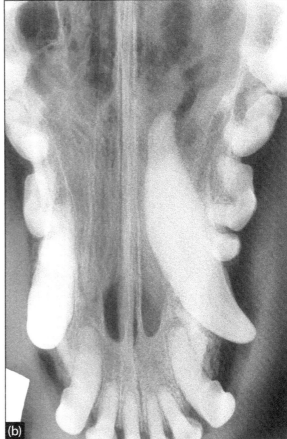

Fig. 9.26 This patient had chronic unilateral nasal discharge that had been treated for 3 years with different antibiotics. (a) Partially retained 104 with hair and debris packed into the periodontal pocket. (b) Radiograph confirming retention of 104 and destruction of caudal nasal structures.

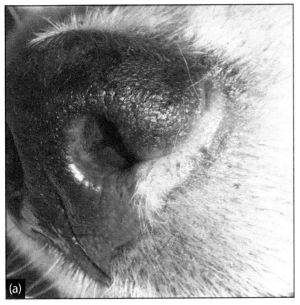

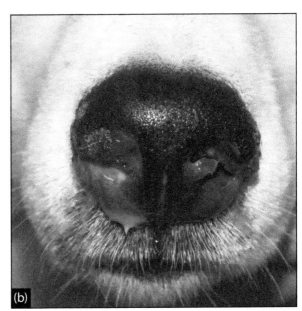

Fig. 9.27 (a, b) Bilateral nasal discharge with ulceration of the nasal area caused by sinonasal aspergillosis.

Radiography often shows asymmetric changes in the radiodensity, with irregular borders of the nasal cavities (**Figure 9.30**). In aspergillosis it is important additionally to obtain frontal sinus projections (**Figures 9.31, 9.32**).

In cats the most common systemic fungal disease is cryptococcosis, which can be present in the nasal

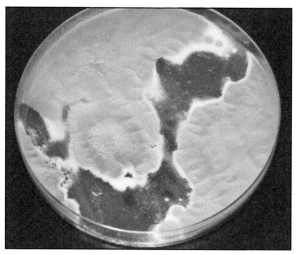

Fig. 9.28 **Mycological culture after 48 hours incubation confirming aspergillosis.**

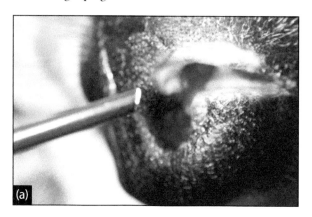

cavity and produce similar radiographic and clinical signs to other infections.[14]

Pseudomonas, spirochetes (Vincent disease), *Chlamydia* infections

These infections do not produce a specific clinical or radiographic appearance, therefore diagnosis requires in-vitro culture and sensitivity. The sensitivity test may provide crucial information (e.g. *Pseudomonas* spp. are often widely resistant).

Inflammatory
Feline idiopathic rhinitis

This condition has a wide range of possible etiologies, which include dental, immune system dysfunction, chronic oral inflammation, chronic nasal infection, and nasal injuries. One of the lasting complications of high-rise syndrome injuries in cats is chronic rhinitis.[15] However, the cause of idiopathic rhinitis in cats is currently unknown. The radiographic appearance is either asymmetry between the right and left sides of the nasal cavity (**Figures 9.33, 9.34**) or, in more advanced cases, absence of nasal turbinates unilaterally or bilaterally (**Figures 9.35, 9.36**).

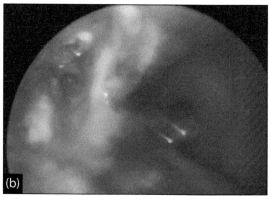

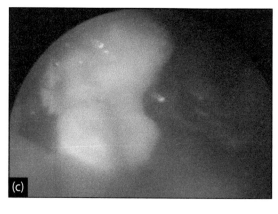

Fig. 9.29 **Preparation for rhinoscopy in a patient infected by *Aspergillus* spp. (a) and images obtained via rhinoscopy (b, c).**

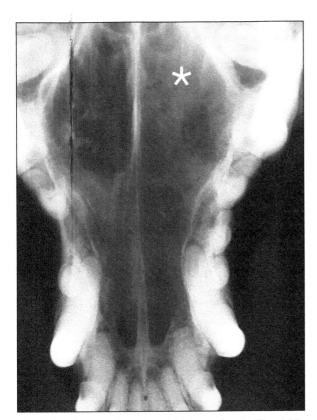

Fig. 9.30 Extraoral radiograph of the dog in Figs 9.27 and 9.29 revealing bilateral destruction of the rostral parts of the nasal cavity and the right caudal nasal cavity, with radiopacity likely caused by exudate (asterisk).

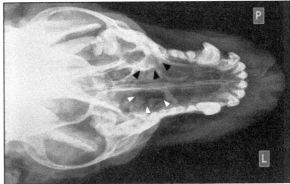

Fig. 9.31 Extraoral VD projection of the nasal cavity in a Labrador retriever with *Aspergillus* infection. The assymmetric appearance of the structures of the left and right nasal cavities is visible, with radiolucent (white arrowheads) and radiodense (black arrowheads) lesions in the caudal part of the nasal cavity.

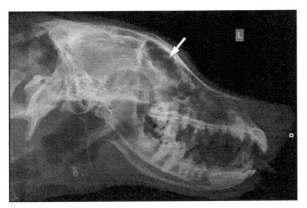

Fig. 9.32 Lateral skull radiograph of the dog in Fig. 9.31. Note the frontal sinus without septa and filled with radiopaque material (arrow).

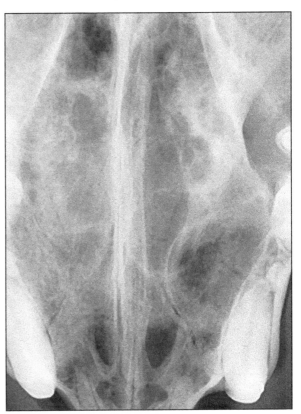

Fig. 9.33 Feline idiopathic rhinitis. There are slight differences in the structures of the left and right nasal cavities with loss of nasal turbinate detail and destruction of nasal bones. To visualize the entire nasal cavity, a size 4 film or PSP plate is appropriate. The presented radiograph is a size 2, therefore the lateral and caudal parts of the nasal cavities are missed.

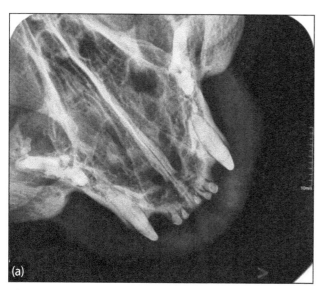
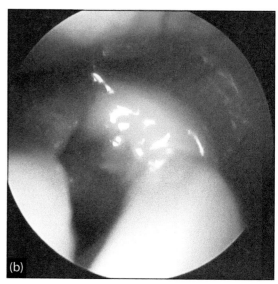

Fig. 9.34 Feline idiopathic rhinitis. Slight differences in the structures of the left and right nasal cavities. The right cavity is more affected, with more significant loss of turbinate details. (a) Note the missing right maxillary first incisor 101. (b) Rhinoscopy reveals exudate in the right nasal cavity.

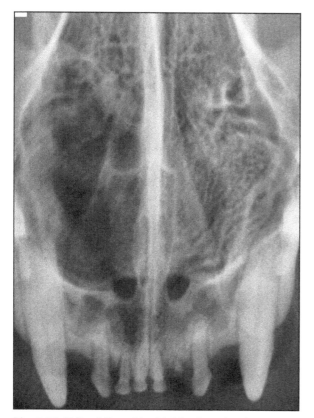
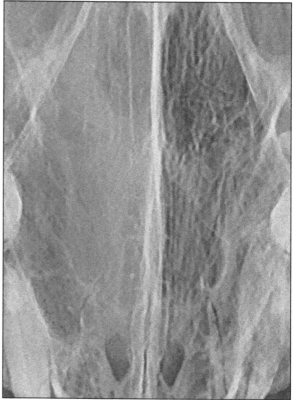

Fig. 9.35 Feline idiopathic rhinitis. Complete lack of nasal turbinates in the right nasal cavity. To visualize the entire nasal cavity, a size 4 film or sensor is appropriate. The presented radiograph is a size 2 and it misses the lateral and caudal parts of the nasal cavities.

Fig. 9.36 Feline idiopathic rhinitis. Right nasal cavity with invisible nasal structures and soft tissue opacity likely caused by exudate.

Diagnosis requires histhopathologic assessment of nasal biopsies. During the biopsy procedure, the typical appearance of the nasal mass is not tumor-like, but more like gray/green masses present amongst atrophic nasal conchae (**Figure 9.37**).

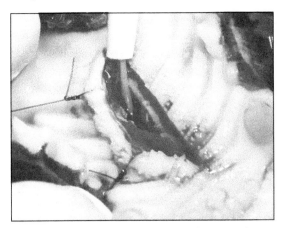

Fig. 9.37 **Palatal access to the nasal cavity of a cat affected by feline idiopathic rhinitis. The typical appearance of the nasal cavity is the presence of gray/green exudate amongst atrophic nasal conchae.**

Other

Some immune mediated diseases, such as uveitis-dermatitis syndrome or discoid lupus erythematosus, can also affect the nasal cavity or its surroundings, but they have no typical radiographic appearance.

Proliferative lesions
Non-neoplastic
- Odontogenic cyst (see Chapter 8, Part G).
- Eosinophilic granuloma complex. These lesions occasionally occur in the nasal cavity and, if not treated, may destroy the nasal structures, which can be seen radiographically. Siberian huskies and Cavalier King Charles spaniels have breed predilections to this condition and a diagnosis can occasionally be made on tissue/exudate cytology.[16] Stained smears of the nasal discharge reveal an overrepresentation of eosinophils and can provide a presumptive diagnosis for preliminary symptomatic treatment (**Figure 9.38**).

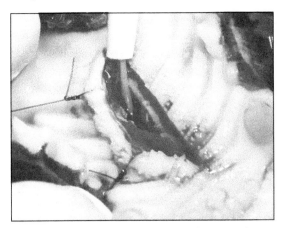

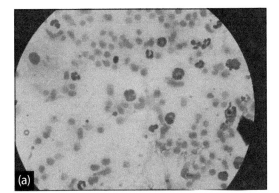

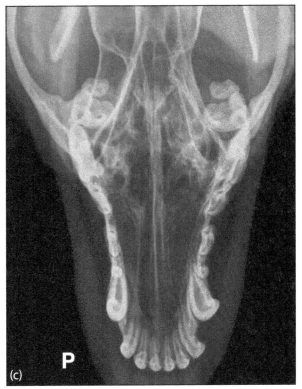

Fig. 9.38 **(a, b) Stained smears from the nasal discharge show overrepresentation of eosinophils. This can be helpful for preliminary symptomatic treatment. (c) In this dog (a Siberian husky, which has breed predisposition for eosinophilic granuloma complex) the extraoral VD radiograph of the nasal cavity appears normal.**

Neoplastic

Benign nasal cavity lesions may still be harmful and require treatment. It is uncommon to diagnose polyps in the nasal cavity, but their excision is curative. Tumors of the turbinates, nasal mucosa, and palatal bone, as well as sinus tumors, can have various causes and pathophysiology, but they have a similar radiographic appearance (**Figures 9.39, 9.40**). Due to the presence of many glandular cells in the nasal cavity, adenocarcinoma is a common neoplasm diagnosed in the nose and sinuses. In cats, nasal lymphoma is the second most diagnosed nasal tumor.[17] As mentioned previously, 3D imaging of the nose can provide precise evaluation of tumor size and extent, and is very helpful in determining the treatment plan (**Figure 9.41**). Many nasal tumors are impossible to excise completely and therefore only palliative treatment is recommended (radiation, chemotherapy, or both) depending on patient status and available effective treatment modalities.

Deformations located on the dorsal part of the maxilla are very often associated with a growth infiltrating the nasal cavity (**Figures 9.42**).

Tumors affecting the rostral part of the nose or nasal planum are mostly soft tissue in origin and may not change the radiographic image. However, imaging is required to rule out infiltration and to have a preoperative record for later follow-up (**Figures 9.43, 9.44**). There are also tumors that primarily affect the incisive and maxillary bones (**Figures 9.45, 9.46**).

Other

Oronasal fistulas

Oral fistulas form as the consequence of periodontal disease or iatrogenic complications of poorly performed extractions. On radiographs, the bone is barely visible or its radiodensity is decreased compared with the normal bone (**Figures 9.47, 9.48**). In chronic cases, visible destruction of nasal structures can also be seen.

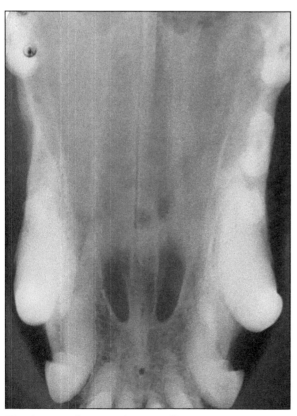

Fig. 9.39 **Radiopaque lesions affecting both nasal cavities in a dog.**

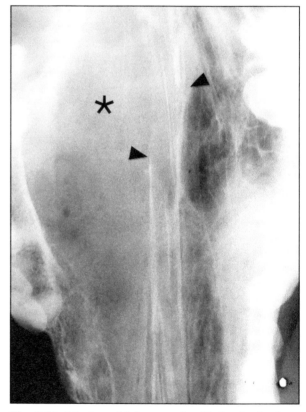

Fig. 9.40 **A lesion with increased radiodensity in the right nasal cavity (asterisk), with lysis of the midline nasal structures (arrowheads).**

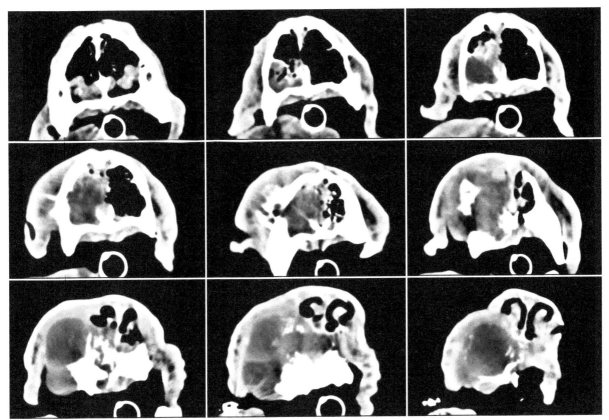

Fig. 9.41 CT scan of a dog with a tumor of the rostral part of the maxilla. Selected nine frames taken every 10 mm from the affected area (rostral 8 cm of the muzzle is presented). Scans show that the tumor crosses the nasal septum at the rostral part. The last frame does not show any pathology, indicating the caudal margin of tumor. Margin sections will be selected based on histopathological diagnosis of biopsy. (Courtesy Dr Lisa Mestrinho.)

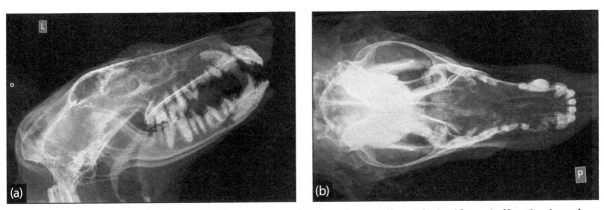

Figs 9.42 (a, b) Radiographs showing a fibrosarcoma affecting the maxilla, with significant infiltration into the nasal cavity and frontal sinus.

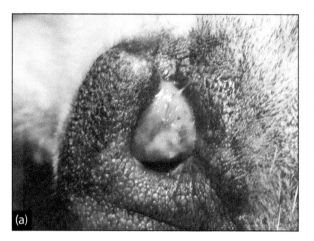

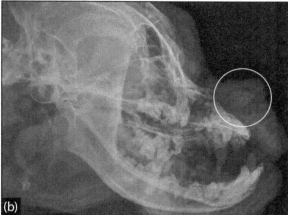

Fig. 9.43 Histiocytic sarcoma in the left nostril (a), which is obliterating the air passage in the left nostril. The radiographs reveal that there are no radiographic changes (b, lateral view highlighting [circle] an area of the soft tissue tumor that is not causing any bone reaction; c, VD view showing the delicate radiopacity of the tumor but no bone reaction [arrows]). Note the supernumerary maxillary incisors in this dog.

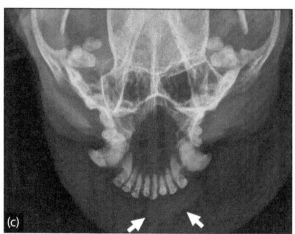

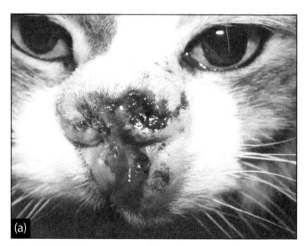

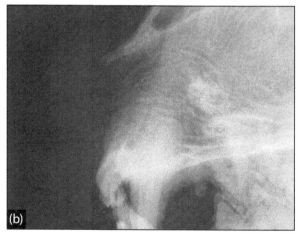

Fig. 9.44 (a) Squamous cell carcinoma of the nasal planum in a cat. (b) The lateral extraoral projection radiograph shows no visible bony reaction.

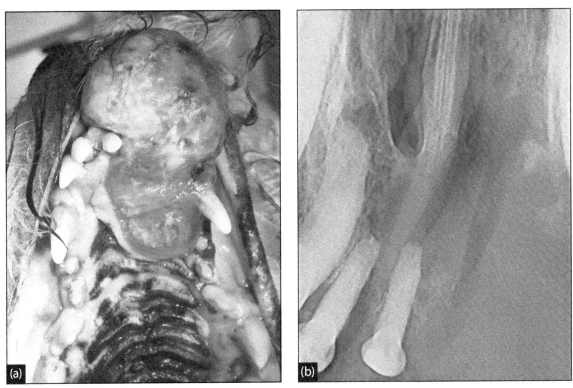

Fig. 9.45 **Soft tissue sarcoma of the rostral maxilla (a) in a dog with infiltrative growth (b).**

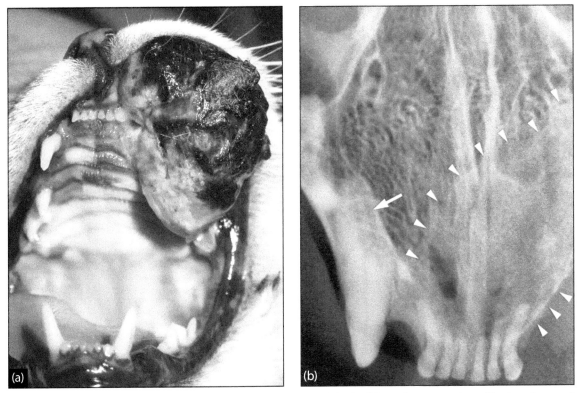

Fig. 9.46 **Osteosarcoma of the rostral left maxilla in a cat (a) with significant bone reaction affecting the nasal cavity (arrowheads) (b). Note the type 2 TR in the right maxillary canine (104) (arrow).**

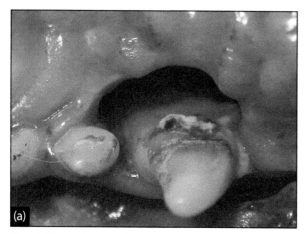

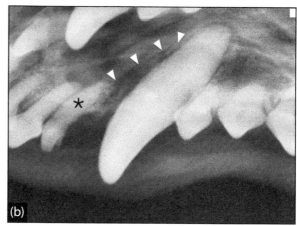

Fig. 9.47 (a) Oronasal fistula associated with severe periodontal disease of the palatal aspect of the left maxillary canine (204). (b) Radiographic features of periodontal disease are present, particularly at the mesial aspect of 204 (arrowheads). Note the presence of a persistent deciduous 603 (asterisk) and missing 203.

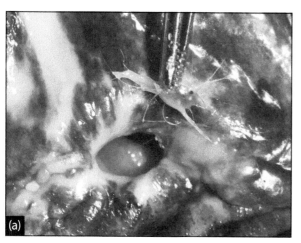

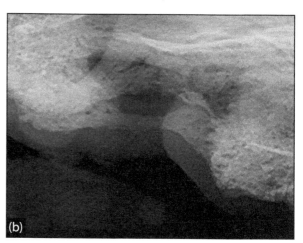

Fig. 9.48 (a) Oronasal fistula in a dog that had lost teeth due to periodontal disease. Debris is present in the fistula. (b) Radiograph showing bone loss at the affected area.

Congenital and acquired cleft palate or palatal defect

Cleft palates are typically associated with other anatomic problems, therefore it is important to evaluate the entire head, preferably with the use of 3D diagnostic imaging technologies.[18] Assymmetry or additional pathologies can be distinguished clinically and radiographically (**Figures 9.49–9.52**).

Malocclusion

Linguoversion of mandibular canines causes the crown tips to occlude with the palatal mucosa. If the canine teeth are fully erupted and the dog is relatively large, such a situation may create an oronasal fistula. This is created not only by the continuous traumatization of the palate by the crown, but also by packing material into the defect followed by its fermentation, infection, and inflammation of the affected area (**Figure 9.53**).

Post-traumatic disorders

Fractures of the bones, wounds (**Figure 9.54**). These are discussed in Chapter 8, Part F.

Brachycephalic airway syndrome

Narrowed nostrils cause mouth breathing, which predisposes to periodontal disease and possible infectious extension to the tonsils (**Figure 9.55**).

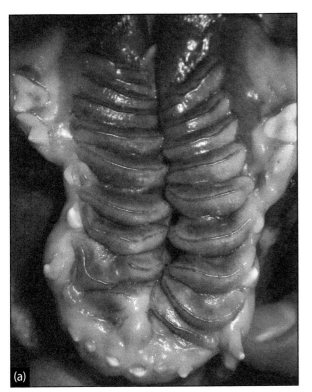

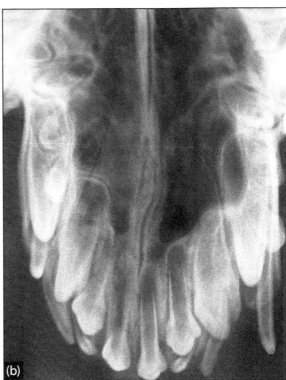

Fig. 9.49 (a) Cleft of the secondary palate in a boxer puppy with slight asymmetry and skeletal malocclusion. (b) Radiograph confirms distortion of the nasal septum.

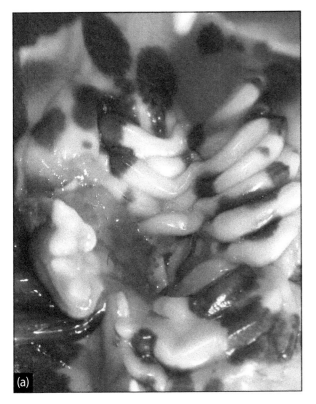

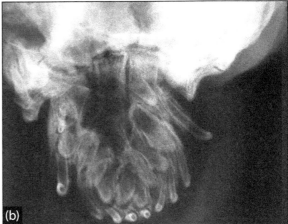

Fig. 9.50 (a) Congenital secondary cleft palate in a boxer associated with cleft lip and severe skull asymmetry causing malocclusion. (b) Radiograph confirms the severe asymmetry and malalignment of the deciduous and permanent dentition.

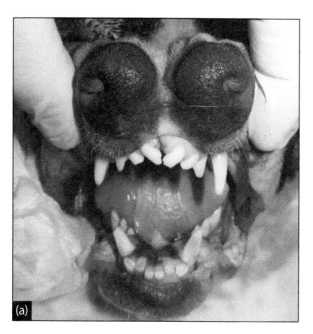

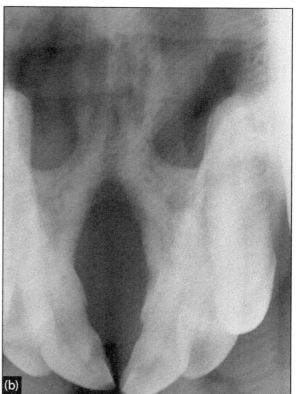

Fig. 9.51 (a) Primary cleft palate with philtrum dividing the nose into two parts. (b) The incisive bones are missing the rostral part of the interincisive suture.

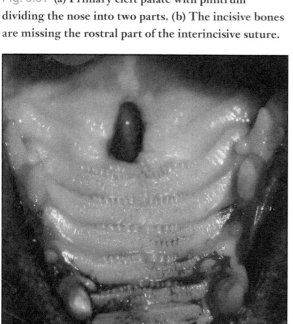

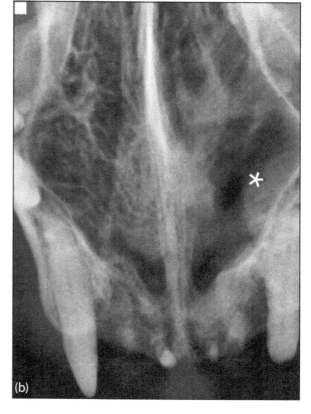

Fig. 9.52 (a) Palatal defect in a cat causing chronic rhinitis. (b) Radiographically visible destruction of the nasal structures of the left nasal cavity (asterisk).

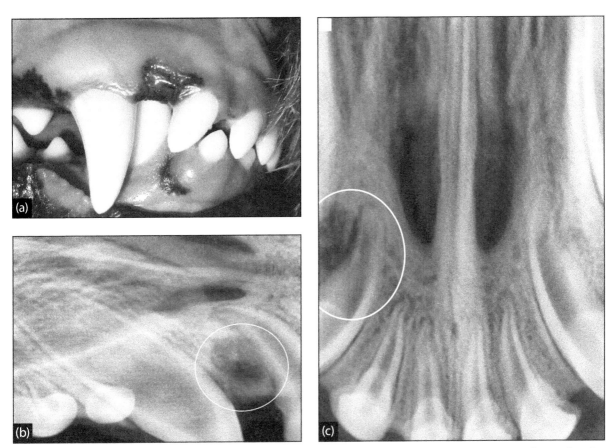

Fig. 9.53 (a) Linguoversion of the right mandibular canine (404) creating palatal trauma. (b, c) Radiographs of the area reveal radiolucency at the diastema between the right maxillary third incisor and canine (103 and 104) where 404 is creating occlusal trauma (circle).

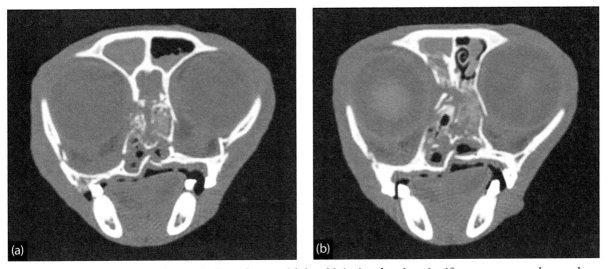

Fig. 9.54 (a–c) CT scan with bone window of a cat with head injuries showing significant trauma to the nasal conchae as well as the palatal, lacrimal, and vomer bones. Most of these injuries were not visible on conventional radiographs. (Courtesy Dr Seth Wallack.)

(Continued)

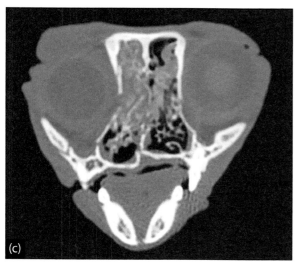

Fig. 9.54 *(Continued)*

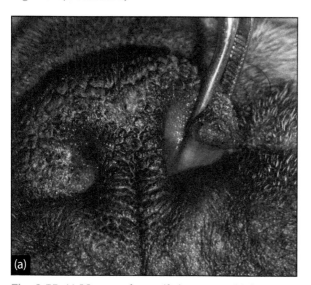

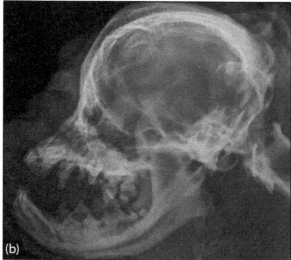

Fig. 9.55 **(a) Narrowed nostrils in a pug, which is a common feature of brachycephalic obstructive airway syndrome. (b) Radiograph of a brachycephalic dog revealing a shortened maxilla, which further affects normal nasal function.**

DIAGNOSIS

Diagnosis of secondary nasal issues starts with a conscious examination, but always requires a detailed examination under general anesthesia. Prior to anesthesia, a preanesthetic laboratory examination should be performed to ensure that the patient is a good anesthetic candidate. In addition, while under anesthesia for radiography, rhinoscopy or other imaging methods (CT or MRI) can be performed along with biopsy and/or collection of material for cytology and cultures.

Collection of material for cytology and culture can be performed even in a conscious patient if he/she is calm.

REFERENCES

1 Gawor J (2012) Coincidental pathology of nasal cavity and oral structures. *Proceedings of the 21st European Congress of Veterinary Dentistry*, Lisbon, pp. 157–158.
2 Bissett SA, Drobatz KJ, McKnight A *et al.* (2007) Prevalence, clinical features, and causes of epistaxis in dogs: 176 cases (1996–2001) *J Am Vet Med Assoc* **231**:1843–1850.

3   Stiles J, Weil AB, Packer RA *et al.* (2012) Post-anesthetic cortical blindness in cats: twenty cases. *Vet J* **193(2):**367–373.

4   Evans HE, de Lahunta A (2013) Skull. In: *Miller's Anatomy of the Dog*, 4th edn. Elsevier, St. Louis, p. 112.

5   da Silva RF1, Prado FB, Caputo IG *et al.* (2009) The forensic importance of frontal sinus radiographs. *J Forensic Leg Med* **16(1):**18–23.

6   CR Lamb, Richbell S, Mantis P (2003) Radiographic signs in cats with nasal disease. *J Feline Med Surg* **5:**227–235.

7   Carle DS, Shope BH (2012) Diagnostic imaging in veterinary dental practice. *J Am Vet Med Assoc* **241(3):**323–325.

8   Wallack S (2003) *Handbook of Veterinary Contrast Radiography*. San Diego Veterinary Imaging, San Diego pp. 137–140.

9   Maretta SM (1992) Chronic rhinitis and dental disease. *Vet Clin North Am Small Anim Pract* **22:**1101–1117.

10 Gawor J (2013) Hereditary oral disorders in pedigree dogs. Proposals for their evidence and assessment. Special issue of European Journal of Companion Animal Practice, Genetic/Hereditary Disease and Breeding. *EJCAP Online* **23(3)**.

11 Hintze S, Oechtering GU (2011) An invisible risk: embedded teeth in brachycephalic dogs. *Proceedings of the 21st European Congress of Veterinary Dentistry*, Chalkidiki, pp. 90–93.

12 Cohn LA (2014) Canine nasal disease. *Vet Clin North Am Small Anim Pract* **44(1):**75–89.

13 Sharman MJ, Mansfield CS (2012) Sinonasal aspergillosis in dogs: a review. *J Small Anim Pract* **53(8):**434–444.

14 Pennisi MG, Hartmann K, Lloret A (2013) Cryptococcosis in cats. ABCD guidelines on prevention and management. *J Feline Med Surg* **15:**611–618.

15 Gawor J (2014) Challenges in diagnostic and treatment in feline high rise syndrome. *Proceedings of the 23rd European Congress of Veterinary Dentistry*, Costa Luminosa, pp. 110–111.

16 Niemiec BA (2010) Pathologies of oral mucosa. In: *Small Animal Dental, Oral and Maxillofacial Disease: A Color Handbook*. (ed. BA Niemiec) Manson Publishing, London, pp. 184–197.

17 Mortellaro CM (2002) The nasal cavity and paranasal sinuses. In: *Clinical Atlas of Ear, Nose and Throat Diseases in Small Animals*. (eds. C Hedlund, J Taboada) Schlutersche, Hanover, pp. 61–111.

18 Nemec A, Daniaux L, Johnson E *et al.* (2015) Craniomaxillary abnormalities in dogs with congenital palatal defects: computed tomographic findings. *Vet Surg* **44(4):**417–422.

FURTHER READING

Brockman DJ, Holt DE (2005) *BSAVA Manual of Canine and Feline Head, Neck and Thoracic Surgery*. British Small Animal Veterinary Assosiation, Gloucester.

Hedlund C, Taboada J, Merchant S, Mortellaro C (2002) *Clinical Atlas of Ear, Nose, and Throat Diseases in Small Animals: The Case-Based Approach*. Schlutersche, Hanover.

Fossum TW (2007) (ed.) *Small Animal Surgery*, 3rd edn. Mosby, St. Louis.

Slatter D (2003) *Textbook of Small Animal Surgery*, 3rd edn. WB Saunders, Philadelphia.

Venker-van Haagen, AJ (2005) *Nose, Throat and Tracheobronchial Diseases in Dogs & Cats*. Schlutersche Hanover.

CHAPTER 10

RADIOGRAPHY OF THE TEMPOROMANDIBULAR JOINT AND MANDIBULAR SYMPHYSIS

Jerzy Gawor

INTRODUCTION

Dysfunction of chewing, jaw opening, or pain occurring with normal movements of the temporomandibular joint (TMJ) can be related to luxation, dislocation, fracture, or other disease affecting this joint.[1]

In dogs, the most commonly diagnosed TMJ pathology is osteoarthritis. In cats, TMJ fracture is the most common; however, osteoarthritis is second and this condition usually coexists with many other pathologies. Pathologic findings were more common on the medial than the lateral aspect in one study.[2]

With regard to the TMJ, the clinical signs of most of its common pathologies (luxation, intraarticular fractures, and/or periarticular fractures) are similar. These include pain, dysfunction, decreased jaw opening, problems with jaws closing, crepitation in the TMJ area, and abnormal movements of the jaws. Even if the symptoms are indicative for luxation, the fact that caudal mandibular fractures can mimic luxations must be taken into account. Therefore, prior to empiric management of the problem, a complete diagnostic plan must be performed.

DIAGNOSIS

Proper management of TMJ problems depends on an accurate diagnosis. Actions based on assumption only can lead to severe complications, such as further damage of injured joint structures, its ankylosis, or other malfunction. Diagnosis is based on a series of well positioned radiographs or, ideally, 3D imaging. CT is superior for TMJ evaluation than standard radiography,[3] whereas MRI provides more accurate evaluation of the soft tissues (**Figures 10.1–10.5**).[4] CT is the preferred diagnostic imaging modality for bony lesions.

Attempts to obtain diagnostic quality 3D TMJ imaging in dogs using ultrasound technology have

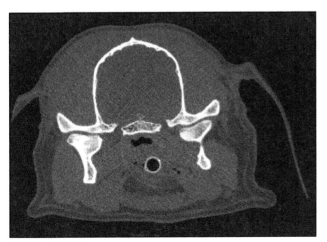

Fig. 10.1 **CT scan of a canine TMJ, transverse view.**

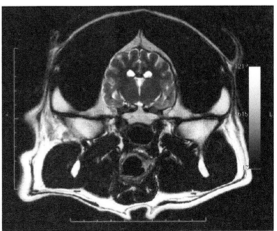

Fig. 10.2 **MR image of a canine TMJ, transverse view. (Courtesy Dr Seth Wallack.)**

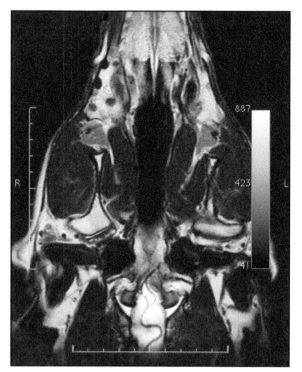

Fig. 10.3 **MR image of a canine TMJ, horizontal view. (Courtesy Dr Seth Wallack.)**

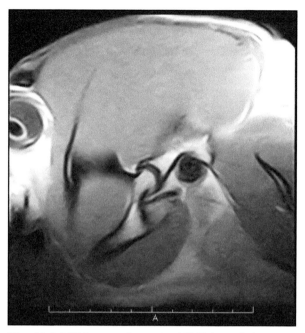

Fig. 10.4 **MR image of a canine TMJ, lateral view.**

not yet provided satisfactory results and will require further refinement before this technique is clinically relevant (**Figure 10.6**).

RADIOGRAPHY

In standard 2D radiographic diagnostic imaging of the TMJs, the mandibular area is visualized by performing three projections: lateral oblique, dorsoventral (DV), and oblique DV.

In the lateral oblique projection it is possible to evaluate the shape of the articular surface of the temporal bone and the condylar process. The vertical projections (DV and ventrodorsal [VD]) provide visibility of the relationships between the condylar process and the articular surface of the temporal bone. Finally, the oblique sagittal (DV) projection further evaluates the bony structures forming the articular surfaces.

Temporomandibular joint projections

Every anatomic structure creating the TMJ should be visualized on the obtained radiographs. There is

no single projection in 2D radiology that provides a complete image of the TMJ. The endotracheal tube may interfere with the image so either it can be removed or positioned in such a way that it is not superimposed on the TMJ area.

- **Lateral oblique view**. The patient is positioned in lateral recumbency and the head is positioned as follows. The palate is angulated approximately 80° to the table plane and the nose elevated from horizontal by 10–25° depending on head type – in general, 10° for dolichocephalic breeds, 15° for mesocephalic, and up to 25° for brachycephalic breeds.[5] The x-ray beam is directed perpendicular to the film/sensor. Because of the anatomic variations listed above, values are only a guide (**Figures 10.7–10.9**).
- **Dorsoventral view**. The body and head are positioned in sternal recumbency and the x-ray beam is directed perpendicular to the film. This position is easier to obtain and more stable as the mandibles stabilize the position of the head if they are symmetrical. If they are not symmetrical, more effort is required in patient

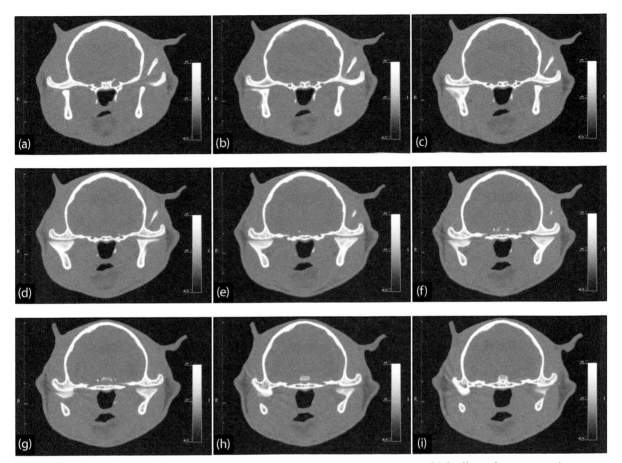

Fig. 10.5 CT scan. (a–i) Series of feline TMJs showing slices every 0.62 mm, which allows for very precise evaluation of the entire structure of both TMJs.

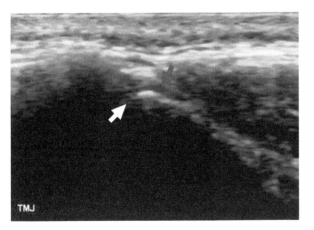

Fig. 10.6 Ultrasound image of the TMJ. White arrow, condylar process; red arrow, articular space.

positioning to obtain optimal projection, with the film parallel to the plane of the articular surfaces (**Figures 10.10–10.12**).

- **Ventrodorsal**. The body lies in dorsal recumbency and the x-ray beam is directed perpendicular to the film. There are no particular benefits from this view as the radiographed object (TMJ) is further from the film/plate in this position.[5] Additionally, in brachycephalic breeds this position

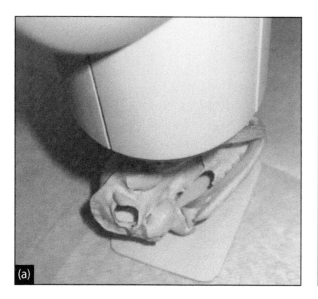

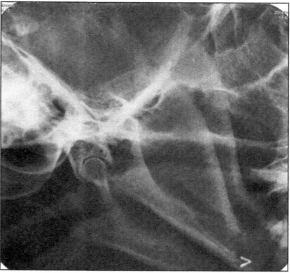

Fig. 10.8 Lateral oblique radiograph of a feline TMJ.

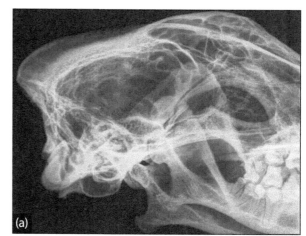

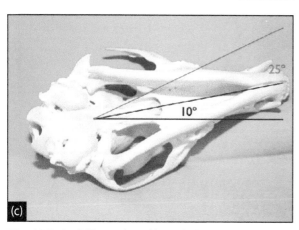

Fig. 10.7 (a–c) Examples of lateral oblique views. Note that the x-ray beam is perpendicular to the film and the head is correctly positioned.

Fig. 10.9 (a) This lateral oblique radiograph of a canine TMJ is not diagnostic. (b) The more lateral position provides a better image of the articular space.

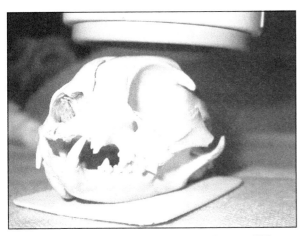

Fig. 10.10 **Model demonstrating that the mandibles stabilize the position of the head (if they are symmetrical), making it easier to obtain the ideal position for a DV projection.**

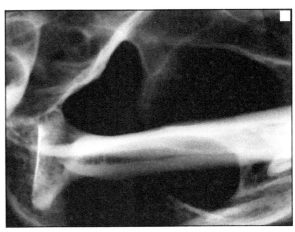

Fig. 10.11 **DV radiograph of a feline TMJ. This radiograph was exposed on a size 2 sensor. Ideally both TMJs should be visible, but this requires a size 4 film or plate.**

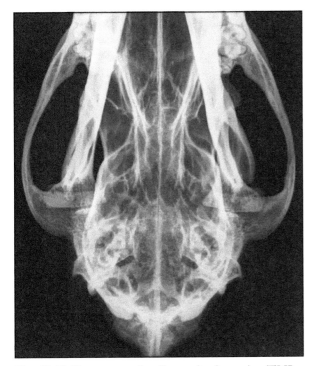

Fig. 10.12 **Dorsoventral radiograph of a canine TMJ.**

is harder to stabilize. Nevertheless, it is occasionally preferable to have both vertical views for comparison (**Figure 10.13**).

- **Dorsoventral oblique**. The body lies in sternal recumbency and the x-ray beam is pointed at the TMJ through the orbit at an 80° angle to the film. Because of the angulation of the x-ray beam, there is elongation of some structures; however, the TMJ is adequately imaged (**Figures 10.14–10.16a**).

New technologies (e.g. cone-beam CT) provide the possibility to present both TMJs in lateral views in a panoramic projection (**Figure 10.16b**).

Symphyseal projections

Cats and dogs have a Class I symphysis, as described by Scapino (1981).[6] This is best imaged in a series using 3D imaging (**Figure 10.17**). In classic radiography of the symphysis, it is important to position the head, film, and x-ray beam in the most symmetrical way possible. The x-ray beam should also be perpendicular to the hypothetical axial line of the symphysis, otherwise the symphyseal space (if present) will not be visible (**Figure 10.18**). The tongue should be pushed towards the pharynx so as not to extend it between the object and the film. To obtain more information about the symphyseal structure, at least two images with two different exposures (lighter and darker) are required (**Figure 10.19**).

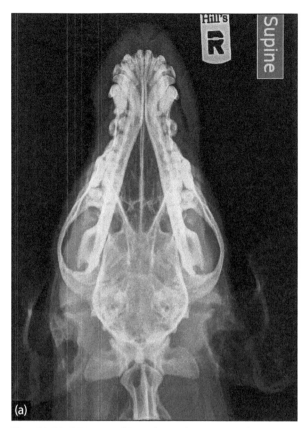

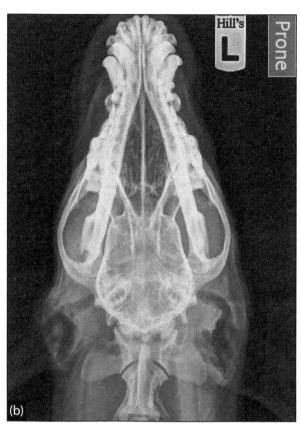

Fig. 10.13 DV (a) and VD (b) projections of the TMJ demonstrating that there is no significant difference for the TMJ visualization.

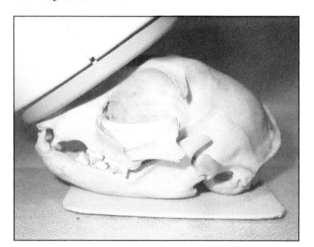

Fig. 10.14 Model demonstrating the position for a DV oblique projection where the patient is placed in sternal recumbency and the x-ray beam is directed at the TMJ through the orbit.

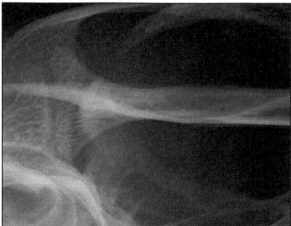

Fig. 10.15 DV oblique radiograph of a feline TMJ. This radiograph was exposed on size 2 sensor. Ideally both TMJs should be visible, but this requires a size 4 film or plate.

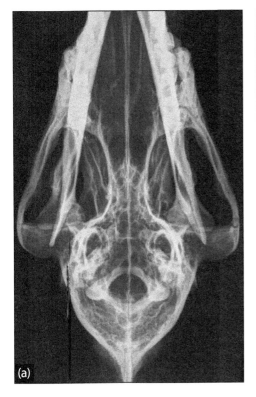

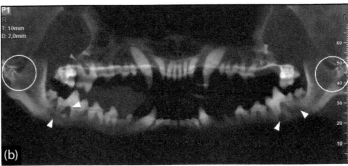

Fig. 10.16 (a) DV oblique radiograph of a canine TMJ.
(b) Panoramic cone-beam CT projection of the dog showing
both TMJs in lateral view (circles). There are additional
pathologies in the maxilla (blue arrowheads) and mandible (white
arrowheads). Note that teeth 306, 311, 406, and 411 are missing.
(Courtesy Dr Nicolas Girard.)

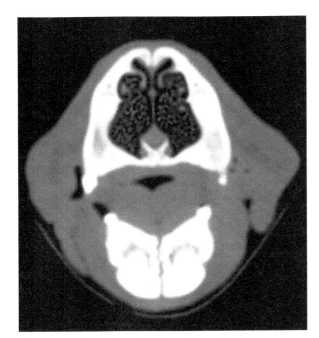

Fig. 10.17 Example of 3D imaging of the
mandibular symphysis, which provides the most
accurate evaluation.

CLINICAL CONDITIONS AFFECTING THE TEMPOROMANDIBULAR JOINT

Trauma

- **TMJ subluxation**. Appears as a widened joint space, but without dislocation of the jaws (**Figure 10.20**).
- **TMJ luxation**. Luxation is the result of separation of the condylar process from the articular surface of the temporal bone and mandibular fossae.[7] Rostrodorsal luxation is the most common presentation (**Figures 10.21, 10.22**). Caudal luxation is almost always associated with fracture of the retroarticular process (**Figure 10.23**).[8] Clinically, unilateral rostral TMJ luxation results in a shift of the rostral mandible in a contralateral direction to the affected side. Caudal unilateral luxation causes a shift of the mandible in the same direction as the affected side (**Figure 10.24**). It is therefore important to obtain diagnostic views of both TMJs.

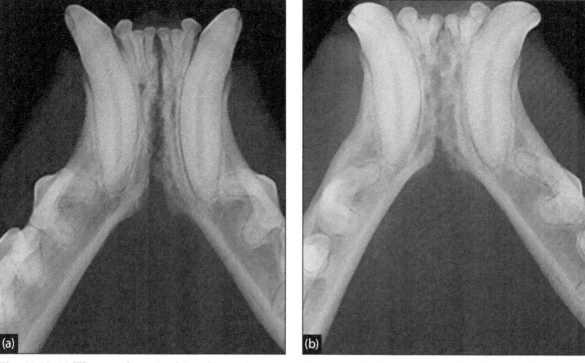

Fig. 10.18 (a) The x-ray beam in this radiograph is perpendicular to the hypothetical axis of the symphysis. (b) In this radiograph the symphyseal space is not visible.

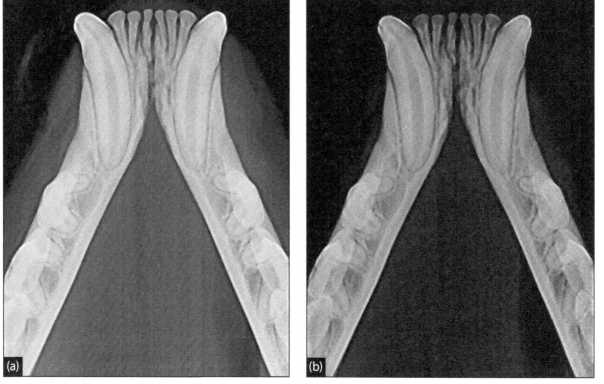

Fig. 10.19 Radiographs of the symphyseal structure with (a) slight underexposure (lighter) and (b) increased exposure (darker).

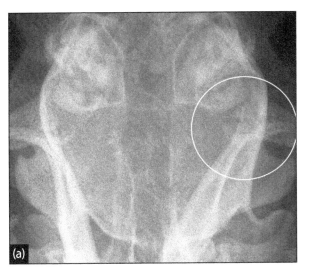

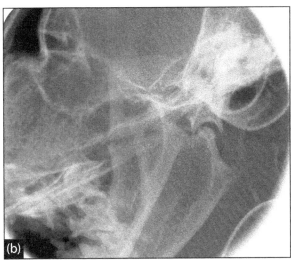

Fig. 10.20 TMJ subluxation. Although these radiographs are not symmetrical, the joint space on one side is widened in both the DV view (a, circle) and the lateral oblique view (b).

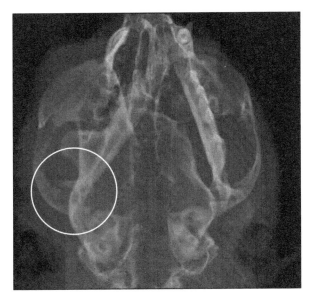

Fig. 10.21 Extraoral DV view of the entire head revealing rostral luxation of the right TMJ (circle).

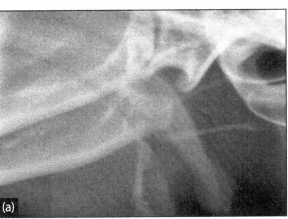

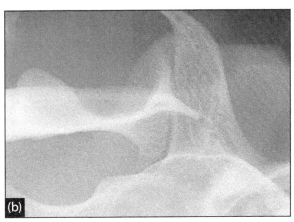

Fig. 10.22 Rostrodorsal luxation of the right TMJ. (a) Extraoral lateral oblique view; (b) DV view.

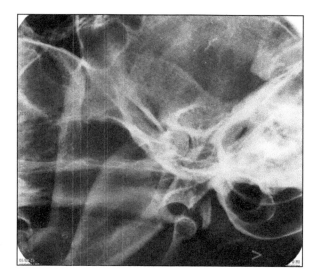

Fig. 10.23 **Caudoventral luxation of the TMJ with fracture of the retroarticular process.**

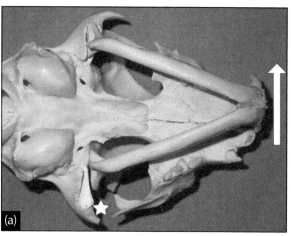 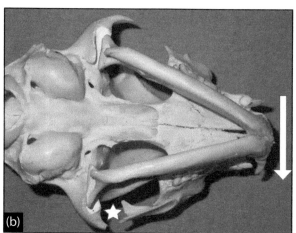

Fig. 10.24 **(a) Pathologic shift of the mandible caused by rostrodorsal TMJ luxation. Star, affected TMJ; arrow, direction of the mandibular shift. (b) Pathologic shift of the mandible caused by ventrocaudal TMJ luxation. Star, affected TMJ; arrow, direction of the mandibular shift. (From Gawor J (2011) Zwichnięcie stawu skroniowo-żuchwowego u kotów. Rozpoznanie i leczenie. [Feline temporomandibular joint luxation. Diagnosis and management.]** *Weterynaria w Praktyce* **11-12:34–39, with permission.)**

- **Lateral displacement of the coronoid process.** This condition is not directly linked to TMJ pathology; however, there are two reasons for placing this problem in the TMJ and symphysis chapter. First, it affects the TMJ, and secondly the excessive symphyseal laxity has been mentioned as a possible factor in open mouth jaw locking syndrome (**Figure 10.25**).[9]
- **Fractures.** Periarticular and intra-articular (**Figures 10.26–10.28**).

Inflammatory and dysplastic conditions
- **Osteoarthritis (OA).** Although OA is the most common disease of the TMJ in dogs and the second most common in cats, it is accepted that this is typically secondary to TMJ dysplasia, trauma, or sporadically unilateral mandibulectomy.[10] Characteristic radiographic changes of TMJ OA are joint space narrowing, ankylosis, periarticular new bone formation, and subchondral bone sclerosis or lysis (**Figure 10.29**).[2]

Fig. 10.25 Lateral displacement of the coronoid process in a dog.

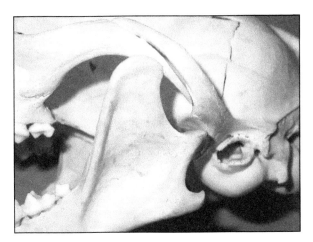

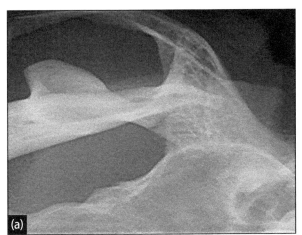

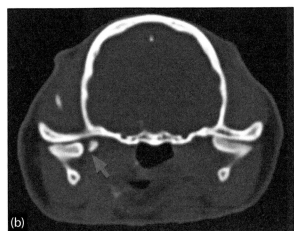

Fig. 10.26 Intra-articular fracture of the condylar process on a standard skull radiograph (a) and a CT scan (arrow) (b).

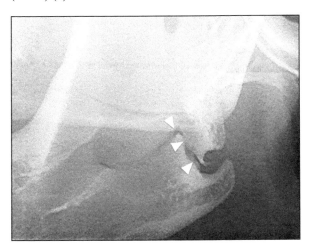

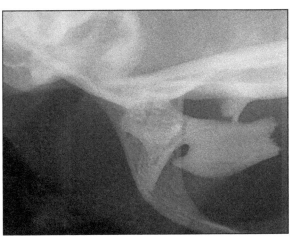

Fig. 10.27 Fracture of the condylar process (arrowheads). This condition appears clinically similar to rostrodorsal luxation.

Fig. 10.28 Fracture of the mandibular coronoid process. This condition appears clinically similar to caudoventral luxation.

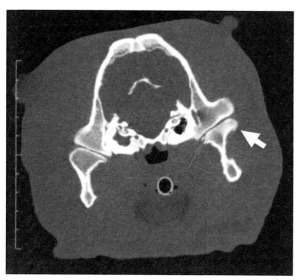

Fig. 10.29 Features of osteoarthritis of the left TMJ. Note the uneven articular surface (red arrow) and the periosteal reaction (white arrow). The patient (a French bulldog) had pain on opening the jaws.

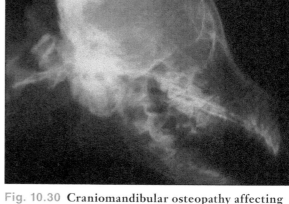

Fig. 10.30 Craniomandibular osteopathy affecting the area of the TMJ in a West Highland white terrier puppy.

- **Craniomandibular osteopathy**. This condition is described in Chapter 8, Part G and **Figure 10.30**.
- **Ankylosis**. This condition has been described as a pseudoankylosis caused by extracapsular changes, which is reflected in the limited mobility of the joint. True TMJ ankylosis is caused by intracapsular lesions and results in bony union of the joint surfaces. Many different conditions, such as trauma, inflammation, infections, degenerative diseases, or cancer, were misdiagnosed as ankylosis prior to advanced diagnostic techniques (**Figure 10.31**).
- **TMJ dysplasia**. This complex problem is associated with open jaw locking syndrome in Basset hounds, Irish setters, Weimaraners, Akitas, and Shiba Inus. Breed predilection to

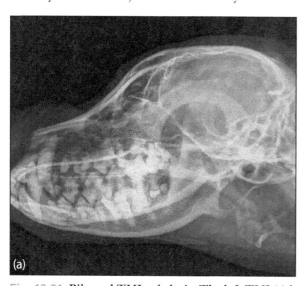

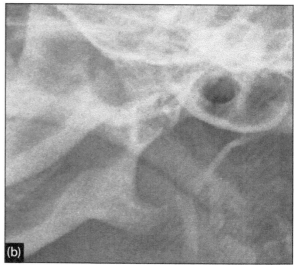

Fig. 10.31 Bilateral TMJ ankylosis. The left TMJ (a) has a narrowed and invisible articular space, even with magnification (b).

(Continued)

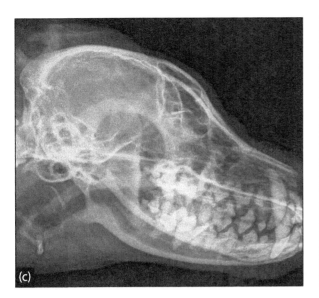

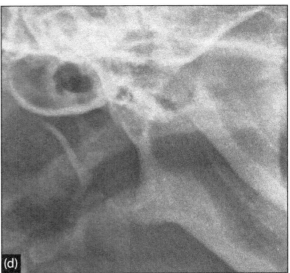

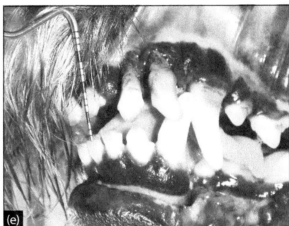

Fig. 10.31 *(Continued)* **Bilateral TMJ ankylosis. The right TMJ in the same patient (c) and its magnification (d). The dog clinically could only open its jaws 4 mm (distance measured from the tip of the crown of 301 to the tip of the crown of 201) (e).**

TMJ dysplasia is also reported in American cocker spaniels, Cavalier King Charles spaniels, and Labrador retrievers.[11,13] Jaw locking syndrome has been reported in cats (Persians were predominant). It may suggest that brachycephalism can be a predisposing factor in cats.[10] The most common sign of TMJ disease is problems with or inability to open the jaws (**Figure 10.32**).

Neoplasms

Tumors near and within the TMJ affect the function and comfort of the patient. Pain and problems with jaw opening are the first symptoms. The radiographic characteristics are discussed in Chapter 8, Part G and in **Figures 10.33, 10.34**.

CLINICAL CONDITIONS AFFECTING THE MANDIBULAR SYMPHYSIS

Dogs and cats have two mandibles (right and left), which are joined at the symphysis. The symphysis is a synarthrosis, which is defined as "a form of articulation in which the bony elements are united by continuous intervening fibrous tissue". In Nomina Anatomica Veterinaria (2005) this structure is called articulate intermandibularis or intermandibular suture (sutura intermandibularis).[12] Between the rostral ends of the two mandibles, there is a plate of fibrocartilagenous tissue. This tissue is radiolucent, therefore radiographs of the rostral mandible in dogs and cats with an intact symphysis will always have a lucent line running down the midline.

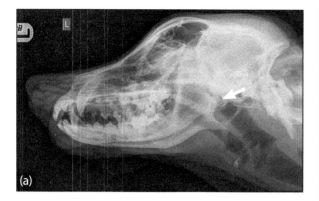

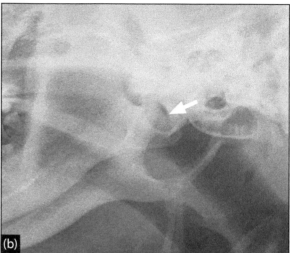

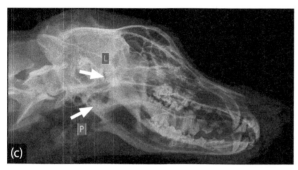

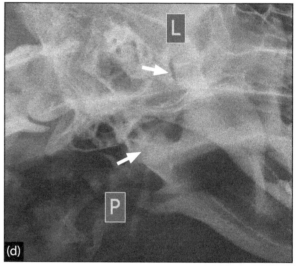

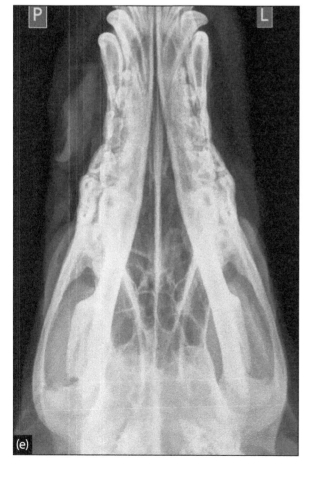

Fig. 10.32 TMJ bilateral dysplasia in 9-month-old Irish setter. Note the visible imperfect condylar surface and the uneven articular space of both TMJs: left (a, b) and right (c, d) sides. DV view (e). The patient had clinically abnormal lateral shifts of the mandibles.

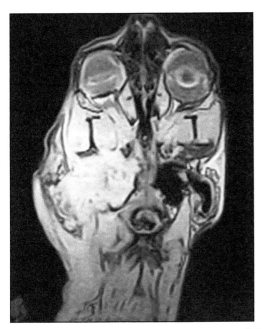

Fig. 10.33 **MR image of a cat showing a tumor of the right tympanic bullae affecting the right TMJ. The patient could not open his mouth.**

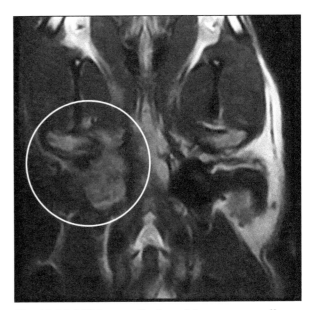

Fig. 10.34 **MR image of a dog with squamous cell carcinoma in the right tympanic bullae, which is very slightly affecting the caudal part of the right TMJ (circle). The patient evidenced pain while yawning.**

A single, large, fibrocartilage pad lies between and is anchored to the smooth areas of the symphyseal plates. The pad has its greatest dorsoventral height in the rostral part of the joint. The fibrocartilagenous pad is typically cuneiform in coronal section, being wider above than below. In cats, the pad is asymmetrical.[6]

In large, young healthy dogs, the symphysis is a narrow firm union with virtually no mobility between the two mandibles. In smaller dogs, especially the brachycephalic breeds, the symphysis is normally quite wide and will have varying degrees of mobility.

The symphysis area undergoes changes with age and is under the continued influence of forces of mastication and many other processes acting in this area. Conditions such as trauma, inflammation, resorption, infection, or proliferation can change the radiographic appearance of the symphysis. This influence may lead to a slight or even complete change of shape, length, and radiodensity of the intermandibular space as well as affect its mobility, which was reported in cats.[13]

Trauma

Separation of the symphysis and parasymphyseal fracture are the most common injuries in the feline mandible and the second most common in canines.[14] Occasionally, this separation is precisely at the area of the fibrocartilage pad, but perisymphyseal fractures may also occur. These can be less stable than symphyseal separation and require additional fixation to obtain stability (**Figures 10.35, 10.36**).

Periodontal disease or tooth resorption of mandibular incisors and canines

In cats with healthy teeth and periodontium, the symphysis often looks wider and more regular (**Figure 10.37**). Old cats with incisors or mandibular canines affected by resorption or periodontal disease have a narrower symphysis with rough surfaces (**Figures 10.38, 10.39**).[15] Occasionally, the space is barely visible or even completely invisible (**Figure 10.40**). In dogs with severe periodontal disease, the typical appearance is alveolar bone loss, which can be very significant and weaken the area, predisposing to pathologic fracture (**Figures 10.41, 10.42**).

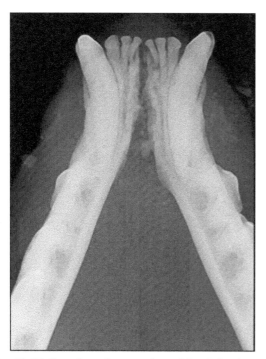

Fig. 10.35 **Symphyseal separation with minimal dislocation of the mandibles in a cat.**

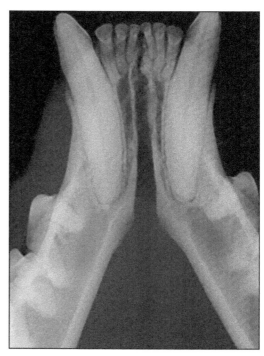

Fig. 10.37 **Radiograph showing a wide symphysis with an irregular surface in a cat with healthy teeth and periodontium.**

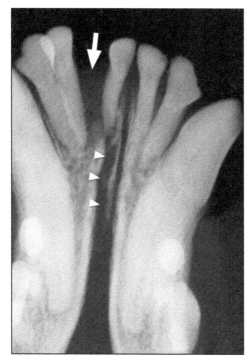

Fig. 10.36 **Symphyseal separation with parasymphyseal fracture (arrowheads) of the right rostral mandible. Note the missing left incisor (arrow).**

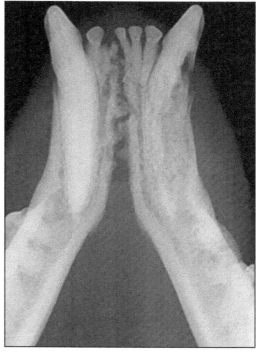

Fig. 10.38 **Irregular symphyseal surface in a cat with fractured incisors and a left mandibular canine (304) with a type 2 tooth resorption.**

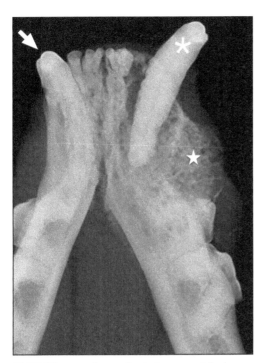

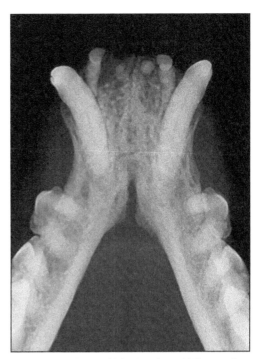

Fig. 10.39 Narrowed symphysis in a cat with the left mandibular canine (304) affected by periodontal disease and type 1 tooth resorption (TR) (asterisk), histopathologically confirmed osteomyelitis (star), and a type 2 TR on the right mandibular canine (404) (arrow).

Fig. 10.40 Fused mandibles in the middle portion of the symphysis in a cat with clinically present chronic stomatitis.

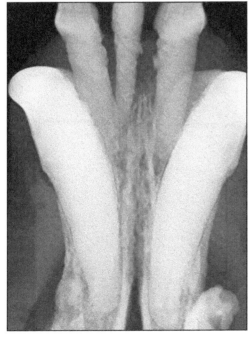

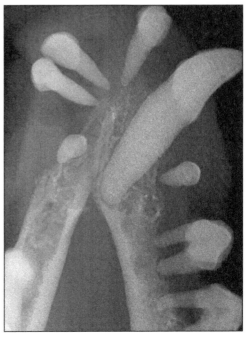

Fig. 10.41 Alveolar bone loss in a Yorkshire terrier causing loss of space in the rostral portion of symphysis.

Fig. 10.42 Radiograph showing severe periodontal disease with almost complete alveolar bone loss weakening the symphyseal area.

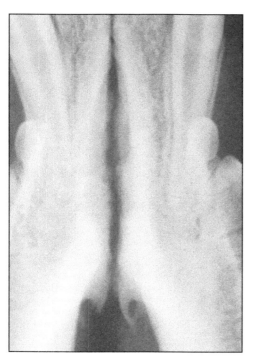

Fig. 10.43 Radiograph of a 10-month-old West Highland white terrier with craniomandibular osteopathy, showing periosteal reaction of the mandible.

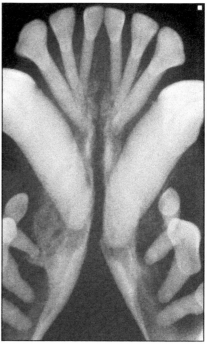

Fig. 10.44 Renal secondary hyperparathyroidism associated with renal insufficiency affecting a 10-year-old dog. Demineralization of the alveolar bone and widening of symphysis is visible. (Courtesy Dr Brook Niemiec.)

Metabolic and inflammatory diseases affecting the symphyseal area

- **Craniomandibular osteopathy (CMO).** CMO creates a massive periosteal reaction, which makes the symphyseal space narrower as the adjacent cortical bone proliferates. It can also compromise the mobility of the symphysis (**Figure 10.43**).
- **Hyperparathyroidism**. Appears as severely demineralized bone, and in these cases the symphyseal space appears widened (**Figure 10.44**).

Neoplasms

Some neoplasms are destructive to adjacent bone; however, others are not. Nondestructive lesions do not normally change the position of the symphysis. Because there are blood vessel anastomoses coming through the symphysis, even perisymphyseal lesions can easily be transmitted to the contralateral mandible (**Figures 10.45–10.47**).[6]

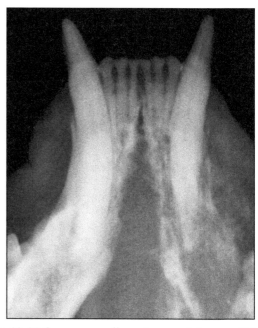

Fig. 10.45 Squamous cell carcinoma of the mandibles in a cat. The bony reaction affecting the left mandible is severe and has crossed the midline to affect the right mandible. The radiograph is elongated to obtain a more accurate picture of the distal part of the symphysis.

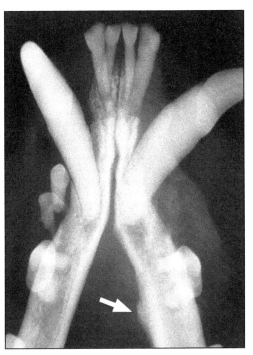

Fig. 10.46 **Histopathologically confirmed fibroma in the left rostral mandible. There is visible alveolar bone loss associated with periodontal disease, which may have been accelerated by the tumor, as well as a small area of periosteal new bone formation (arrow).**

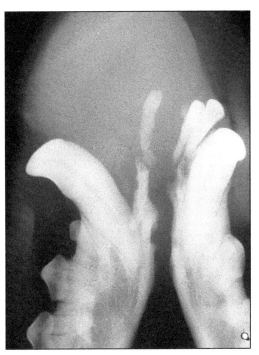

Fig. 10.47 **Fibrosarcoma causing severe bone loss and enlargement of the symphyseal area.**

Other conditions

Missing teeth, supernumerary teeth, as well as other breed specific conditions can result in symphyseal changes. The number of mandibular incisor teeth can change the shape, location, and direction of the symphysis. However, this does not seem to affect its mobility or functionality (**Figures 10.48, 10.49**).[15] In brachycephalic breeds, the symphysis is wide and loose and is assumed to be a predisposing factor to jaw lock syndrome, as it has been suggested that a certain degree of mobility in symphysis is required for the open jaw locking (**Figures 10.50, 10.51**).[11]

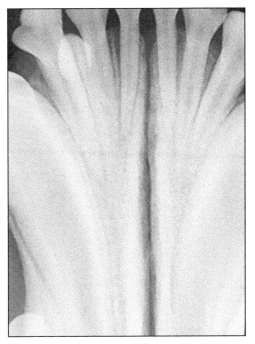

Fig. 10.48 **Supernumerary right mandibular second incisor causing slight change of symphyseal shape in its rostral portion.**

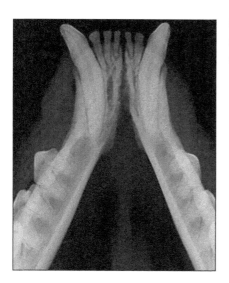

Fig. 10.49 Missing left mandibular third incisor causing slight change of symphyseal shape.

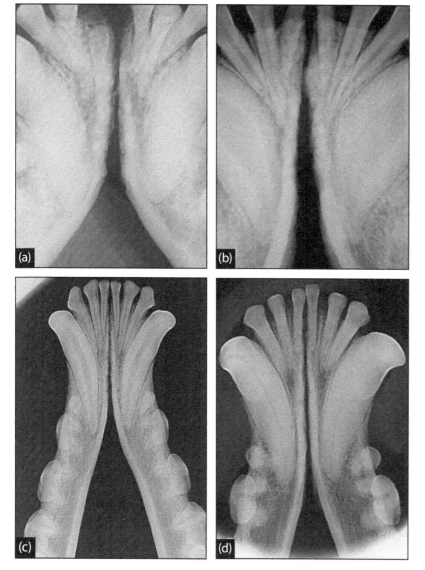

Fig. 10.50 Characteristic shorter symphysis in a pug (a) and an even shorter and wider symphysis in an English bulldog (b). For comparison, the symphysis in a dolichocephalic dog (c) and a mesocephalic dog (d).

REFERENCES

1 Lantz GC, Verstraete FJM (2012) Fractures and luxations involving the temporomandibular joint. In: *Oral and Maxillofacial Surgery in Dogs and Cats*. (eds. FJM Verstraete, M Lommer) Saunders Elsevier, St. Louis, pp. 321–332.

2 Arzi B, Cissel D, Verstreate F *et al.* (2013) Computed tomographic findings in dogs and cats with temporomandibular joint disorders: 58 cases. *J Am Vet Med Assoc* **242(1)**:69–75.

3 Soukup J, Snyder C, Gengler W (2009) Computed tomography and partial coronoidectomy for open mouth jaw locking in two cats. *J Vet Dent* **26(4):** 226–233.

4 Eubanks D (2013) Advanced imaging of the temporomandibular joint and other oral structures. *J Vet Dent* **30(3)**:180–182.

5 Morgan JP, Doval J, Samii V (1998) Head. In: Radiographic Techniques: The Dog. Schlutersche, Hanover, pp. 53–72.

6 Scapino R (1981) Morphological investigation into functions of the jaw symphysis in carnivorans. *J Morphol* **167(3)**:339–376.

7 Taney K, Smith M (2010) Problems with muscles, bones and joints. In: *Small Animal Dental, Oral and Maxillofacial Disease: A Color Handbook*. (ed. BA Niemiec) Manson Publishing, London, pp. 199–224.

8 Verstraete FJM (2003) Maxillofacial fractures. In: *Textbook of Small Animal Surgery*. (ed. D Slatter) WB Saunders, Philadelphia, pp. 2190–2207.

9 Reiter A (2004) Symphysiotomy, symphysiectomy, and intermandibular arthrodesis in a cat with open mouth jaw locking: case report and literature review. *J Vet Dent* **21(3)**:147–158.

10 Legendre L (2008) Diagnosis and treatment of temporomandibular joint problems. *Proceedings of 17th European Congress Veterinary Dentistry*, Uppsala, pp. 81–83.

11 Gatineau M, El-Warrack AO, Maretta SM *et al.* (2008) Locked jaw syndrome in dogs and cats: 37 cases. *J Vet Dent* **25(1)**:16–22.

12 Evans HE, de Lahunta A (2013) Skull. In: *Miller's Anatomy of the Dog*, 4th edn. Elsevier, St. Louis, p. 112.

13 Gawor JP, Czopowicz M, Jank M *et al.* (2015) Mandibular symphysis in cats. Radiographic appearance and mobility. *Proceedings of World Veterinary Dental Congress*, Monterey. http://vdf2015. conferencespot.org

14 Lopes FM, Gioso MA, Ferro D *et al.* (2005) Oral fractures in dogs of Brazil: a retrospective study. *J Vet Dent* **22(2)**:86–90.

15 Gawor J (2013) Symphysis mandible radiographic appearance in different conditions. *Proceedings of 22nd European Congress Veterinary Dentistry*, Prague, pp. 121–122.

CHAPTER 11

RADIOGRAPHY IN PET RABBITS, FERRETS, AND RODENTS

PART A

RABBITS

Vladimír Jekl

INTRODUCTION

Oral and dental pathology is one of the most common disorders encountered in rabbits.[1-3] An ability to recognize anatomic and physiologic variations is necessary in order to understand disease pathophysiology and assess minor changes. This is particularly important when dealing with diseases of the oral cavity and helps ensure optimal treatment of common conditions. Proper oral cavity examination and accurate diagnosis are the keys to appropriate treatment planning and prognosis. For an exact diagnosis and proper therapy, a combination of a thorough oral cavity examination under general anesthesia (**Figures A11.1–A11.4**) and skull/dental radiography and/or computed tomography (CT) is recommended.[4] Without a clear understanding of the normal structures, interpretation of radiographs of the maxillary teeth can be difficult due to the superimposition of other bony structures of the skull.

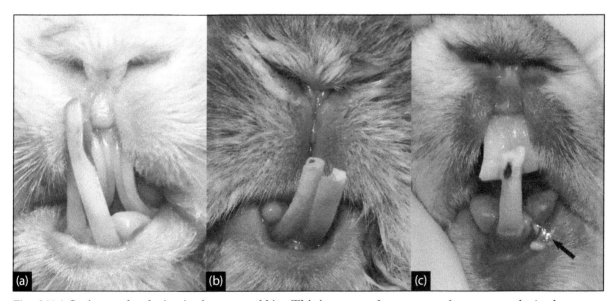

Fig. A11.1 **Incisor malocclusion in three pet rabbits. This is commonly seen secondary to premolar/molar malocclusion (a), but it can also be associated with the use of improper tools for clinical crown height correction (e.g. nail trimmers, scissors [b, c]). Commonly encountered pathologies associated with this condition are clinical crown elongation (a–c), tooth dislocation (a, c), enamel/tooth fractures, damage of the germinative tooth center, pulp exposure (b), and odontogenic abscess formation (c, pus is coming from the alveolar socket of the mandibular left incisor, arrow).**

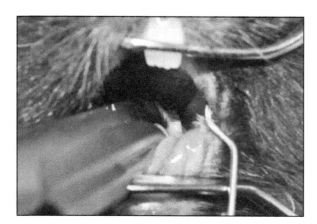

Fig. A11.2 Cheek teeth malocclusion in a 3-year-old rabbit. Note the spike formation on the lingual aspect of the mandibular left first molar.

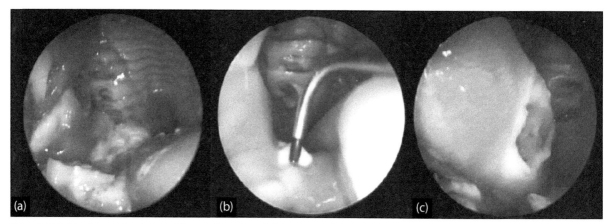

(a) (b) (c)

Fig. A11.3 Endoscopic views of the oral cavity of three pet rabbits showing purulent material in the oral cavity (a), probing of the periodontal space of the mandibular right third premolar (b), and the presence of sharp spikes on the mandibular first molar causing tongue ulceration (c).

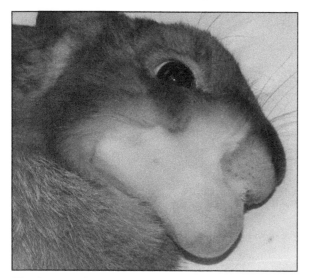

Fig. A11.4 Odontogenic abscess in a 4-year-old rabbit associated with periapical abscessation of the mandibular right third and fourth premolars.

Pet rabbits (*Oryctolagus cuniculus*) belong to the family Leporidae of the order Lagomorpha. They are strictly herbivorous mammals with a highly specialized digestive tract.

ANATOMY

The rabbit skull, excluding the mandible, is an elongated structure that is approximately twice as long as it is wide and three times as long as it is high (**Figures A11.5–A11.7**). The brain is situated within the caudal third. The orbits take up the middle third and almost half its volume, and the nasal chambers occupy the rostral third.[5] The craniotemporal region is composed of occipital bone (sometimes divided into the supraoccipital, exoccipital, and basioccipital regions), basisphenoid, temporal, and parietal bone. The lateral

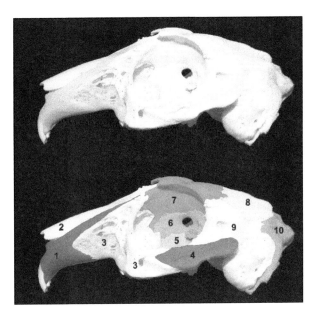

Fig. A11.5 **Skull anatomy: lateral view.** 1, incisive bone; 2, nasal bone; 3, maxilla; 4, zygomatic bone; 5, palatine bone; 6, presphenoid bone; 7, frontal bone; 8, parietal bone; 9, temporal bone; 10, occipital bone.

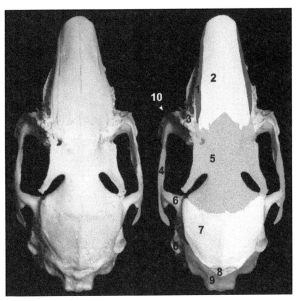

Fig. A11.6 **Skull anatomy: DV view.** 1, incisive bone; 2, nasal bone; 3, maxilla; 4, zygomatic bone; 5, frontal bone; 6, tympanic bone; 7, parietal bone; 8, interparietal bone; 9, occipital bone; 10, tuber faciale.

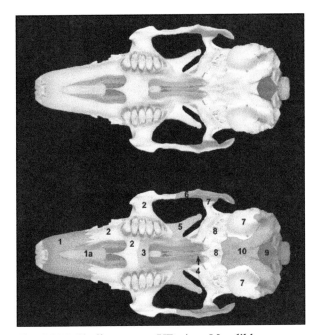

Fig. A11.7 **Skull anatomy: VD view. Mandible was removed for illustrative purposes.** 1, incisive bone; 1a, palatinal process; 2, maxilla; 3, palatine bone; 4, presphenoid bone; 5, frontal bone; 6, zygomatic bone; 7, temporal bone; 8, basisphenoid; 9, foramen magnum; 10, occipital bone.

margins of both exoccipitals extend ventrally into prominent jugular processes. These processes are in close proximity to the tympanic bullae, which are formed by the temporal bones. The deep condyloid fossa is situated between the occipital condyle and the jugular process. It shows a double hypoglossal canal. The frontal segment of the cranium is formed by the presphenoid, orbitosphenoid, and frontal bones. The frontal bones extend bilaterally and taper anteriorly where they meet to form an inverted V-shape between the two nasal bones (**Figure A11.6**).[6]

The nasal bones are notched rostrally and form the dorsal boundary of the osseous nasal apertures. The nasal cavity is divided into symmetrical halves by a vertical cartilaginous nasal septum. Thin extensions of the nasal, maxillary, and ethmoid bones in the nasal passages constitute the dorsal turbinate, ventral turbinate, and ethmoturbinate, respectively. The small dorsal turbinates form the dorsal nasal concha. The ventral turbinates are bony structures that occupy the rostral portion of the lateral wall of the nasal cavity, forming the ventral nasal concha, while the ethmoturbinates form the middle nasal concha and the ethmoidal conchae. The ethmoid bone is located rostral to the cranial cavity and separates it from the nasal cavity. It is represented by the cribriform plate, a sieve-like bone through which the olfactory nerve fibers pass, and a small perpendicular plate that forms the caudodorsal part of the osseous nasal septum. The lacrimal bones are small bones on the rostral surfaces of the orbit, which extend laterally a little beyond the orbital rim. Each one contains a nasolacrimal canal, which allows passage of the lacrimal duct on either side.

The paired incisive bones form the lateral and ventral wall of the nasal cavity rostral to the maxillary bones, each containing two incisors. Incisive bones have frontal and palatine processes (**Figures A11.5–A11.7**). The latter fuse and form the rostral part of the hard palate. The rostral part of the maxilla is pitted and possesses numerous foramina, which provides its typical radiographic appearance. The caudal half of the maxillary bone bears a maxillary tuber medially and a facial tuber laterally. The former projects into the ventrorostral part of the orbit, while the latter extends caudally into the zygomatic process, which fuses with the zygomatic process of the temporal bone as well as the zygomatic bone to form the zygomatic arch.

Temporomandibular joint

The mandibular condylar process articulates with an articular disk in the articular fossa of the temporal zygomatic process, immediately caudal to the orbit. The cartilaginous and fibrous articular disk divides the synovial joint into two independent compartments, but is not radiographically visible (**Figure A11.8**). The shape of the temporomandibular joint (TMJ) allows considerable lateral movement but very little rostrocaudal movement.

Maxillary and palatine bones

The alveolar process of the ventral portion of the maxillary bone contains the reserve crowns of three premolar and three molar teeth within the alveolar sockets (**Figure A11.9**). The palatine bone has a perpendicular part forming the lateral boundary of the choanae and a horizontal part forming the caudal narrow portion of the hard palate. The greater palatine foramen is localized at the level of the 3rd premolar and the first molar teeth (**Figure A11.10**).

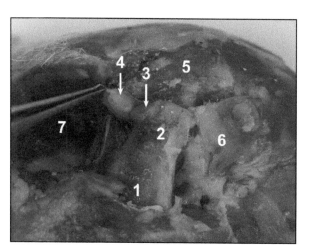

Fig. A11.8 **Anatomy of the rabbit TMJ area: specimen after TMJ luxation. 1, mandibular ramus; 2, condylar process; 3, facies articularis; 4, articular disk; 5, temporal bone; 6, osseous part of the external ear canal; 7, orbit. The mandibular condylar process (2) articulates with an articular disk (4) in the articular fossa of the temporal zygomatic process, immediately caudal to the orbit (7). (Courtesy Michal Kyllar.)**

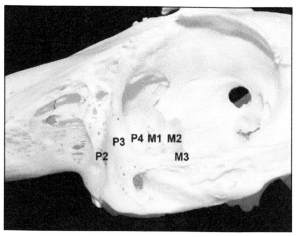

Fig. A11.9 **All maxillary premolars and molars are located in the alveolar process/alveolar bulla. Due to the proximity and relationship of the reserve crown and very thin alveolar bones, periodontal inflammation (periapical abscess) frequently involves surrounding bone and soft tissues.**[2]

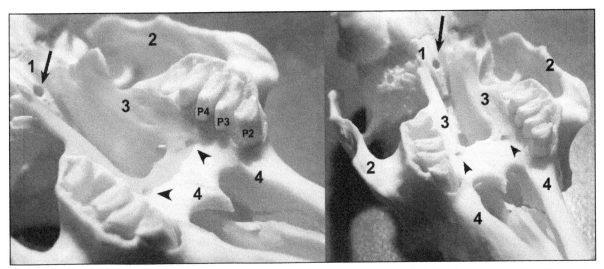

Fig. A11.10 Skull anatomy: VD view of the maxillary and palatine bones. The mandible has been removed for illustrative purposes. The maxillary left first molar and both maxillary third molars are missing. The greater palatine foramina (arrowheads) are localized at the level of the 3rd premolar and the first molar teeth. The large craniopharyngeal canal is located at the ventral aspect (arrow). 1, basisphenoid, 2, zygomatic arch, 3, palatine bone, 4, maxilla.

Mandibles

The mandibles are united rostrally by the cartilaginous mandibular symphysis. The mandibular body is the thick horizontal part that contains alveoli that accommodate the teeth. It is divided into two parts: incisive and premolar/molar. The incisive area forms the symphysis and contains an alveolus each for the paired incisors. The premolar/molar part is continuous caudally with the ramus. It includes five alveoli that hold the two premolar and three molar teeth on each side (**Figure A11.11**). Just caudal to the last molar is a large retroalveolar foramen, which passes from the dorsolateral margin to the medial side of the mandible (**Figure A11.11**). The ramus is a thin and flat expanded bony plate for the attachment of masticatory muscles.[6] The ramus contains the condylar process as a caudodorsal protuberance for articulation with the condylar fossa of the zygomatic process of the temporal bone. The mandibular condylar process is positioned dorsally on the ramus, above the occlusal line. Just rostral to the condylar process is the shallow mandibular notch demarcating the condyloid process from the short, blunt coronoid process. The caudoventral margin of the ramus is rounded and angles dorsally to form the angular process. The canine teeth are absent, resulting in a large gap between the incisors and premolars,

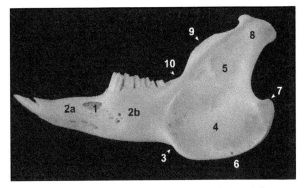

Fig. A11.11 Mandibular anatomy: lateral view. The mandible contains alveoli for the incisor, two premolar, and three molar teeth. 1, mental foramen; 2a, incisive and 2b, premolar/molar parts of the mandibular body; 3, incisura vasorum facialium (facial notch); 4, masseteric fossa; 5, mandibular ramus; 6 mandibular angulus; 7, angular process; 8, condylar process; 9, coronoid process; 10, retroalveolar foramen.

known as the interalveolar margin or diastema. The mandibular foramen is present on the medial surface caudoventral to the last molar tooth, while the mental foramen is situated on the body just craniolateral to the first premolar. The hyoid bone in the rabbit is formed of the body (or basihyoideum) and lingual process as well as the paired greater and lesser cornua.

RABBIT DENTITION

Rabbits have diphyodont and heterodont dentition. Deciduous maxillary incisors may be present up to 14 days of age, but most commonly they are shed *in utero*. Deciduous cheek teeth have short crowns and are shed during the first few days of life. The permanent dentition is present from 35 days of age[7] and there is a total of 28 teeth (*Tables A11.1, A11.2*, **Figure A11.12**). As is true for all true herbivores, the natural diet of rabbits tends to have a low energy content requiring the intake of large quantities of food, which results in constant grinding of the vegetation and rapid wear of the premolars and molars.[8] As a result, all teeth are elodont, aradicular, and hypsodont (i.e. erupting throughout life with high crowns and no true roots). Two studies revealed that tooth eruption and wear rates are variable depending on the type of diet.[9,10] The growth rate of the incisors is 2.0–4.0 mm/week and 1.4–3.2 mm/week for the cheek teeth.[10] Feeding whole hay, which needs more gnawing compared with pellets, creates increased incisor wear, whereas this does not appear to be the case for cheek teeth.

Rabbits have two pairs of maxillary incisors, which are situated in the respective incisive bone, and therefore belong to the mirorder Duplicidentata. Maxillary incisors are C-shaped (i.e. they form a large segment of small circle). The apex/germinal center of the maxillary incisors lie rostral to the first cheek teeth (second premolar). Maxillary incisors, in contrast to those in the mandible, have one longitudinal groove on the labial surface that runs longitudinally along the length of the tooth. Peg teeth are smaller than the major incisors and their apex/germinative centers are localized at about half the length of the major incisor. Peg teeth may be of different size in different breeds, but there is no rule to recognize the breed based on this particular anatomic feature (**Figure A11.13**).

Mandibular incisors are longer than the maxillary incisors and their radius of curvature is larger.

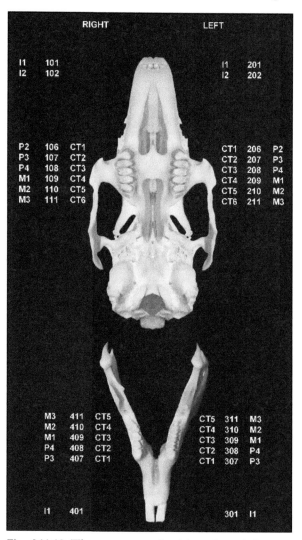

Fig. A11.12 The permanent dentition of an adult rabbit is comprised of incisors (I), premolars (P), and molars (M). Premolars and molars are also called cheek teeth (CT), due to their similarity in form and function. The modified Triadan system is commonly used by veterinary dentists for tooth description.

Table A11.1   Deciduous dentition of the rabbit

	INCISORS	CANINES	PREMOLARS
Upper dental arch	2	0	3
Lower dental arch	1	0	2

Table A11.2   Permanent dentition of the rabbit

	INCISORS	CANINES	PREMOLARS	MOLARS
Upper dental arch	2	0	3	3
Lower dental arch	1	0	2	3

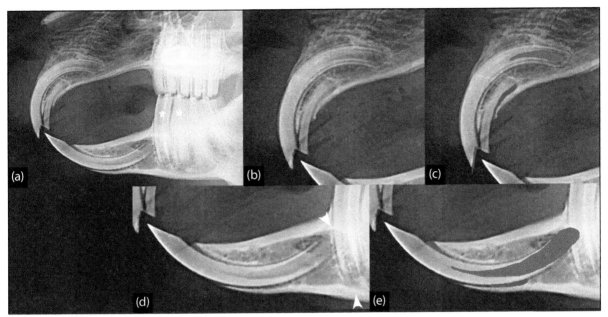

Fig. A11.13 Lateral view of the rostral part of the skull (a) with detailed illustrative evaluation of the maxillary (b, c) and mandibular (d, e) incisors. The apices of all incisors should be rounded (red line, c). The pulpal cavity is more radiolucent than the surrounding dental tissue (red colour, c, e). The occlusal surface of maxillary first incisors is not completely chisel-like, suggesting slight mandibular protrusion due to a disorder of the cheek teeth or TMJ. The periodontal space (blue) is widened on the lingual aspect of the maxillary second and mandibular incisors. This feature is seen when abnormal forces are produced on the mandibular incisor and slight orthodontic tooth movement in a linguolabial direction is seen. The mandibular incisors and cheek teeth are slightly apically elongated (arrowheads). The cheek teeth show slight step-mouth patterns (e.g. clinical crowns of mandibular premolars [asterisks] are slightly higher than mandibular molars). These are features of a mild stage of dental disease.

The apex/germinal center of the mandibular incisors is located linguorostrally to the first mandibular cheek teeth (third premolar). All incisors have one pulp cavity (**Figure A11.13**).

Under normal circumstances, the major incisor teeth wear to a chisel-like shape. This is the result of two separate but connected factors. First, the enamel is thicker on the labial surface than on the lingual/palatal surface and tends to wear more slowly than the rest of the occlusal surface. Additionally, there is active tooth on tooth grinding activity in the rabbit, as during gnawing the mandibular condyle shifts rostrally with rostral mandibular displacement.[5]

Rabbits have no canines and a large diastema separates the rostral part of the oral cavity, which is used for food slicing and biting, from the caudal part which is used for chewing.

Premolars and molars have similar structure in each quadrant of the oral cavity and create a uniform functional grinding unit – in horses this is known as the 'cheek tooth battery'. In English literature they are commonly known as 'cheek teeth'. The cheek teeth in each jaw are in close contact and surrounded by thin alveolar bone. Both maxillary and mandibular teeth are arranged in a straight line, with the palatal/labial profile of the maxillary dental arch being slightly convex (**Figures A11.7, A11.10**).[11] Each tooth is curvilinear and cylindrical. Enamel is thicker on the lingual aspect of the mandibular cheek teeth and the buccal aspect of the maxillary cheek teeth; this is where the larger enamel ridges are present, which could also imitate spikes. Third molars are usually curved caudally. The apices/germinal centers of mandibular cheek teeth are arranged in a divergent fan-shape, while those of the maxillary cheek teeth are located closer to each other.

All premolars as well as the first and second molars consist of two longitudinal parts (*lamellae dentis*), which are separated by a large groove that is lined by enamel. These two parts are firmly connected with cellular cementum and a buccal enamel bridge in the maxilla and a lingual enamel bridge in the mandible (bilophodonty).[3] For most of the length of the tooth the dentin of each lamina encloses a separate pulp chamber; however, the two chambers merge near the apical/germinative part of the tooth.[12] The pulp cavity extends coronally approximately three-quarters the length of the tooth. Each conical pulp chamber tapers towards the occlusal surface.[8] There is a deep longitudinal fold of enamel in the center of the premolars as well as the first and second molars, which can be seen as a radiopaque line running longitudinally on lateral radiographs of the skull. The last maxillary and mandibular molars have only one pulp chamber and are much smaller than other cheek teeth. The circumference of all teeth is made up of enamel covered by a layer of acellular cementum in which the fibers of the periodontal ligament are embedded.[3]

The occlusal surface (**Figure A11.14**) is made up of layers of dentin, enamel, and cementum of various thickness, which are arranged in transverse occlusal enamel ridges (lophodont dentition).[13] These transverse enamel ridges occlude with the opposite teeth during chewing, and provide an efficient surface for

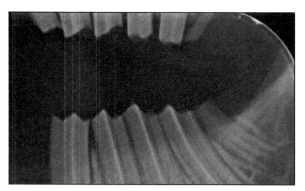

Fig. A11.14 **The occlusal surface is not an even plane, as transverse enamel ridges form a zig-zag pattern. The premolars and molars are grouped as a functional unit with a relatively horizontal occlusal surface with transverse enamel folds (i.e. lophodont teeth). The enamel folds correspond to deep invaginations of the enamel on the palatal side of the maxillary cheek teeth and the buccal side of the mandibular cheek teeth.**

grinding and crushing plant material. This arrangement can be seen on lateral radiographs of the skull as a zig-zag line between the upper and lower cheek teeth.[14]

The mandibular dental arches are narrower than the maxillary arches (anisognathia), therefore the palatal edges of the maxillary cheek teeth oppose the buccal edges of the mandibular cheek teeth.[14]

POSITIONING AND RESTRAINT FOR RADIOGRAPHY OF THE SKULL

Radiography of the head should be performed in all cases of suspected dental or skull disease. An understanding of the anatomy of the skull and teeth structure is crucial. Radiographs can only be obtained with the rabbit under general anesthesia, because even small movements or obliqueness can cause severe anatomic distortion and misinterpretation. It is important that a standard film marking location is established that is known to anyone who might interpret the radiographic images, especially in lateral oblique and intraoral views.

Conventional dorsoventral (DV), right lateral, two lateral oblique, and rostrocaudal (RC) views are usually performed. Digital dental radiographs are also very useful. A combination of intraoral and extraoral views is preferred as this provides the ability to interpret even subtle pathologic changes. If a facial mass is present, a cotton ball or wedge of foam can be used for proper positioning or a ventrodorsal (VD) view should be obtained.

Obtaining a VD view with the patient in dorsal recumbency may impair respiration and therefore rabbits should be repositioned in sternal recumbency as soon as possible. Maintaining patient oxygenation throughout the procedure is essential.

Assessment of the tympanic bullae, TMJs, and teeth is possible using standardized oblique angles. Tympanic bullae are best examined using DV and left/right 40° lateral oblique views. The TMJ is best visualized in a 90° RC view and in 70° and 90° lateral oblique/lateral views.[15,16] The DV, VD, and left lateral views allow evaluation of the relationship between the mandible and maxilla and the integrity of the margins of the mandibles and maxillary bones. Complete symmetry on the radiograph indicates optimal positioning.

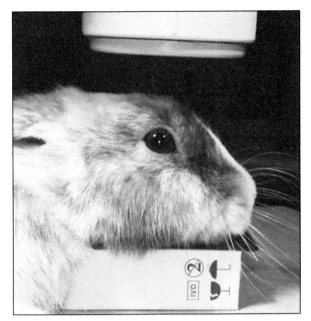

Fig. A11.15 **Positioning of a rabbit for a DV view. For optimal positioning, the head is slightly elevated (in this case with the use of the box for microscope slides).**

RADIOGRAPHIC VIEWS[4]

Dorsoventral and ventrodorsal views

The DV view is preferred over the VD view because respiration may be impaired in rabbits while in dorsal recumbency.[17]

For the DV view, the patient is placed in sternal recumbency with the mandible resting on the cassette or sensor (**Figure A11.15**). The position of the head is maintained by using a small sandbag placed over the dorsal cervical region. Alternatively, a small box can be placed beneath the mandibles to support the head. The pinnae need to be positioned away from the area of interest. The forelimbs are taped cranially or left without any fixation. Exact positioning is achieved by gentle head manipulation, until the incisor interdental space, nasal philtrum, and the middle of the area between the eyes are in a straight line. The x-ray beam is centered on the middle of the line connecting the medial eye canthi. Complete symmetry of structures on the radiograph indicates optimal positioning (**Figures A11.16, A11.17**).

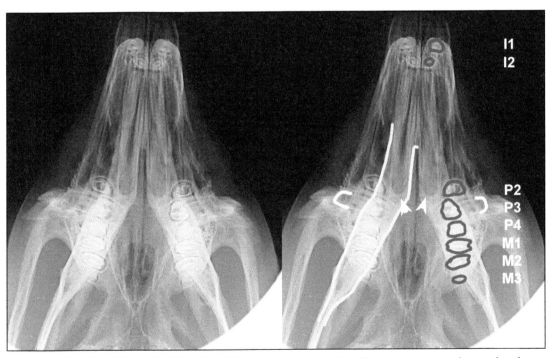

Fig. A11.16 **DV view of an 18-month-old-rabbit with normal dentition. Maxillary incisors, premolars, and molars are seen on the radiograph as ovoid structures surrounded by the radiolucent periodontal apparatus (blue) and radiopaque alveolar bone. Premolars and the first two molars have a central enamel ridge, which is radiopaque and is seen as horizontal line in the middle of the tooth. Apices of the maxillary third premolars are indicated by white lines. The mandibles (yellow line) should be symmetrical and the apices of mandibular incisors (arrowheads) should be visible.**

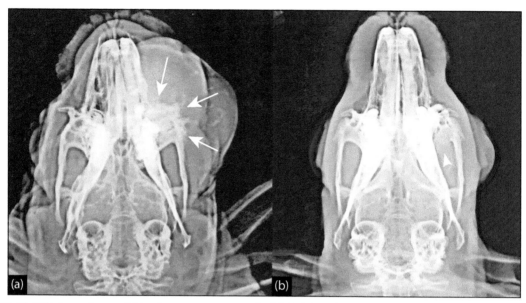

Fig. A11.17 DV view of two rabbits that were presented with left facial swelling. The radiographs reveal extensive lysis of the maxilla and new bone formation (arrows) secondary to third and fourth premolar apical infection and osteomyelitis of the alveolar bulla (a) and maxillary zygomatic process (b, arrowhead). Osteomyelitis of the zygomatic arch can be missed, therefore optimal positioning (assessment of symmetry) and careful radiographic interpretation is crucial. (Courtesy Vladimír Jekl and Karel Hauptman.)

The VD view is performed with the patient in dorsal recumbency. The head is extended and taped or held in place with a bandage with the ventral margins of the mandible parallel to the cassette. Symmetry between the right and left sides should always be evaluated. The x-ray beam is centered on the middle of the line connecting the medial canthus of each eye. If the rostral part of the nasal cavity or the maxillary incisors and premolars needs to be evaluated, the mandible is gently displaced laterally to prevent superimposition over the area of interest.

Rostrocaudal view

The patient is placed in dorsal recumbency with the nose pointing upwards and the long axis of the head perpendicular to the x-ray film. It may be helpful to place the patient in a trough. The head is supported using a wedge of foam or a bandage. The mouth is closed as an open-mouth view does not provide additional information. The forelimbs are positioned parallel to the thorax. The x-ray beam is centered between the eyes (**Figures A11.18, A11.19**).

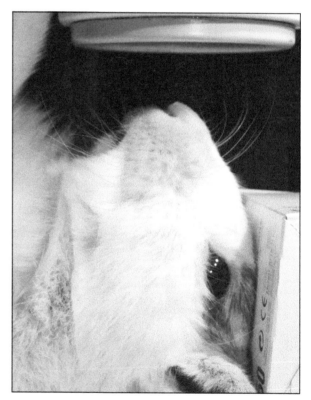

Fig. A11.18 Positioning of a rabbit for a RC view. The x-ray beam is centered between the eyes in the area just dorsal to the nostrils.

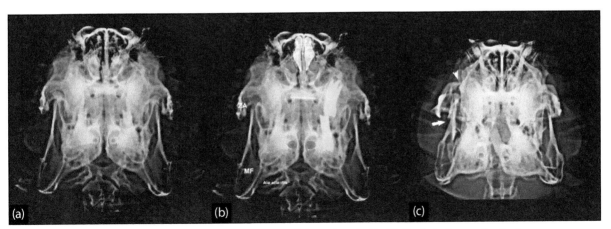

Fig. A11.19 **RC view of a 2 year-old-rabbit with normal dentition (a, b). (b) Red circles, major incisors; green, cheek teeth; yellow line, hard palate; ZA, zygomatic arch. The nasal cavity is divided by the vomer bone into two symmetrical parts. The nasal passages (light blue) are localized medially to the maxillary recess. The TMJ is well visualized on this view (dark blue, condylar processes of the mandible). The mandibular fossa (MF) is a very thin part of the mandible and in some cases, post-processing image adjustments could imitate mandibular decalcification. (c) RC view of a rabbit with multiple fractures of the zygomatic arch (arrowhead) and mandibular ramus (arrow) and mandibular symphysis separation (red).**

Lateral view

The lateral view of the head is performed with the patient in right or left lateral recumbency, depending on the locality of the lesion. If the study is only general screening for dental pathology, the right lateral position is recommended as the standard view (**Figure A11.20**). Cotton wool or a foam wedge can be used to support the nose and keep the head in position. Proper positioning is where the nasal philtrum is parallel to the x-ray film and the rami of the mandibles, tympanic bullae, incisors, and all the bilateral anatomic structures are superimposed on their opposite structures. During inspection, the vertical alignment of the

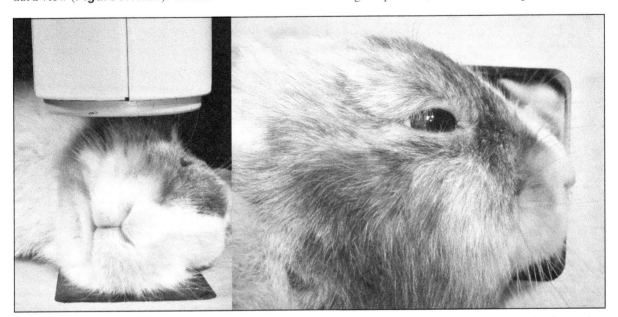

Fig. A11.20 **Positioning of a rabbit for lateral view. The disadvantage of using dental plates for extraoral radiographs is that in larger rabbits, the smaller plate size requires multiple images to allow for whole skull assessment.**

two eyes provides a pair of useful points of orientation, as the globes should be aligned in views from above or from the front. Alternatively, the ventral margins of the two mandibles can be palpated, as the two should be exactly opposite each other.[3] The pinnae and forelimbs must not be superimposed on the area of interest and should be left in their natural position or taped away from the skull. For the assessment of the occlusal surfaces of the premolars and molars, the mouth can be held open slightly by placing a customized syringe body or piece of cork between the incisors. Alternatively, this can be performed with a gauze attached to the incisors, which is taped to the table. The x-ray beam is centered on the medial canthus of the eye. Exact superimposition of the tympanic bullae and mandibles on the final radiograph indicates optimal positioning (**Figures A11.21, A11.22**).

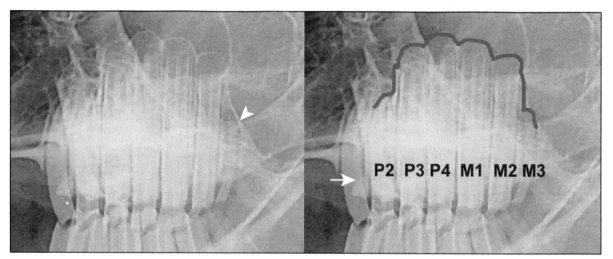

Fig. A11.21 Extraoral lateral view of the alveolar bulla in a 3-month-old rabbit. Improper positioning makes interpretation more problematic. The rabbit was positioned in lateral recumbency; however, the long axis of the head was not positioned parallel to the radiographic plate with the nose very close to the cassette. This is a common artifact. Therefore one premolar (P2, arrow) is visible, which is not superimposed on the contralateral tooth and seven cheek teeth can be counted. Apices of premolars and molars are not elongated; the alveolar bone is of high density and rounded (blue line). Normal apical pulp is visible as a radiolucency between the alveolar bone and enamel folds, which are radiopaque. Note also the slight widening of the periodontal space surrounding the last molar (arrowhead).

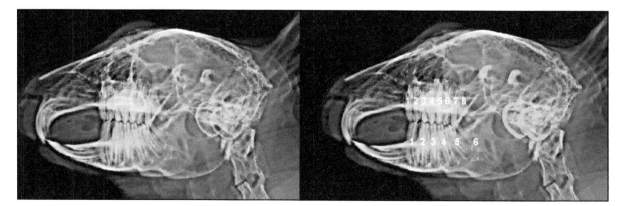

Fig. A11.22 Lateral view of a rabbit with improper positioning, where the nostrils are very close to the sensor/cassette. Due to resulting angulation, a false polyodontia is seen (normal dentition is six cheek teeth in each maxilla and five in each mandible). Tympanic bullae (green color), mandibular coronoid process (yellow color), zygomatic process (blue color), and the ventral margins of the mandibles are not superimposed. (Courtesy Vladimír Jekl.)

Lateral oblique view

For lateral oblique views, the patient is placed in right or left lateral recumbency depending on the part of the head to be imaged (**Figures A11.23, A11.24**). The mouth is closed or held open with an appropriately sized syringe body inserted between the incisors or with a gauze attached to the incisors and taped to the table. A foam wedge can be placed under the mandible to slightly elevate the nose. The head is rotated to an angle of 30–40° or the x-ray tube is adjusted to the desired angle (this is preferred by the author). To minimize image distortion, the rotation should not be excessive. The x-ray beam is centered at the medial canthus of the eye.

Intraoral and extraoral views

Intraoral dental radiography has significant advantages over conventional radiography due to the enhanced image resolution and detail. Small sized dental films or digital sensors can be used for intraoral radiography (20 × 30 mm; 20 × 40 mm; 27 × 54 mm). The use of special rabbit intraoral plates is recommended for mandibular cheek teeth radiography; however, these can only be used in

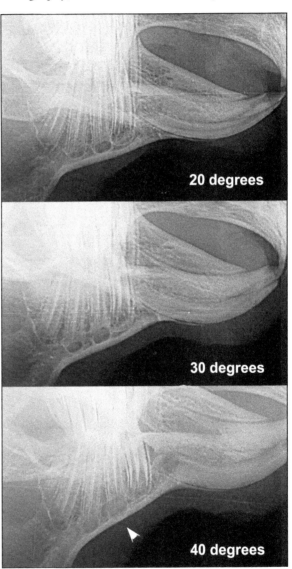

Fig. A11.24 Set of lateral oblique radiographs of the rabbit in Fig. A11.23 taken at different angles. The mandibular reserve crowns and apices are best viewed at an angle of 30–40 degrees. In the 40-degree lateral oblique view, apical elongation of the mandibular fourth premolar can be seen (arrowhead). Opaque horizontal lines going through the radiographs are artifacts, which are caused by errors of reading the plate by the scanner or by fine plate scratches. (Used with permission from Vladimír Jekl.)

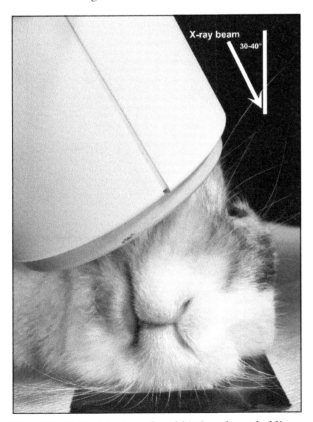

Fig. A11.23 Positioning of a rabbit for a lateral oblique view. The head is positioned in the same manner as for the lateral view, and the x-ray beam angled into the desired position. (Courtesy Vladimír Jekl.)

larger rabbits. Larger films are used for extraoral radiography to achieve proper position and teeth examination (30 × 40 mm; 57 × 76 mm; 57 × 94 mm). Correct film placement within the oral cavity is difficult in rabbits less than 1 kg. However, using small x-ray films or special rabbit intraoral sensors, as well as obtaining additional views, it is possible to evaluate all the incisors, premolars, and molars precisely, even in small rabbits (**Figures A11.25, A11.26**). More radiographs of a particular region are usually needed as not all the teeth fit on the film.[4]

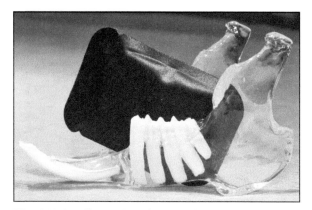

Fig. A11.25 Illustrative photograph of the placement of the radiographic plate/sensor for the intraoral view using the parallel technique.

The parallel technique, which is performed with the rabbit in lateral recumbency, requires that the film and long axis of the tooth are parallel to each other with the x-ray beam directed perpendicularly to both the teeth and x-ray film/sensor. This technique may be used for the assessment of the occlusal surface of the maxillary and mandibular premolars and molars. It is also possible to evaluate the entire crown of mandibular molars by this method.

The bisecting angle technique can be performed with the patient in sternal (**Figures A11.27**) or lateral recumbency. Only the mandibular incisors can be examined with the patient in dorsal recumbency (**Figure A11.28**). The bisecting angle technique overcomes the difficulties of obtaining accurate images of teeth with different shapes and superimposing surrounding structures. In rabbits, it is impossible to place a film parallel to the maxillary incisors, premolars, and molars so the x-ray beam is centered on the area of interest and is placed perpendicular to the bisecting angle, which is the line that bisects the angle created by the long axis of the sensor and the long axis of the tooth (**Figures A11.28–A11.30**).

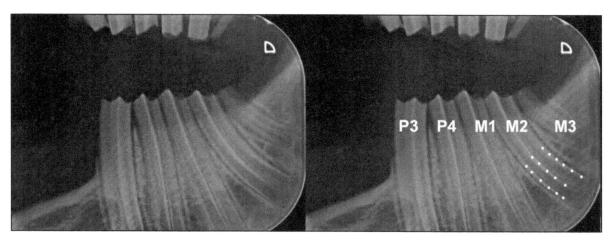

Fig. A11.26 Intraoral view using the parallel technique. With this technique, it is possible to obtain a diagnostic lateral view of the mandible and, to a certain extent, the maxillary premolars and molars. The last two molars can be visualized along with their apices. The apices of the premolars and first molar are not visible, therefore an extraoral oblique view is necessary to asses these anatomic locations. The normal 'zig-zag' occlusal pattern is present. Under normal circumstances, each premolar and molar tooth should have three enamel folds, which are visible as high density parallel lines along the longitudinal tooth axis (dotted lines). Alveolar bone and lamina dura should be visible surrounding all teeth.

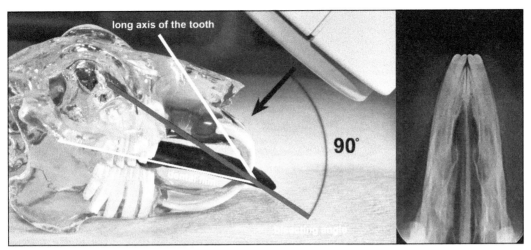

Fig. A11.27 Bisecting angle technique for the maxillary incisors. To use the bisecting angle technique, the x-ray tube is adjusted so that the central beam of the x-ray bisects the angle between the long axis of the film and the tooth. Due to the relatively high curvature and very long reserve crowns of the maxillary incisors, the final image may be foreshortened.

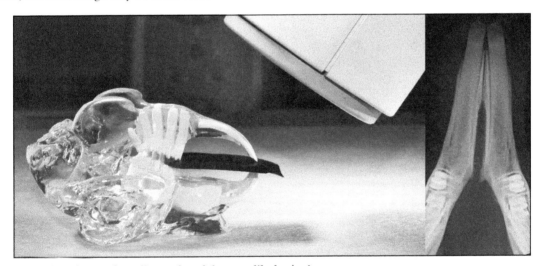

Fig. A11.28 Bisecting angle radiography of the mandibular incisors.

Fig. A11.29 Radiography of the maxillary premolars and molars using the bisecting angle technique. The x-ray beam is directed approximately 45 degrees to the plate.

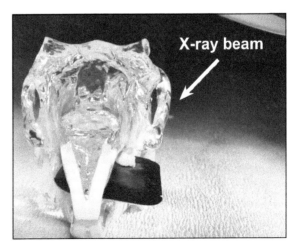

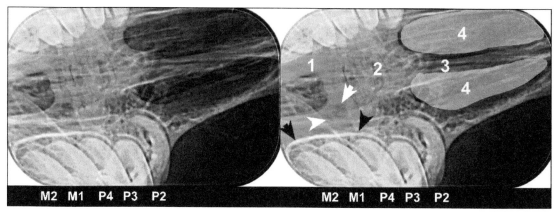

Fig. A11.30 **Radiography of the maxillary premolars and molars using the bisecting angle technique. Even in healthy dentition, the reserve crown of the second premolar can be seen partially distorted due to its larger degree of curvature, which is normal. Black arrowheads indicate the margins of the alveolar bulla. 1, palatine bones with major palatine foramen (white arrowheads); 2, maxilla; 3, vomer; 4, nasal cavity.**

RADIOGRAPHIC INTERPRETATION

Proper interpretation of skull and dental radiographs is based on a sound knowledge of normal anatomy. When assessing the teeth on a radiograph, the following should be evaluated: position, size and shape, contour, internal structure, density, occlusal surface, reserve crown, periodontal space, and alveolar bone.

SPECIFIC ANATOMIC REFERENCE LINES

Böhmer and Crossley (2009)[18] acquired, by comparing prepared skulls with the radiographs of identical animals, specific anatomic reference lines that facilitate the objective assessment of the severity of dental disease. Using these reference lines, the extent of malocclusion in rabbits can be determined more exactly and the results are reproducible by different examiners. These findings can be easily demonstrated to owners (**Figures A11.31, A11.32**). This author finds these reference lines particularly helpful in rabbits with moderate to severe dental disease and for demonstrating dental findings to owners. However, if minor changes are found, it is recommended to obtain different radiographic views and/or use other imaging modalities to more precisely differentiate pathologic lesions.

Various dental pathologies in rabbits are demonstrated in **Figures A11.33–A11.50**.

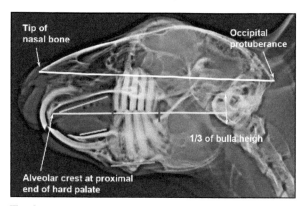

Fig. A11.31 **Lateral view of a rabbit head. In clinically healthy rabbits, no dental structure should extend dorsal to a reference line that connects the proximal end of the nasal bone with the tip of the occipital protuberance on the lateral view Another reference line runs parallel to the one previously mentioned, beginning at the rostral end of the hard palate (yellow line) mostly immediately caudal to the second incisor and extending caudally to pass through the tympanic bulla at approximately one-third of its height. This line matches the occlusal plane in healthy rabbits. The maxillary and mandibular dental arches are approximately the same length (red lines). The apices of the mandibular cheek teeth should not penetrate the ventral mandibular cortex, which should have a near even thickness beneath the first three cheek tooth apices (blue line). Remodeling of the ventral cortex adjacent to the tooth apices indicates that there is retrograde elongation of the mandibular premolars and molars teeth. The palatine and mandibular bone plates should slightly converge rostrally in normal rabbits (green lines), the amount of convergence varying somewhat with breed skull type.[18]**

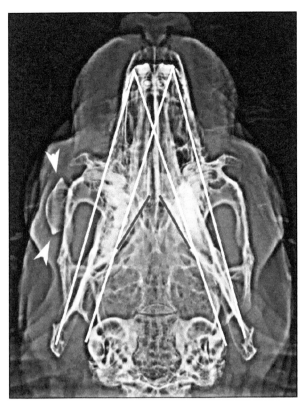

Fig. A11.32 **DV view of a rabbit head. The first anatomic reference line connects the lateral margin of the maxillary first incisor's tip with the medial edge of the mandibular ramus on the same side caudally. Another line, which diverges slightly from the previous one, runs from the lateral border of the tympanic bulla to the lateral rim of the contralateral maxillary incisor. With the exception of the tips of the apices of the significantly curved maxillary third and fourth premolar teeth (see Fig. A11.16), no part of any tooth should be located outside these two lines. The two blue lines indicate the medial cortex of the mandible. This should be almost straight, smooth, and even.**[18] **Note the calcified lens with a hypermature cataract (arrowheads).**

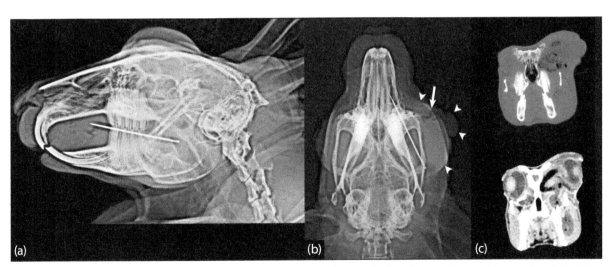

Fig. A11.33 A 5-year-old rabbit with early stage dental disease and a retrobulbar abscess of nonodontogenic origin. Note the presence of a foreign body (sewing needle) stuck in the soft tissue of the cheek (a, lateral view; b, DV view). Note the obvious exophthalmos with soft tissue swelling due to the retrobulbar infection seen on the DV view (b, arrowheads) and axial CT slices (c, bony and soft tissue window, the needle was removed prior to the CT). The arrow in b demonstrates radiolucent areas associated with gas-producing bacterial pathogens. The presence of gas (radiolucent rounded areas) and gas accumulation surrounding the optical nerve is an indication for orbit evisceration. This case demonstrates the importance of performing CT, as the retrobulbar abscess was associated with spreading of the infection from the ventral part of left masseter muscles to the retrobulbar region. (Courtesy Vladimír Jekl and Karel Hauptman.)

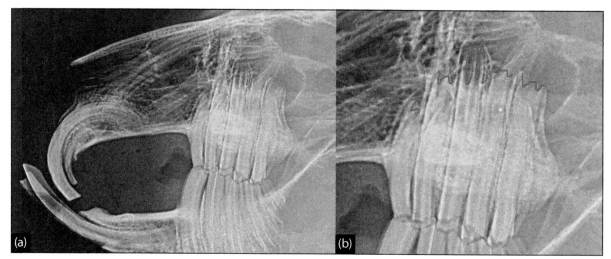

Fig. A11.34 (a) Extraoral lateral view of a 4-year-old rabbit with severe incisor malocclusion as well as apically and coronally elongated cheek teeth. Cheek teeth occlusion is also abnormal. (b) Marked up view of the maxillary cheek teeth reveals the irregular shape of the molars, with barely visible enamel folds. The apices are elongated and apical alveolar bone is not visible due to alveolar bulla 'perforation'. Normal 'germinal centers' have been obliterated. These signs of maxillary premolar and molar apical elongation are easy to interpret, but the reference lines for normoclussion could be also used.[18] (Courtesy Vladimír Jekl and Karel Hauptman.)

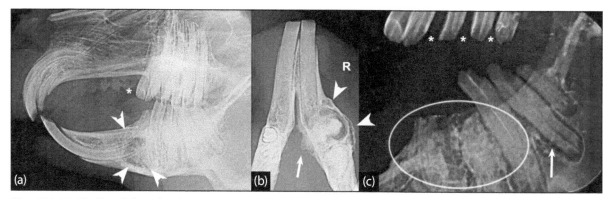

Fig. A11.35 Skull and dental radiography of a 4-year-old rabbit with severe dental disease. (a) Extraoral lateral view. Note the radiolucent area close to the apex of the mandibular incisors and third premolars (arrowheads). Apical elongation of all teeth, loss of normal 'zig-zag' occlusal pattern, and clinical crown elongation of the maxillary second premolars (asterisk) is apparent. (b) Intraoral radiograph of the mandible with the bisecting angle technique. Note the periodontal alveolar bone lysis around the mandibular right third premolar (arrowheads), with loss of normal tooth structure, periosteal reaction from the medial side (arrowheads), and apical tooth elongation (long arrow). The right incisors appear not to be affected. The mandibular left incisor and premolars have normal structure. (c) Complete loss of normal dental structure of both mandibular right premolars (white oval), irregular shape of all the mandibular molars with widening of the periodontal space (arrow). Also note loss of normal 'zig-zag' occlusal pattern and widening of the interdental spaces of the maxillary premolars and molars (asterisks). (Courtesy Vladimír Jekl and Karel Hauptman.)

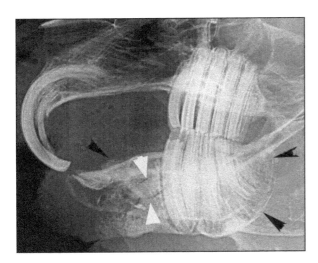

Fig. A11.36 A 6-year-old rabbit with severe dental disease and osteomyelitis associated with improper mandibular incisor extraction. Clinical crowns and the apices of the maxillary incisors and peg teeth are elongated. All the premolars and molars are apically elongated with formation of diastemas. The maxillary premolars and molars also have minimal volume of dental pulp. The white arrowheads indicate the apical part of one partially extracted mandibular incisor with a retained tooth root, which was associated with extensive osteomyelitis. The calcified wall of the abscess is indicated by the black arrows.

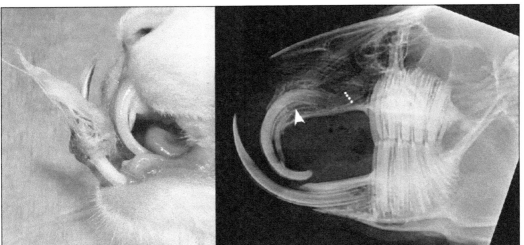

Fig. A11.37 Severe incisor malocclusion in a non-dwarf breed rabbit. Abnormal tooth shape (bending) (arrowhead) on the lateral radiograph suggests a traumatic origin of this lesion. Apical elongation of all the incisors and cheek teeth is also visible. The nasolacrimal duct (lumen indicated with white dots) is widened due to elongation of the maxillary incisor apices.

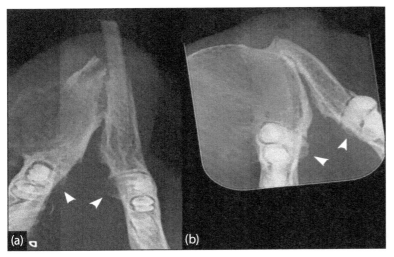

Fig. A11.38 Intraoral mandibular radiographs of two rabbits. A 2-year-old male after unilateral (a) and a 4-year-old female rabbit after bilateral mandibular incisor extraction (b). Intraoral radiography is extremely valuable in cases of incisor postextraction osteomyelitis. In these two cases, the premolars are not affected. The arrowheads indicate apical elongation of the third mandibular premolars and widening of the periodontal spaces. Slight periapical lysis of the above described premolars can also be seen in (b).

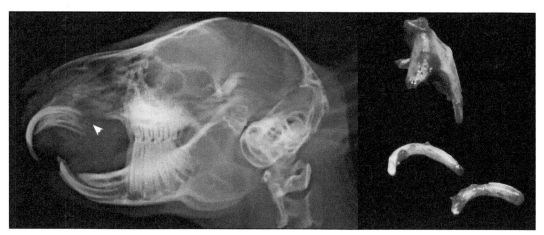

Fig. A11.39 A 6-month-old rabbit with traumatic fracture and dislocation of the incisive bone (arrowhead) and incisors. The incisive bone was surgically excised and all the incisors extracted.

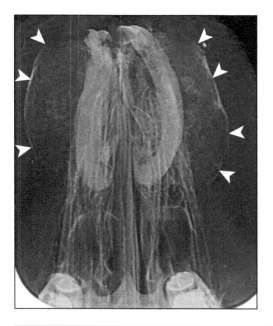

Fig. A11.40 Maxillary osteosarcoma in a 6-year-old rabbit. Note the extensive osteoproliferation (arrowheads) and loss of incisival bone detail.

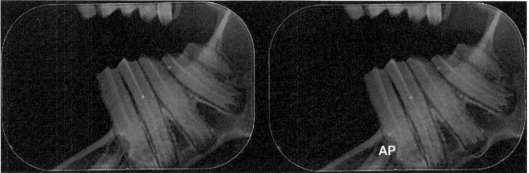

Fig. A11.41 Intraoral view: parallel technique. Dental disease in this 4-year-old rabbit is characterized by an irregular occlusal margin, loss of enamel folds, apical premolar and molar elongation (b, blue line), as well as narrowing of pulp cavities (b, red line). The apical part of the mandibular incisor (b, AP) is superimposed with a small part of the reserve crown of the mandibular third premolar.

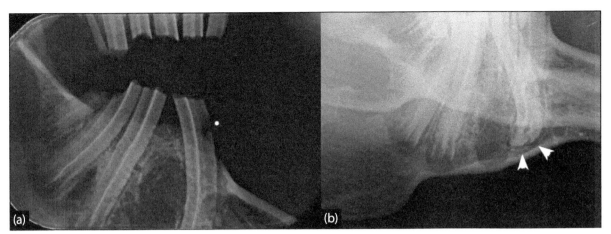

Fig. A11.42 Radiographs of a 4.5-year-old rabbit 3 months following extraction of the mandibular fourth premolar. Using a combination of intraoral parallel technique (a) and extraoral lateral oblique (b) views gives the best results. The free space following extraction was bridged by the surrounding premolar and molar teeth and the extraction site is well healed. The cheek teeth are apically elongated. The mandibular third premolar has a lytic lesion (a, white dot) due to dental caries and its apex shows dysplastic changes (b, arrowheads). All the mandibular molars are bent with irregular enamel folds. (Courtesy Vladimír Jekl and Karel Hauptman.)

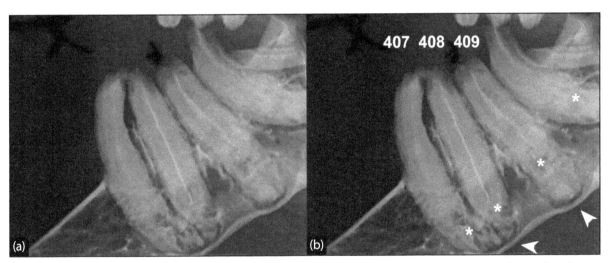

Fig. A11.43 Severe dental disease in an 8-year-old rabbit (a, b). All the mandibular right premolars and molars are of abnormal shape and are apically elongated (b, arrowheads) and show structural changes with loss of enamel folds. The dental pulp is not visible, and the apical parts of the premolars and molars show tooth resorptive lesions associated with ischemic pulp necrosis (b, asterisks). In the premolars, alveolar bone and lamina dura are not visible, suggesting ankylosis of these teeth. (Courtesy Vladimír Jekl and Karel Hauptman.)

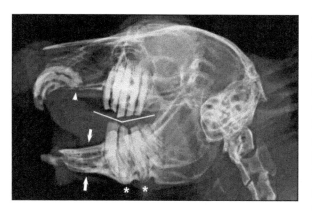

Fig. A11.44 Lateral oblique (20°) skull radiograph of a 7-year-old rabbit with severe dental disease. The maxillary and mandibular incisors have very small clinical crowns and their labial surface is rough. These incisors have obliterated pulp cavities and the reserve crowns are apically elongated with perforation of the incisive bone (arrowhead). The radiolucent area in the middle of the reserve crown of the mandibular incisors is indicative of osteomyelitis with tooth lysis (arrows). The cheek teeth are maloccluded with an uneven occlusal plane (white line). The maxillary cheek teeth have increased opacity due to the structural changes of the enamel and dentin as well as tooth calcification. Enamel folds are not present. There is also apical elongation of all the premolars and molars. Obvious apical elongation of the mandibular fourth premolar and molar are marked with asterisks. (Courtesy Vladimír Jekl and Karel Hauptman.)

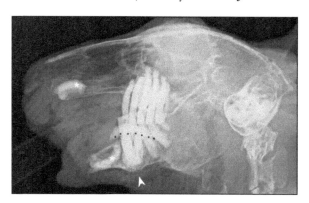

Fig. A11.45 End-stage dental disease in a 5-year-old rabbit. Note the dysplastic changes of the apical parts of all incisors (asterisk). No clinical crowns of the incisors are present. The number of cheek teeth is also reduced. Additionally, there is obvious premolar and molar malocclusion with coronal elongation (especially of the second molar, which is deviated rostrally (black dots). The apices of the mandibular third and fourth premolars perforate the ventral mandibular cortex and are in close proximity to each other, which could be a sign of severe dysplasia or inflammatory changes (arrowhead). The overall skull opacity is very low, which indicates metabolic bone disease. In this case the diagnosis was chronic renal failure with secondary renal hyperparathyroidism. (Courtesy Vladimír Jekl and Karel Hauptman.)

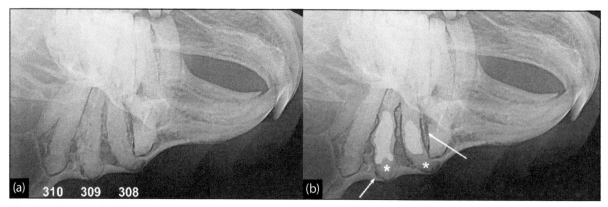

Fig. A11.46 Lateral oblique view of the left mandible of a rabbit with advanced dental disease. Note the obvious ventral mandibular cortex thinning and deformation ('bumps') due to apical premolar and molar elongation. Enamel folds, lamina dura, and teeth pulps are not present. The mesial and distal parts of the mandibular premolars and molar reserve crowns have an uneven surface (b, red) with the fourth premolar and first molar showing small radiolucent areas associated with dental lysis (b, yellow). There is dilaceration of the reserve crowns of the fourth premolar and first molar (b, asterisks). The last molar is thickened (b, blue). The widened periodontal space (b, arrows) can be due to periodontitis or alveolar bone lysis due to ischemic causes. (Courtesy Vladimír Jekl and Karel Hauptman.)

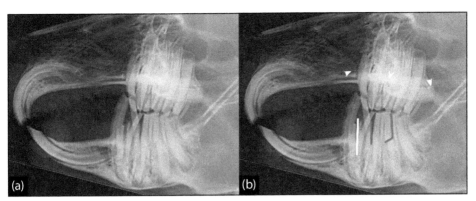

Fig. A11.47 Lateral radiograph of a rabbit with longitudinally fractured (spited) mandibular premolars (b, white and red lines) and first molar (b, blue). Insufficient mineralization of the dental substance, enamel and dentin hypoplasia, and structurally altered cementum are the predisposition for these types of pathologic fractures. The arrowheads (b) show the radiopaque line (an artifact) associated with the presence of hair inside the scanner or the sensor envelope. (Courtesy Vladimír Jekl and Karel Hauptman.)

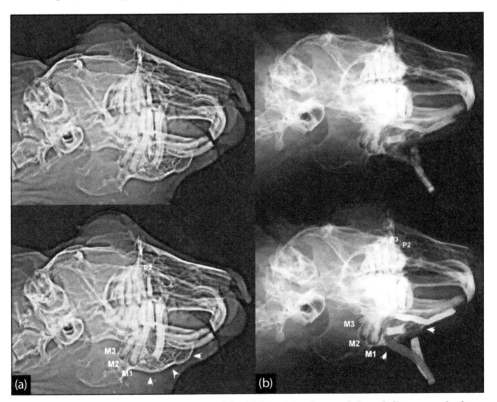

Fig. A11.48 Lateral oblique views of two 3.5-year-old rabbits with advanced dental disease and odontogenic abscesses. In both rabbits, all the premolars and molars are structurally changed with loss of interdental enamel folds, almost missing pulpal cavities, and loss of lamina dura. The periodontal space is widened (blue color). (a) Obvious mandibular cortex osteoproliferation (arrowheads) with inner bone lysis associated with periapical inflammation of the incisor and mandibular third (green) and fourth premolar (red). The mandibular fourth premolar is lytic and only a small tooth remnant is present. (b) The mandibular third (green) and fourth (red) premolar migrated in the osteomyelitic mandible and aberrantly erupted through its ventral part. The mandibular third premolar is fractured. Note also the obvious deformation (dilaceration) and loss of tooth structure of the mandibular incisor (yellow). (Courtesy Vladimír Jekl and Karel Hauptman.)

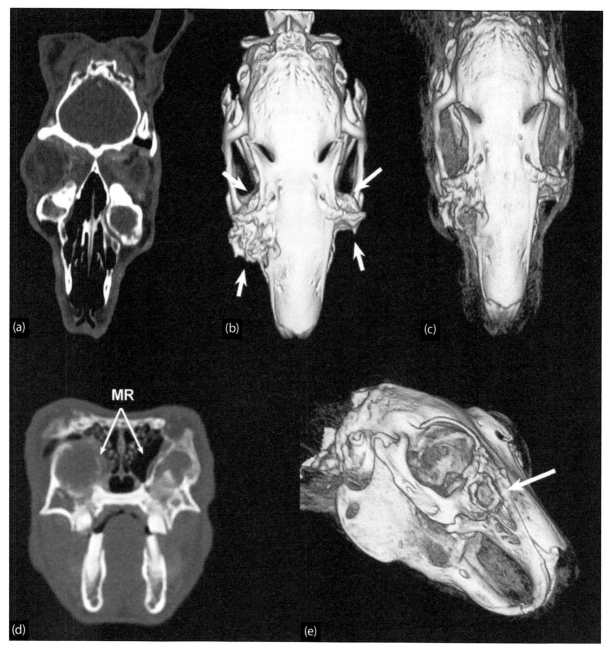

Fig. A11.49 CT of the skull of a 3.5-year-old rabbit with maxillary odontogenic abscesses and unilateral right maxillary recess empyema. Coronal (a) view at the area of maxillary premolars and molars reserve crown and axial (d) view at the area of the maxillary second premolars. (d) The reserve crowns of both maxillary second molars are missing or lytic and the alveolar bulla and the right maxillary recess (MR) are filled with hypodense material (pus). Different CT 3D models (b, c, DV view; e, lateral view) show extensive bone lysis and osteoproliferation dorsal to the maxillary premolars (arrows). In both maxillae, all the premolars were affected. (Courtesy Vladimír Jekl and Karel Hauptman.)

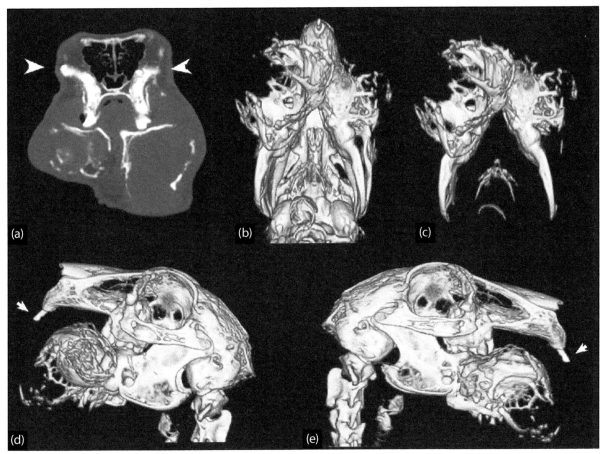

Fig. A11.50 **Axial (a) CT image and 3D CT models (b–e) of a rabbit skull with extensive osteomyelitis of both mandibles. The axial image also demonstrate marked elongation and dental lysis of the maxillary third premolars (arrowheads). The isolated image of the mandible (c) shows in detail the extensive lysis and periosteal reaction, including total lysis of all the mandibular teeth. Incisors were previously extracted; however, peg teeth regrowth was evident (d, e, arrows). (Courtesy Vladimír Jekl and Karel Hauptman.)**

CONTRAST EXAMINATION OF THE NASOLACRIMAL DUCT

The rabbit has only a single lacrimal punctum, located in the anteriomedial aspect of the lower eyelid. The nasolacrimal duct is very slender and has a tortuous route, where the duct passes close to the apices of the maxillary premolars and incisors. It has a rich vascular and lymphatic supply, epithelium with undulations, and a small opening into the nasal vestibule. The maxilla, lacrimal bone, and maxilloturbinates form the osseous boundary of the nasolacrimal duct. Each nasolacrimal duct contains a proximal enlargement (lacrimal sac) located in the funnel-shaped fossa near the rostromedial orbital margin and then tapers. Another area of normal anatomic attenuation is located close to the maxillary incisor apices.

Epiphora, an abnormal overflow of tears down the cheek or face, is caused by an overproduction or an inadequate drainage of tears. In rabbits, it is frequently caused by blockage of the nasolacrimal duct secondary to apical incisor elongation or premolar apical inflammation. Due to the chronic obstruction, the nasolacrimal duct becomes dilated and therefore predisposed to bacterial infection.

Contrast examination of the nasolacrimal duct is easy to perform and may reveal the severity of distension and the area of obstruction, which is typically extraluminal. A complete clinical examination (including intraoral and ophthalmologic examination) should be performed prior to the procedure. In addition, cytology and culture/sensitivity should be performed. Nasolacrimal duct flushing can precede dacryocystorhinography.

General anesthesia in combination with local analgesic (topical eye analgesics [e.g. oxybuprokain]) is recommended for the initial examination and irrigation of the nasolacrimal duct. The patient is placed in lateral recumbency with the head in a slightly oblique position and with the nares located ventrally to prevent aspiration of the flushed material. A lacrimal, intravenous, or metal irrigation cannula (24–27 gauge) with a blunt end can be used for irrigation (**Figure A11.51**).

The convoluted course of the nasolacrimal duct prevents complete duct cannulation, so gentle manipulation is critical. The lower eyelid is pulled away from the cornea and the nasolacrimal punctum is located. A 2 ml syringe is filled with sterile saline and the cannula is inserted into the nasolacrimal duct. If the nasolacrimal duct has a small diameter, an eye needle with a blunt end (olive) is positioned very close to the nasolacrimal punctum. Gentle pressure is applied during flushing of the duct. Milky fluid or pus should exude from the ipsilateral nostril if the procedure is successful. In some cases, gentle digital pressure in the area of the lacrimal sac is necessary to force the fluid to flush the blockage.

For a contrast nasolacrimal duct examination, the patient is placed in lateral recumbency with the affected side away from the x-ray film to facilitate contrast administration. The patient is placed on the x-ray cassette prior to initiating the procedure, with its head fixed in the lateral position.

Dacryocystography with the use of 0.3–0.8 ml of contrast iodine media (300 mg of iodine) is a very useful method for visualization of the nasolacrimal duct.[4] The concentrated solution gives better images than diluted preparations. Only gentle pressure should be applied during nasolacrimal duct irrigation. The contrast administration follows the same principles as described in nasolacrimal duct flushing. Initial administration of a small amount of contrast (0.3–0.5 ml) is recommended to prevent contrast media inhalation and further superimposition with the nasolacrimal duct. Then lateral and DV radiographs are taken. The intraoral views are performed with the use of dental films, which will supplement the contrast study.

The use of an eye lubricant or tear replacement and anti-inflammatory drugs after each procedure is recommended to protect the superficial eye structures and reduce any potential inflammatory response after the nasolacrimal duct cannulation. There is a risk of nasolacrimal duct rupture if high pressure is applied during the procedure.

Abnormal findings commonly include partial or complete obstruction of the nasolacrimal duct, duct distension, or irregular borders (**Figures A11.52–A11.55**).

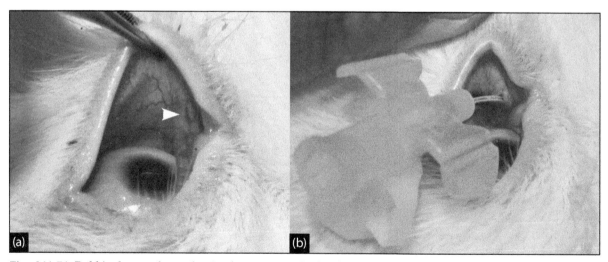

Fig. A11.51 **Rabbits have only one lacrimal punctum, which is located close to the medial canthus of the eye (a, arrowhead). (b) Cannula inserted in the lacrimal punctum. (Courtesy Vladimír Jekl and Karel Hauptman.)**

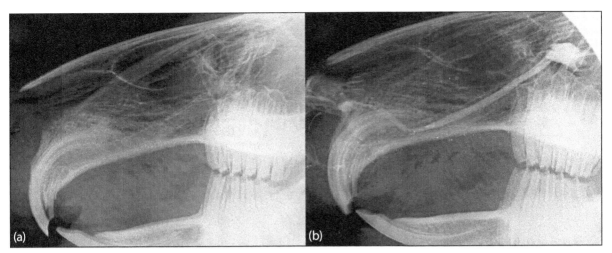

Fig. A11.52 Lateral views of the maxilla of a 1-year-old rabbit. Due to its convoluted path, the nasolacrimal duct is predisposed to obstruction at the area of the incisor apices. Survey radiograph (a) and contrast dacryocystography (b) of a normal nasolacrimal duct.

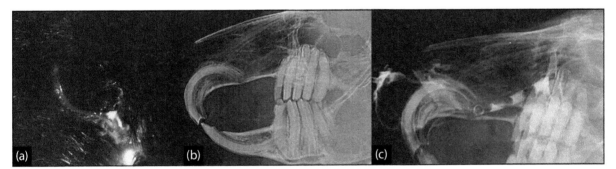

Fig. A11.53 Epiphora in rabbits is a very common problem (a) and is mostly associated with dental disease, particularly apical incisor elongation (b, c). Radiolucent areas in the nasolacrimal duct are caused by the presence of air in the cannula. Therefore, it is recommended that the cannula is filled with contrast media just prior to contrast administration. (Courtesy Vladimír Jekl and Karel Hauptman.)

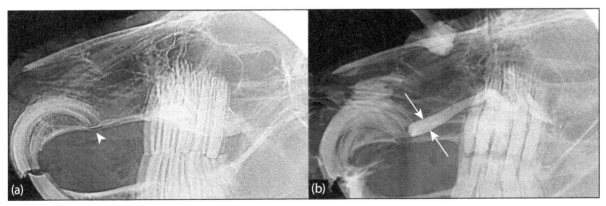

Fig. A11.54 Obvious maxillary incisor apical elongation with narrowing of the pulpal cavity. (a) The incisive bone is almost perforated by the apices of the maxillary incisors (arrowhead). (b) Contrast nasolacrimal duct examination reveals obvious duct enlargement associated with extraluminal obstruction by elongated maxillary incisor apices (arrows). (Courtesy Vladimír Jekl and Karel Hauptman.)

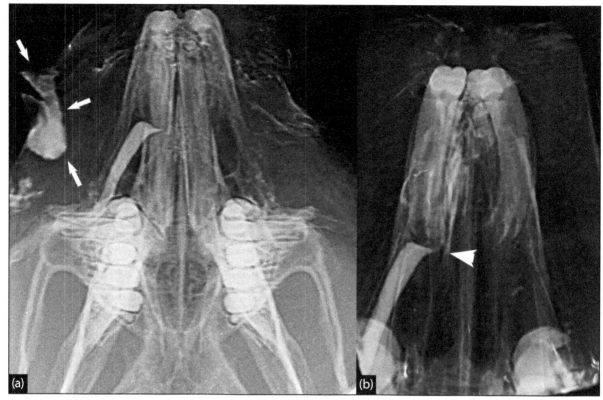

Fig. A11.55 DV extraoral (a) and intraoral (b) views of the rabbit in Fig. A11.53 with epiphora. The elongated apex of the maxillary right incisor caused partial nasolacrimal duct obstruction (b, arrowhead). The arrows (a) indicate contrast media leakage from the conjunctival sac. Contrast media is also present at the area of lips due to nasal leakage of the media. (Courtesy Vladimír Jekl and Karel Hauptman.)

REFERENCES

1 Jekl V, Hauptman K, Knotek Z (2008) Quantitative and qualitative assessments of intraoral lesions in 180 small herbivorous mammals. *Vet Rec* **162:**442–449.

2 Capello V, Lennox AM (2012) Small mammal dentistry. In: *Ferrets, Rabbits, and Rodents. Clinical Medicine and Surgery*, 3rd edn. (eds. KE Quesenberry, JW Carpenter) WB Saunders, St. Louis, pp. 452–471.

3 Böhmer E (2015) *Dentistry in Rabbits and Rodents.* Wiley and Sons, Chichester.

4 Jekl V (2013) Principles of radiography. In: *BSAVA Manual of Rabbit Imaging, Surgery and Dentistry.* (eds. FM Harcourt-Brown, J Chitty) British Small Animal Veterinary Association, Gloucester, pp. 39–58.

5 Crossley DA (2003) Oral biology and disorders of lagomorphs. *Vet Clin North Am Exot Anim Pract* **6:**629–659.

6 Farag FM, Daghash SM, Mohamed EF *et al.* (2012) Anatomical studies on the skull of the domestic rabbit (*Oryctolagus cuniculus*) with special reference to the hyoid apparatus. *J Vet Anat* **5:**49–70.

7 Horowitz SL, Weisbroth SH, Scher S (1973) Deciduous dentition in the rabbit (*Oryctolagus cuniculus*): a roentgenographic study. *Arch Oral Biol* **18(4):**517–523.

8 Ali ZH, Mubarak R (2012) Histomorphological study of dentine pulp complex of continuously growing teeth in the rabbits. *Life Sci* **9:**3.

9 Schulz E, Piotrowski V, Clauss M *et al.* (2013) Dietary abrasiveness is associated with variability of microwear and dental surface texture in rabbits. *PLoS One* **8(2):**e56167.

10 Müller J, Clauss M, Codron D *et al.* (2014) Growth and wear of incisor and cheek teeth in domestic rabbits (*Oryctolagus cuniculus*) fed diets of different abrasiveness. *J Exp Zoo* **321A:**283–298.

11 Capello V, Gracis M (2005) *Rabbit and Rodent Dentistry Handbook*. Zoological Education Network, Lake Worth.

12 Bishop MA (1995) Is rabbit dentine innervated? A fine-structural study of the pulpal innervation in the cheek teeth of the rabbit. *J Anat* **186:**365–372.

13 Michaeli Y, Hirschfeld Z, Weinrub MM (1980) The cheek teeth of the rabbit: morphology, histology and development. *Acta Anat (Basel)* **106(2):**223–239.

14 Harcourt-Brown FM (2009) Dental disease in pet rabbits 1. Normal dentition, pathogenesis and aetiology. *In Pract* **31:**370–379.

15 King AM, Cranfield F, Hall J *et al.* (2010a) Radiographic anatomy of the rabbit skull with particular reference to the tympanic bulla and temporomandibular joint: Part 1: Lateral and long axis rotational angles. *Vet J* **186(2):**232–243.

16 King AM, Cranfield F, Hall J *et al.* (2010b) Radiographic anatomy of the rabbit skull, with particular reference to the tympanic bulla and temporomandibular joint. Part 2: Ventral and dorsal rotational angles. *Vet J* **186(2):**244–251.

17 Gracis M (2008) Clinical technique: normal dental radiography of rabbits, guinea pigs, and chinchillas. *J Exot Pet Med* **17(2):**78–86.

18 Böhmer E, Crossley D (2009) Objective interpretation of dental disease in rabbits, guinea pigs and chinchillas. Use of anatomical guideliens. *Tierärztliche Praxis Kleintiere* **37(K):**250–260.

PART B

FERRETS

Vladimír Jekl

INTRODUCTION

Ferrets belong to the family Mustelidae and are obligate carnivores with reduced teeth number and size. They are occasionally classified as hypercarnivores, as they lack the ability to efficiently digest significant amounts of plant foods. The ferret dentition lacks appreciable tooth area for crushing and grinding compared with areas reserved for cutting. The jaws are short and the tooth bearing portions of both jaws are about equal in length, but the lower dental arch is narrower than the upper and thus fits within it, providing for a shearing action when chewing.

Ferrets are heterodont, with the deciduous teeth erupting between the 19th and 31st day postnatally, and exfoliating between days 51 and 76 (*Tables B11.1, B11.2*).[1] Deciduous incisors are the only teeth present at birth.[2] At approximately 6–7 weeks of age, the permanent dentition starts to erupt and completely replaces the deciduous dentition by 11 weeks of age (**Figure B11.1a**). The last permanent teeth to erupt are the mandibular fourth premolars. The replacement of deciduous teeth (**Figure B11.2**) is generally faster in females than in males.

Table B11.1 **Deciduous dentition of the ferret**

	INCISORS	CANINES	PREMOLARS	MOLARS
Upper dental arch	3	1	3	0
Lower dental arch	3	1	3	0

Table B11.2 **Permanent dentition of the ferret**

	INCISORS	CANINES	PREMOLARS	MOLARS
Upper dental arch	3	1	3	1
Lower dental arch	3	1	3	2

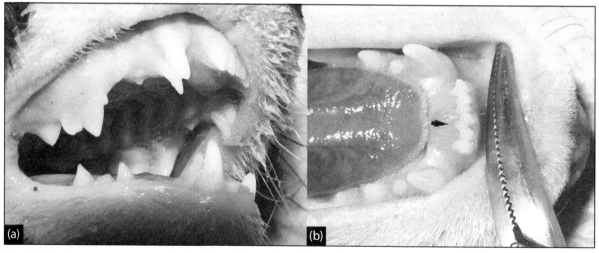

Fig. B11.1 **Supernumerary teeth should be differentiated from the deciduous teeth. (a) An 8-week-old male ferret with a double set of canines caused by the presence of a persistent deciduous (seen distally) and permanent (more mesial/rostral) teeth. Exfoliation of the deciduous canines takes place over a wide range of time – from 57 to 72 days. (b) Supernumerary incisor in a 2-year-old male ferret. The supernumerary incisor is typically found between the first and second maxillary incisor (arrow), which is a very common hereditary condition, especially in males. (Courtesy Vladimír Jekl and Karel Hauptman.)**

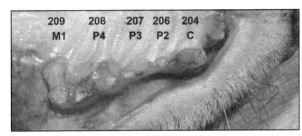

Fig. B11.2 **Intraoral picture of the left maxillary dental arch in a 2-year-old ferret. The single maxillary molar has a specific tooth shape and is wider in the buccolingual direction than in the mesiodistal direction.**

POSITIONING

Patient positioning and the angulation of the x-ray beam are very important, as the head and teeth of ferrets are relatively small. Therefore, even slight mistakes in angulation can lead to foreshortening or elongation of the image as well as superimposition of the hard tissues. A combination of extra- and intraoral techniques is best for radiographic evaluation of the oral cavity and associated structures. Visualization of the entire tooth is ideal, but not always possible due to the tooth size or position (e.g. in ferrets it is difficult to take a radiograph of the maxillary molar due to its very caudal anatomic location [**Figure B11.2**]). Occasionally, more than two views are necessary for evaluation of this tooth.

As ferret heads are comparable to cats, similar radiographic techniques are applied.[3] For the extraoral technique, dorsoventral (DV) and lateral views of the whole skull are obtained (**Figures B11.3–B11.6**). For proper evaluation of the temporomandibular joint (TMJ), a rostrocaudal view should also be taken. Lateral oblique views with the mouth open are best for evaluating the canines, maxillary incisors, premolars, and molars. The lateral oblique view is best

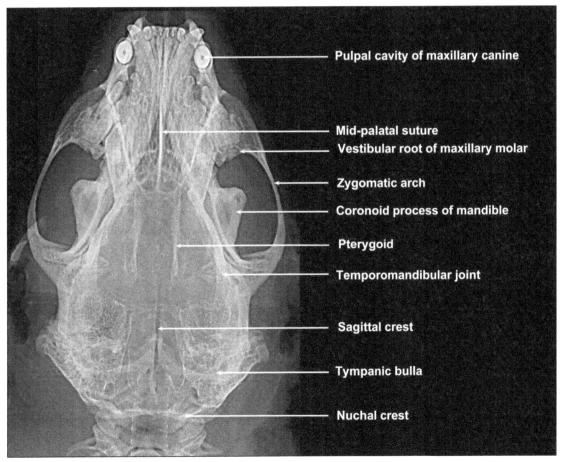

Fig. B11.3 **DV radiograph an adult ferret skull. The skull lacks sutures, which makes it impossible to accurately differentiate individual bones. (Courtesy Vladimír Jekl and Karel Hauptman.)**

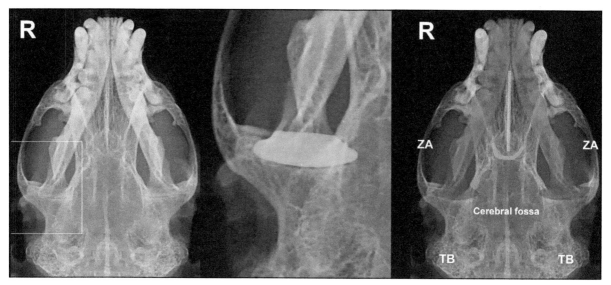

Fig. B11.4 **DV radiograph of a ferret skull with a detailed view of a temporomandibular joint. The mandibular articular condyle is highlighted in blue. The mandible is highlighted in red. Legend: yellow line, vomer; green line, lamina cribrosa; ZA, zygomatic arch; TB, tympanic bulla. (Courtesy Vladimír Jekl and Karel Hauptman.)**

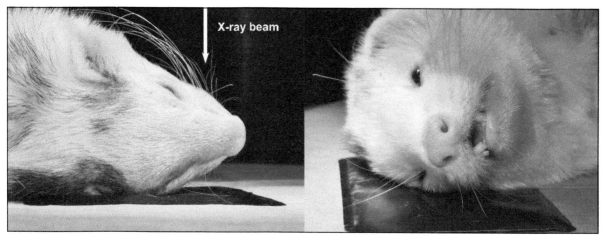

Fig. B11.5 **Proper positioning of a ferret for a lateral view. The long axis of the head should be parallel with the radiographic plate/cassette. The mouth can be open or closed.**

accomplished with the patient in lateral recumbency with the mouth open and the position indicating device adjusted to create an angle of approximately 25–35° as is reported in other companion carnivores (**Figures B11.7, B11.8**). Because of the small oral cavity opening, size 0 (2 × 3 cm), 1 (2 × 4 cm), and 3 (2.7 × 5.4 cm) sensors appear to provide the best images. Maxillary and mandibular incisors and canines, as well as the mandibular premolars and molars, can be evaluated using the parallel or bisecting angle technique (**Figures B11.9, B11.10**).

NORMAL SKULL AND DENTAL ANATOMY AND RADIOGRAPHY

Without a clear understanding of the normal structures, interpretation of radiographs of the maxillary teeth can be difficult due to the superimposition of other bony structures of the skull. Ferret skulls are relatively elongated and flat with a short facial region. The skulls of adult male ferrets are about 17% longer and 22% wider and have more prominent sagittal and occipital crests than those of the females.[4]

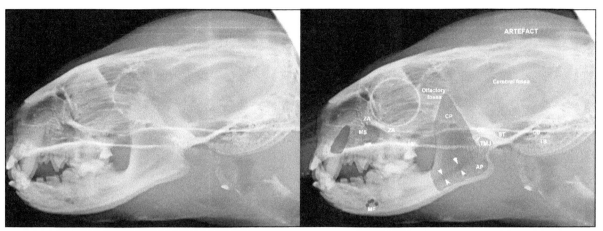

Fig. B11.6 Lateral view. The contour and thickness of most craniofacial bones can be evaluated from this view. The limits between the cranial and facial portions of the skull are clearly defined by the rostrally convex contour projected from the cribriform plate of the ethmoid bone (green line). The petrous portion of the temporal bone is seen as a dense opacity superior to the tympanic bulla. An oblique radiopaque line constitutes the base of the cranium. The maxillary sinus is seen as a radiolucent area above the roots of the upper third and fourth premolars (blue color, MS). The hard palate (HP), which extends from the anterior to the posterior nasal spine, presents as a radiopaque line nearly parallel to the cranial base (CB). Orbita (yellow circle) is not well defined by the zygomatic arch (ZA) as in rabbits. Legend: TB, tympanic bullae; ST, hypophyseal fossa; red color, roots of maxillary canines. The mandibular ramus is very big (purple color) in ferrets, with a prominent coronoid process (CP) and a small temporomandibular joint (TMJ) and angular process (AP). Red dots at the rostral part of the mandible shows mental foramina (MF).

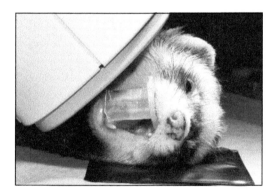

Fig. B11.7 (Left) Positioning for a lateral oblique view. The radiographic cassette/sensor is placed extraorally.

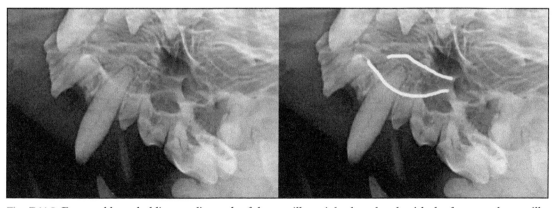

Fig. B11.8 Extraoral lateral oblique radiograph of the maxillary right dental arch with the focus on the maxillary canine. The conchal crest (blue line) and palatine fissures (yellow line) are represented by radiopaque lines and could be misinterpreted as pathology. Note the slight foreshortening of the clinical crowns of the second and third premolars.

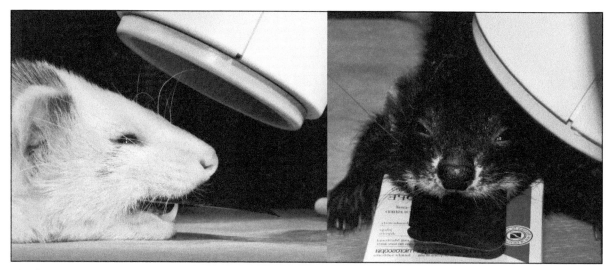

Fig. B11.9 **Proper positioning of a ferret for intraoral radiography of the maxillary left canine.**

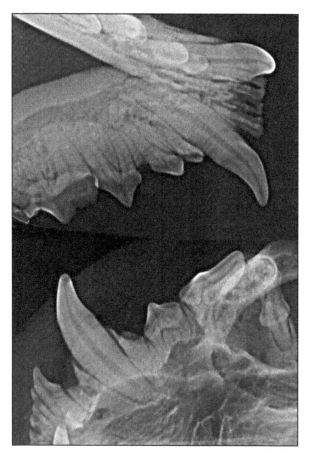

Fig. B11.10 **Bisecting angle view of the maxillary (top) and mandibular (bottom) right canine teeth in a 3-year-old male ferret. (Courtesy Vladimír Jekl and Karel Hauptman.)**

The skull lacks sutures in the adult animal, making it impossible to differentiate individual bones (**Figures B11.3, B11.6**). The brain case is disproportionally large, and caudally there is a prominent nuchal crest extending transversely from one auditory bulla to the other.[5] The widest portion of the skull is between the zygomatic arches. The broad and convex surface on each side of the dorsum of the skull is the temporal fossa, where the strong temporal muscle arises.[6] On the median line is a well-developed sagittal crest that extends from the occipital bone to the orbits. This anatomically obvious structure rostrally splits into a 'V shape', symmetrical divergent lines extending to the postorbital processes of the frontal bones. Symmetrical tympanic bullae and petrous portions of the temporal bones are significantly radiopaque (**Figures B11.3, B11.4**). The sella turcica can be located on the midline as a radiopaque spot.

In the basal parts of the zygomatic processes of the temporal bone there are obvious, transversely wide mandibular fossae. The cerebral fossa can be seen as a large oval radiolucent area in the middle of the calvaria (**Figures B11.3, B11.4**).

The facial region is short and comprises the dorsal surfaces of the maxillary, nasal, and incisive bones as well as the nasal processes of the frontal bones. The longitudinal radiopaque nasal septum divides the facial skeleton into two symmetrical parts (**Figure B11.6**). Two maxillary sinuses with irregular contours are

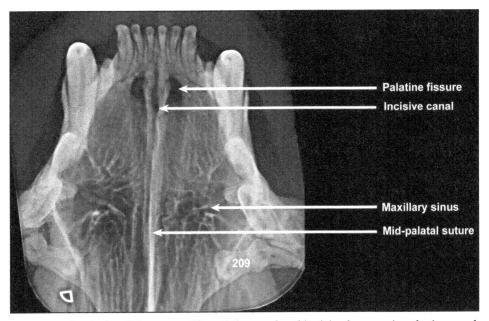

Fig. B11.11 **DV view of an isolated ferret maxilla and the nasal and incisive bones using the intraoral technique. The ferret is positioned as in Fig. B11.3 with the intraoral plate placed in the mouth cavity.**

symmetrically located on either side of the nasal septum between the third and fourth premolars (**Figure B11.11**). Small sphenoid sinuses are located caudoventrally and frontal sinuses caudodorsally in the nasal cavity. The dorsal nasal concha is represented by a well-developed shelf on each side, and the ventral nasal concha (maxilloturbinate) occupies the largest part of the nasal cavity.[5]

The cribriform plate of the ethmoid bones is located at the caudal part of the nasal septum (**Figures B11.3, B11.4**). The incisive bones constitute the most rostral margin of the upper jaw and, together with the nasal bones, border the external nasal opening.

The horizontal parts of the incisive bones, the palatine processes of the maxillae, and the palatine bone form the hard palate, which extends beyond the caudal molars (**Figure B11.6**). The choanae open at the end of the hard palate. The small ventral opening of the incisive canal is found between the palatine processes of the incisive bones and the opening between the first incisors on either side. The paired oval palatine fissures, situated in the incisive bones medial to the third incisors, are separated by the palatine processes of the incisive bones. The major and minor palatine foramina are paired small holes,

usually found medial to the fourth premolars, through which the major and minor palatine arteries emerge (**Figure B11.6**).

Maxillary dental arch

There are normally three incisors situated in each incisive bone, which have slightly longer clinical crowns than the mandibular incisors. The permanent incisors erupt between 42 and 56 days of age.[1] The permanent incisors erupt lingual/palatal to the deciduous incisors and possess a single, simple cusp with laterally compressed roots. The first two maxillary incisors are similar in size with straight roots. The maxillary third incisors are longer and typically wider than the second incisors and have a slight banana-curve shape (**Figures B11.11, B11.12**). Lateral and caudal to the incisive bones are the paired maxillae, each of which contains one canine, three premolars, and one molar.

The maxillary canine tooth is the largest and longest tooth in the jaw (**Figures B11.10–B11.12**). It is slightly curved with approximately 60% of the tooth below the alveolar margin. In cross section it has an ovoid shape. Ferret permanent canines erupt at 55–56 days of age. The crown possesses a single, sharply pointed cusp that projects beyond the lips

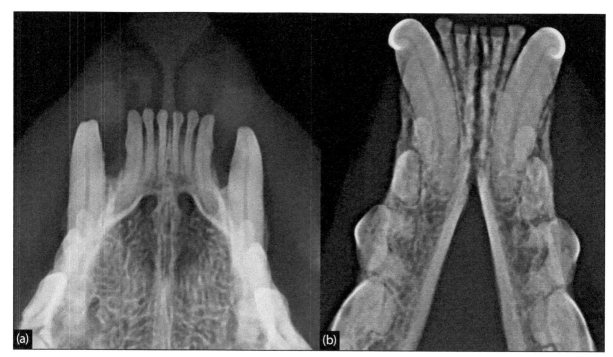

Fig. B11.12 An occlusal view of the permanent maxillary (a) and mandibular (b) incisors and canines can be typically imaged in one radiograph. Bisecting angle view. Note the larger maxillary third incisors, which have a similar shape to the canines. Only 50% of the canine crowns can be properly evaluated in this view, which is why the canines should be evaluated independently on a radiograph directed at the canine tooth (using the bisecting angle technique). Note that the view of the maxillary incisors and canines is slightly elongated. (Courtesy Vladimír Jekl and Karel Hauptman.)

and is visible resting against the lower lip. It erupts rostropalatally to the maxillary deciduous canine. Between the maxillary third incisor and the adjacent canine is a diastema a few millimeters wide that provides space for the mandibular canine to fit into the dental arch when the jaws are closed, ensuring proper occlusion.[7] The maxillary canine fits bucally immediately caudal to the mandibular canine.

Radiographs of the maxillary incisors and canines (**Figures B11.11, B11.12**) often include the palatine fissures, which appear as large symmetrical radiolucent areas in the rostral maxilla near the apical area of the incisors. The conchal crest is visible as a radiopaque line extending from the root of the canine tooth to the mesial root of the third premolar (**Figure B11.8**). There is a radiopaque line extending from the palatine fissures to the caudal maxilla, and this line is typically visible along the apical third of the roots of the maxillary canines and along the apex of the maxillary premolars and molars. This is the line created by the junction of the vertical body of the maxilla and the palatine process, which creates the lateral border of the floor of the nasal cavity, as in dogs and cats.[8,9] The maxillary nasal sinus is also visible in many radiographs of the maxilla (**Figures B11.6, B11.8, B11.11**).

The permanent premolars begin to erupt between 51 and 71 days of age. The premolars are compressed buccolingually and have secodont crowns. The second premolar is the smallest and in some individuals is in direct contact with the adjacent canine tooth. The second premolar has two roots, which may be fused, and erupts palatally to the corresponding deciduous tooth. The maxillary third premolar is larger than the second premolar, has two roots, and erupts rostropalatally to the corresponding deciduous tooth. In crowded jaws, P3 may be rotated buccopalatally within the maxillary dental arch. The maxillary carnassial tooth in ferrets is the fourth premolar, which has three roots. The maxillary fourth premolar erupts caudal to the last deciduous premolar and occludes with the mandibular first molar.

The maxillary first molar has three roots and erupts caudally to the last premolar at approximately 56 days of age. The maxillary molar is wider buccopalatally than rostrocaudally and its long axis is transverse. The clinical crown has two cusps on the buccal and one cusp on the palatal part of the tooth. This tooth also occludes with the mandibular first molar.

Mandible and mandibular dental arches

The mandible consists of a pair of bones that are attached to each other by a fibrocartilaginous junction at the mandibular symphysis. In this author's experience, this intermandibular joint is frequently ossified in older ferrets (this also occurs in cats).[10] From the symphysis, the two bones diverge from each other, forming the 'V'-shaped mandibular space. The body of the mandible holds the mandibular teeth. Rostrally, the body of the mandible looks relatively smooth and rounded and contains several mental foramina, which are the rostral openings of the mandibular canal. The largest and most caudal mental foramen is located ventral to the third and fourth premolars.[6]

The ramus of the mandible resembles a triangle and contains three noticeable processes. Being a relatively high vertical structure, the prominent coronoid process is the largest and occupies most of the ramus. The condylar process and the TMJ are situated at about the level of the last molars. Finally, there is a small angular process.

The angle of the mandible is an inconspicuous eminence ventral to the condylar process. It serves as the insertion of the pterygoid muscle medially and the masseter muscle laterally. The triangular masseteric fossa on the lateral surface of the ramus accommodates the insertion of part of the masseter muscle. The shallowly depressed medial surface of the ramus serves as the insertion of the temporal muscle. Immediately ventral to this insertion is the mandibular foramen.[6] The condyle is small if observed from the lateral view, and most of the condylar surface is surrounded by the mandibular fossa and the postarticular process. The mandibular canal is viewed as a long, narrow radiolucent stripe extending from the mental foramen to the mandibular foramen. It runs directly beneath the roots of the premolars and first molar and nearly parallel to the ventral border of the mandible. The large root of the lower canine extends to the vicinity of the third premolars and its apex is very close to the mandibular canal.

There are three permanent incisors in each mandibular quadrant, one canine tooth, three premolars and one molar. The mandibular incisors are also single rooted teeth, which are all similar in shape but smaller in size in comparison with the maxillary incisors. The first incisor is smaller than the others and its root is localized close to the mandibular symphysis (**Figure B11.12**). There is a peculiarity in the placement of the mandibular incisors in that the second incisors are set more lingual to the others; however, they are slightly labially tilted ensuring the proper alignment for occlusion with the maxillary incisors.

The mandibular canines are long and pointed and lie just mesial to the maxillary canines. They are single rooted and similar in size and shape to the maxillary canines. The mandibular canine may slightly rub against the maxillary canine, creating wear facets on the buccal side of the mandibular and lingual side of the maxillary. These wear facets seem to have no clinical significance. Small diastemata exist between the mandibular canine and second premolar as well as between the third and fourth premolars.

There are three premolars (P2–P4) in the normal ferret mandible. The first two premolars are small single rooted teeth, while the third has two roots (**Figure B11.13**). There is a gradual increase in tooth size from the first premolar towards the molar. Mandibular premolars erupt lingually to the deciduous premolars at 61–71 days of age. Similar to the maxillary premolars, the mandibular premolars are compressed buccolingually and have pointed cusps.

There are two molars in the mandibular dental arch. The mandibular carnassial teeth in ferrets are represented by the first molar, which is the largest tooth in the mandible and has two roots (mesial and distal). However, in this author's experience a slender accessory root is present on the lingual aspect in more than 60% of ferrets). The mesial root is typically larger than the distal root, both

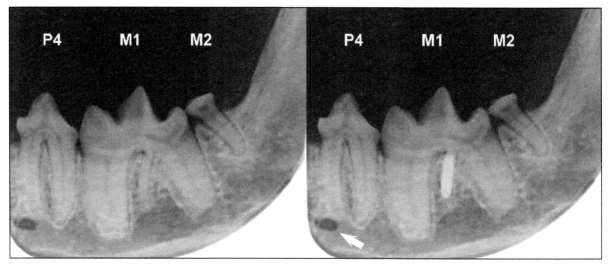

Fig. B11.13 Radiographs of the mandibular fourth premolar and molars of a ferret. The first molar has three roots. The buccal root is the smallest in size (highlighted in blue). This part of the tooth must not be left in place when performing extractions. The last molar is single rooted. Note the radiolucent oval area close to the mesial root of P4 is the caudal mental foramen (arrow). (Courtesy Vladimír Jekl and Karel Hauptman.)

in width and length. The crown of the first molar has three distinct cusps. Two mesial cusps forming the blades of the carnassial tooth. The smaller and lower cusp, in conjunction with the second molar, interlocks with the cusp of the maxillary molar.[7] The maxillary and mandibular carnassial teeth, when in occlusion, create the effective tearing action resulting in the forming of wear facets on the buccal side of the maxillary and lingual side of the mandibular carnassial tooth. The mandibular first molar erupts caudal to the deciduous fourth premolar at 50 days of age. The mandibular second molar is a small, single rooted tooth with a small cusp and is not in occlusion with any of the maxillary molars. It erupts caudally to the first molar at 62 days of age.

DENTAL DISEASE

Dental diseases in ferrets include congenital/hereditary diseases, fractured teeth, dental abrasion, dental caries, periodontal disease, endodontic infection, and neoplasia.[11] It has also been described that teeth may be lost in a variety of systemic disease processes including malnutrition and renal disease;[12] however, this is an uncommon cause of exfoliation.

Supernumerary teeth

The most common hereditary dental disorder is supernumerary maxillary incisors,[2,11] which are seen more commonly in males than females. The incidence of this condition, which commonly has no clinical impact, can be over 12% in particular ferret populations (**Figure B11.1**). Gemini incisors can be also seen (**Figure B11.14**).

Fractures

Traumatic uncomplicated fractures of at least one canine is a very common condition (**Figure B11.15**) with the incidence in the author's clinic more of than 90%. These fractured teeth are typically incidental findings during clinical examination and a fractured tip of the canine is commonly overlaid with tertiary dentin. Pulpitis resulting from direct pulp exposure can destroy the pulp and create a nonvital and infected tooth. However, only in very rare circumstances will radiographic evidence of periapical disease develop.[13] Why periapical disease is less common in ferrets compared with dogs has not been investigated. Lack of radiographic signs of infection should *not* be a reason not to treat the tooth. All teeth with direct pulp exposure should be treated with root canal therapy or extraction. Jaw fractures are extremely rare (**Figure B11.16**).

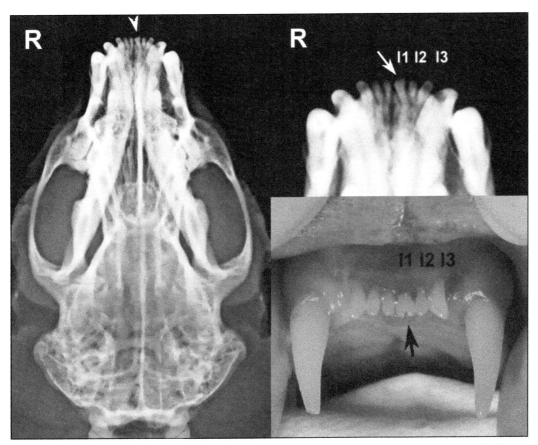

Fig. B11.14 **This gemini maxillary left first incisor (arrow) in a 2-year-old ferret is a rare finding.** (Courtesy Vladimír Jekl and Karel Hauptman.)

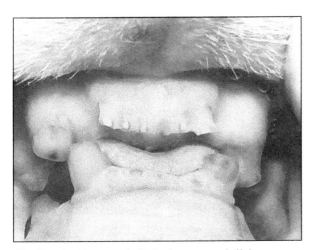

Fig. B11.15 **Fractured clinical crowns of all four canines as well as abrasion of all incisors in a 7-year-old male ferret. (Courtesy Vladimír Jekl and Karel Hauptman.)**

Dental abrasion

Dental abrasion is very common in older ferrets, with the incidence as high as 85%.[7] It appears to be associated with feeding commercial dry diets. Ferrets tend to chew objects in their environment, including cloth bedding and toys. Prolonged chewing on foreign objects, such as cage bars and cloth, can cause significant damage to their teeth (**Figure B11.15**). Kibble abrasion is likely due to a combination of factors, including the abrasive qualities of kibble, the volume of tooth material in ferret teeth, and the biomechanics of shifting from natural food slicing to kibble crushing. Kibble-mediated dental damage exacerbates, contributes to, or is the direct cause of multiple dental pathologies, including teeth worn into the pulp cavity, fractures due to biomechanical stress on worn teeth, avulsed teeth, and abscesses. Also, it likely exacerbates or promotes periodontal disease.[7]

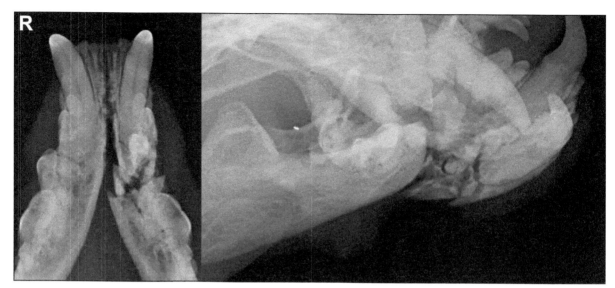

Fig. B11.16 Comminuted fracture of the left mandible. The mandibular left second and third premolars were included into the fracture site. (Courtesy Vladimír Jekl and Karel Hauptman.)

Periodontal disease

Periodontal disease (gingivitis and periodontitis) is one of the most commonly encountered diseases in pet ferrets. In one study[7], dental calculus and periodontitis were encountered in more than 90% of examined ferrets. A further study[11] reported that advanced stages of periodontal disease associated with gingival recession and furcation exposure are rarely seen in ferrets. However, the pet ferrets examined in the first study[7] had a 12.4% dental abscess rate, some associated with extensive bone loss. Therefore, a thorough dental examination should be performed in all cases, as would be the case in dogs and cats. Dental radiography will help in assessing the prognosis and treatment options (**Figures B11.17–B11.20**).

Oral tumors

Oral tumors in ferrets are very rare (**Figure B11.21**) and include maxillary squamous cell carcinoma[14], maxillary osteosarcoma, mandibular liposarcoma[15], lymphoma, and osteoma.[16] Finally, odontogenic cysts may also occur.

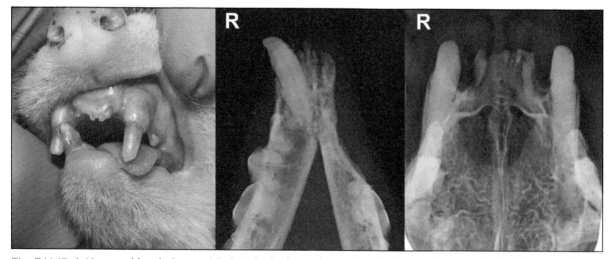

Fig. B11.17 A 10-year old male ferret with dental calculus and periodontal disease. The mandibular left canine had been extracted 4 years previously. Note the mandibular and maxillary lysis of almost all the incisors, old fractures of the remaining canines, and missing mandibular left first premolar. (Courtesy Vladimír Jekl and Karel Hauptman.)

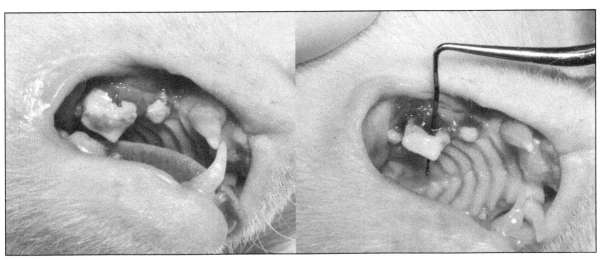

Fig. B11.18 **A 4-year-old female ferret with advanced periodontal disease (dental calculus, gingival recession and furcation exposure). The maxillary right P2 was missing. After dental scaling, furcational exposure and distal root exposure of the fourth premolar was evident. Dental radiographs are still necessary to properly assess the extent of disease. (Courtesy Vladimír Jekl and Karel Hauptman.)**

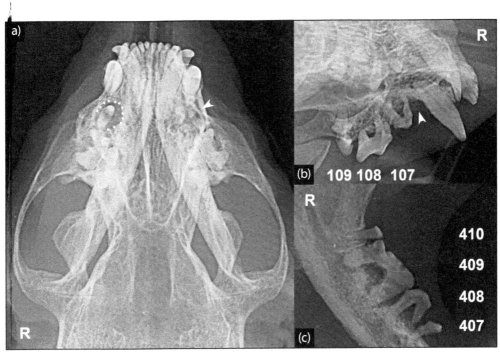

Fig. B11.19 **(a) Extraoral DV, (b) bisecting angle maxillary, and (c) parallel right mandibular radiographs of the 4-year-old female ferret in Fig. B11.18 showing vertical (b) and horizontal (b) bone loss around the right maxillary (b) and mandibular (b) premolars and first molar. Note the maxillary right P3 periapical lucency (a, dotted line) and maxillary right (b, arrow) and maxillary left (a, arrow) P2 lysis. (Courtesy Vladimír Jekl and Karel Hauptman.)**

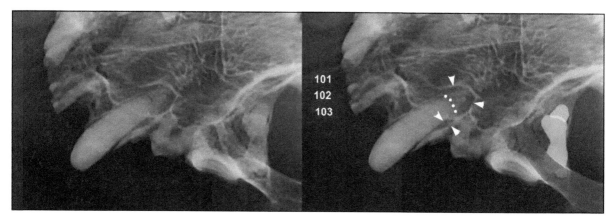

Fig. B11.20 Maxillary right dental arch. Extraoral lateral oblique view. The last maxillary molar crown (blue) and roots (yellow) are superimposed with the zygomatic arch (red). There is also resorption of the maxillary first and second incisors, irregular crown shape of the maxillary third incisor, apical lysis/fracture (dotted line), and widening of the periodontal space surrounding the maxillary right canine apex (arrows) suggestive of periodontal disease. (Courtesy Vladimír Jekl and Karel Hauptman.)

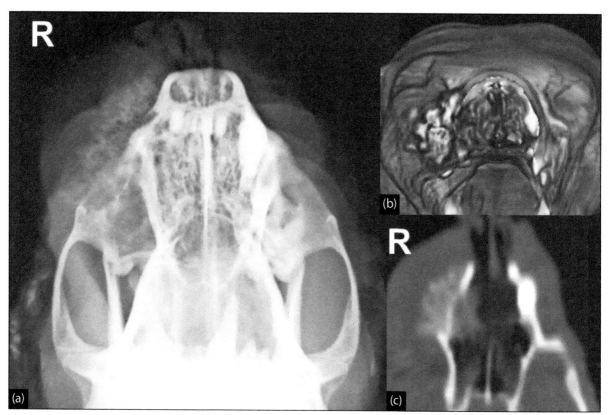

Fig. B11.21 Maxillary osteosarcoma in a 6-year-old ferret. Note the osteoproliferation and osteolysis of the right maxilla seen on the radiographs (a), 3D reconstruction (b) and CT coronal view (c). (Courtesy Vladimír Jekl and Karel Hauptman.)

REFERENCES

1 He T, Friede H, Kiliaridis S (2002) Dental eruption and exfoliation chronology in the ferret (*Mustela putorius furo*). *Arch Oral Biol* **47:**619–623.

2 Berkovitz BKB (1968) Supernumerary deciduous incisors and the order of eruption of the incisor teeth in the albino ferret. *J Zool* **55:**445–449.

3 Coffman CR, Bridgen GM (2013) Oral and dental imaging equipment and techniques for small animals. *Vet Clin North Am Small Anim Pract* **43:**489–506.

4 Lawes INC, Andrews PLR (1987) Variation of the ferret skull (*Mustela putorius furo L.*) in relation to stereotaxic landmarks. *J Anat.* **154:**157–171.

5 Evans H, Quoc An N (2014) Anatomy of the ferret. In: *Biology and Diseases of the Ferret*, 3rd edn. (eds. JG Fox, RP Marini) Wiley Blackwell, Ames, pp. 23–68.

6 He T, Friede H, Kiliaridis S (2002) Macroscopic and roentgenographic anatomy of the skull of the ferret (*Mustela putorius furo*). *Lab Anim* **36:**86–96.

7 Church B (2007) Ferret dentition and pathology. In: *Ferret Husbandry, Medicine and Surgery*, 2nd edn. (ed. JH Lewington) Saunders Elsevier, St. Louis, pp. 467–485.

8 Bannon KM (2013) Clinical canine dental radiography. *Vet Clin North Am Small Anim Pract* **43(3):**507–532.

9 Lemmons M (2013) Clinical feline dental radiography. *Vet Clin North Am Small Anim Pract* **43(3):**533–554.

10 Gioso MA, Carvalho (2005) Oral anatomy of the dog and cat in veterinary dentistry practice. *Vet Clin North Am Small Anim Pract* **35:**763–780.

11 Eroshin VV, Reiter AM, Rosenthal K *et al.* (2011) Oral examination results in rescued ferrets: clinical findings. *J Vet Dent* **28(1):**8–15.

12 Johnson-Delaney CA (2008) Dental disease in ferrets: more serious than we thought. *Proceedings of the North American Veterinary Conference*, Orlando, pp. 1809–1811.

13 Nemec A, Zadravec M, Račnik J (2016) Oral and dental diseases in a population of domestic ferrets (*Mustela putorius furo*). *J Small Anim Pract* **57(10):**553–560.

14 Graham J, Fidel J, Mison M (2006) Rostral maxillectomy and radiation therapy to manage squamous cell carcinoma in a ferret. *Vet Clin North Am Exot Anim Pract* **9(3):**701–706.

15 Fuentealba C, Blue-McLendon A (1995) Liposarcoma arising from the mandibular bone marrow in a ferret. *Can Vet J* **36(12):**779–780.

16 De Voe RS, Pack L, Greenacre CB (2002) Radiographic and CT imaging of a skull associated osteoma in a ferret. *Vet Radiol Ultrasound* **43(4):**346–348.

PART C

SKULL AND DENTAL RADIOGRAPHY IN PET RODENTS

Vladimír Jekl

INTRODUCTION

Amongst mammals, the order Rodentia (rodents) has the largest number of species. Commonly kept pet rodents can be simply divided into three Suborders: Hystricognatha (guinea pigs, chinchillas, degus), Myomorpha (mice, rats, gerbils, hamsters), and Sciuromorpha (prairie dogs, chipmunks, squirrels).

Many exotic pet owners develop a strong emotional bond with their animals and expect appropriate/high-level medical care from the veterinary practitioner. Dental disease makes up a considerable component of the work of any exotic pet practice (**Figures C11.1, C11.2**).[1–3] The clinical crown (which is visible above the gingival margin and thus can be visually examined) represents only a small portion of the tooth as most of the dental tissue, as well as all periapical structures and supporting bone remains hidden to clinical inspection.[4] Therefore, radiography is of particular importance in the evaluation of teeth and surrounding tissue and represents the main diagnostic tool in veterinary dentistry. Skull and dental radiographs should be performed in any patient with suspected or confirmed dental disease. Consequently, in-depth knowledge of rodent skull and dental anatomy is necessary for proper skull/dental radiograph interpretation.

The aim of this chapter is to describe the anatomy, correct radiographic positioning, and radiography of selected rodent species, with the emphasis on guinea pigs, chinchillas, degus, and rats, which are the most commonly kept pet rodents. The skull and

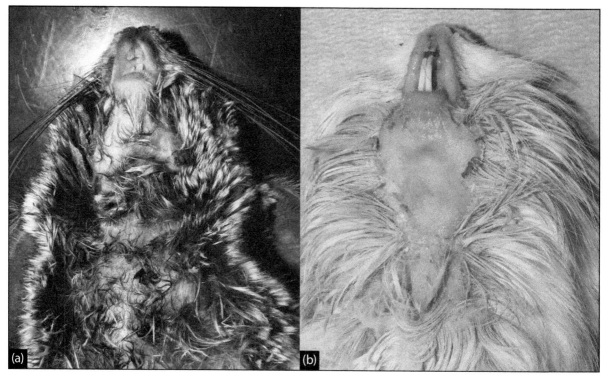

Fig. C11.1 **Ventral view of a head and neck area of a chinchilla (a) and a guinea pig (b). Alopecia and wet dermatitis was associated with excessive salivation due to the dental disease (premolar and molar malocclusion, spike formation, buccal mucosa injury). (Courtesy Vladimír Jekl and Karel Hauptman.)**

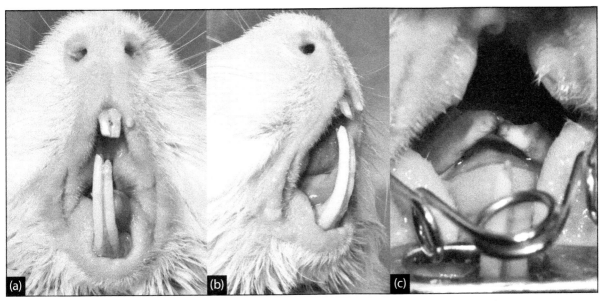

Fig. C11.2 **Incisor malocclusion and elongation of the mandibular incisor clinical crowns (a, b) in a 4-year old male guinea pig presented for anorexia. Right mandibular shift (mandibular displacement) is also visible. Incisor malocclusion in guinea pigs is commonly associated with premolar and molar clinical crown elongation. (c) Oral examination under general anesthesia, with the cheek and mouth dilatator in position. Note the severely elongated mandibular premolars causing a 'bridge'-like structure over the tongue (entrapment), which prevented eating. (Courtesy Vladimír Jekl and Karel Hauptman.)**

dental anatomy described in this chapter are specific to the aforementioned rodent species and should not be applied to all species from other suborders.

ANATOMY

Rodent dentition is monophyodont and heterodont. This means that rodents develop one permanent set of teeth and their teeth have different shape and function. Guinea pigs are diphyodont; however, their deciduous teeth are replaced by the permanent dentition *in utero* or early postnatally.[5] All rodents belong to the mirorder Simplicidentata, with one pair of maxillary and one pair of mandibular incisors.

In general, rodents have reduced numbers of teeth with a long diastema between the incisor and the premolar teeth (if present) and molars. The cheek folds separate the gnawing apparatus from the caudal part of the oral cavity. Each mandibular cheek tooth is in occlusion with the corresponding maxillary tooth. The mandibles and mandibular cheek tooth dental arches are frequently wider in comparison with the maxilla and maxillary tooth dental arches (**Figure C11.3**). This gives rodents their typical head appearance.

A single pair of well-developed incisor teeth is present in in the maxillae and mandibles. Incisors are continuously growing (aradicular hypsodont, i.e. elodont) in all rodent species, with the enamel thickest on the labial surface and thinning as it extends distal and mesial. Opposing aspects have only a dentin and cementum covering.[6] The enamel of the incisor teeth has multiserial Hunter-Schreger bands, which strengthen the enamel, prevent cracks from propagating through the tooth, and provide a higher wear resistance. This arrangement of incisor enamel, in association with the softer underlying dentin, provides a sharp chisel-like occlusal surface.[7] Elodont-type teeth grow on their pulpal axis throughout life; the apex of such teeth never close, resulting in a so-called open-rooted system.[8] The length of the crown of the elodont tooth is maintained by a combination of cell proliferation at the apical end and attrition of the incisal edge. The clinical crown makes up one-third and the reserve crown two-thirds of

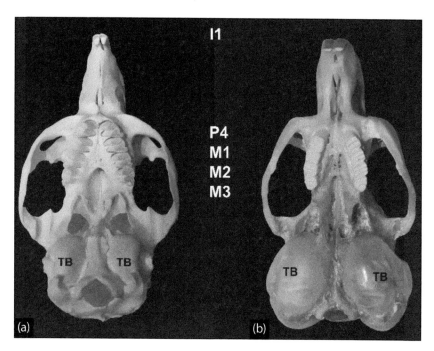

Fig. C11.3 VD views of guinea pig (a) and chinchilla (b) skulls. Both species have in each dental quadrant: one incisor, one premolar and three molars. As premolars and molars form one functional grinding unit, they are commonly named 'cheek teeth'. Tympanic bullae (TB) are very prominent, especially in chinchillas. Maxillary dental arches converge in a rostral direction. (Courtesy Vladimír Jekl and Karel Hauptman.)

the length of the incisors. The clinical crowns of the maxillary incisors are much shorter than those of the mandibular incisors. In guinea pigs and chinchillas, the incisors, premolar, and molar teeth grow approximately 2–7 mm per month; however, eruption rates seem to be related to diet abrasiveness.[9]

Myomorpha (mice-like rodents)

In the Suborder Myomorpha, the labial surface of the incisors is yellow or white in color.[10] Molars have a limited period of growth and are short-crowned with long, narrow tooth roots (brachydont and bunodont dentition). Each mandibular molar is in occlusion with the corresponding maxillary molar. The mandibular symphysis does not fuse completely in some species (hamsters, rats), therefore independent movement of each jaw is possible. Dental formulae, topographic location of maxillary and mandibular incisor apices, incisor clinical crown pigmentation, and number of molar roots in selected Myomorpha species are presented in *Tables C11.1–C11.3*.

In rats and mice, the molar crowns are divided into lobes by transversely oriented enamel folds with enamel-free cusps arranged in three rows of three (**Figure C11.4**). The main cusps are oriented in buccolingual or buccopalatal rows and connected by lower ridges. As the patient ages,

Table C11.1 Dental formula of the Myomorpha (mice-like rodents [e.g. rats, mice, hamsters, and gerbils])

	INCISORS	CANINES	PREMOLARS	MOLARS
Upper dental arch	1	0	0	3
Lower dental arch	1	0	0	3

tooth abrasion causes the formation of enamel ridges. The dentin on the chewing surface of the teeth is exposed unprotected between the multiple enamel ridges, which predisposes the teeth to caries.[11] The size of the teeth decreases from the first to the last molar.

In hamsters, the molar crowns are rectangular and flat with small cusps on the occlusal surface. The cheeks are occupied by the cheek pouches, which are situated between the skin and masticatory muscles.

In gerbils, the molars are arranged in a straight line. The occlusal surfaces of all molars are almost flat and without cusps or fissures.[10]

Sciuromorpha

The teeth of squirrel-like rodents are heterodont with elodont incisors (*Table C11.2*) and brachydont

Table C11.2 Clinical crown pigmentation and topographic location of the maxillary and mandibular incisor apices

	INCISOR PIGMENTATION (LABIAL SURFACE)	LOCATION OF THE MANDIBULAR INCISOR APICES	LOCATION OF THE MAXILLARY INCISOR APICES
Hystricognatha			
Guinea pigs	White	Level of the first mandibular molar	Mesial aspect of the first premolar
Chinchillas	Yellow to orange	Mesial aspect of the premolar	One-half of the diastema
Degus	Yellow to orange	Distal to last molar	Two-thirds of the diastema, close to the apex of the premolar
Myomorpha			
Rat	Yellow to orange	Level of or distally to the last molar	Two-thirds of the diastema
Mice	White		Three-quarters of the diastema
Hamster	Yellow to orange		One-half to two-thirds of the diastema
Gerbil	Yellow to orange		Two-thirds of the diastema
Sciuromorpha	Yellow to orange	Distally to the last molar	Labially of the apex of the first cheek tooth

Table C11.3 Number of molar roots in selected Myomorpha rodent species

	MAXILLARY MOLARS			MANDIBULAR MOLARS		
SPECIES	M1	M2	M3	M1	M2	M3
Rat	4–5	4	3	2	2	2
Mouse	3	3	3	3–4	3	3
Hamster	4	4	3	2	2–3	2
Gerbil	3	2	1	3	2	1

Table C11.4 Dental formula of the Sciuromorpha (squirrel-like rodents [e.g. prairie dogs, chipmunks and squirrels])

	INCISORS	CANINES	PREMOLARS	MOLARS
Upper dental arch	1	0	1–2	3
Lower dental arch	1	0	1	3

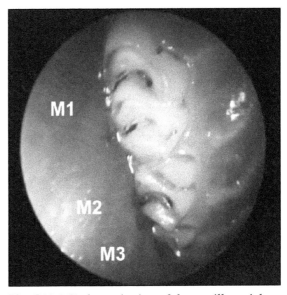

Fig. C11.4 **Endoscopic view of the maxillary right molars of a 1-year-old rat. The molar crowns are divided into lobes by transversely oriented enamel folds with enamel-free cusps. The size of the teeth decreases from the first to the last molar. (Courtesy Vladimír Jekl and Karel Hauptman.)**

premolars and molars (**Figure C11.2**). The mandibular symphysis does not fuse completely, therefore independent movement is possible. This can occur because the mandibular symphysis is not ossified, rather the two mandibles are connected by a muscle.

The cheek teeth are squared with rounded, blunt, cone-shaped bunodont marginal cusps and a concave central area on their occlusal surfaces (*Table C11.4*). Each mandibular cheek tooth is in occlusion with the corresponding maxillary cheek tooth.

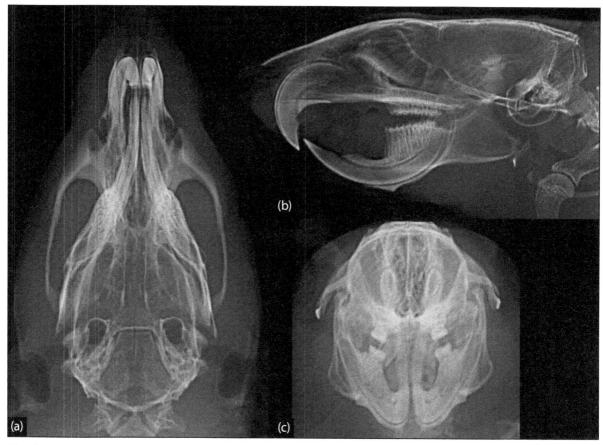

Fig. C11.5 DV (a), lateral (b), and rostrocaudal (c) views of an adult rat with normal dentition. On the lateral view, there are radicular cheek teeth with enamel cusps, with the apices of the long mandibular incisors being located a long way distally to last molar. (Courtesy Vladimír Jekl and Karel Hauptman.)

Hystricognatha (porcupine/guinea pig-like rodents)

Hystricognathous rodents have a strongly deflected angular process and a flange-like or ridged mandible. The masseter inserts ventral and caudal to the teeth, and the coronoid process is greatly reduced. The skull is elongated rostrocaudally, with prominent zygomatic arches, deep pterygopalatinae fossae, and large orbits (**Figures C11.6–C11.11**). The infraorbital canal is short and markedly large. The dorsal surface of the skull is slightly curved rostrocaudally and relatively smooth, with an exception of low temporal lines, which extend from the external occipital protuberance to the orbital crests of each side, and a lacrimal tubercle on the rostral margin of the orbit. The ventral surface of the skull is characterized by small paired slit-like palatine fissures, prominent tympanic bullae (especially in chinchillas, **Figure C11.3**), and large rounded lacerated foramen.

Guinea pigs, chinchillas, and degus are true herbivores with incisors (*Tables C11.2, C11.5*) and all the premolars and molars continuously growing (elodont) throughout life. Elodont teeth never form true anatomic roots. Tooth substance above the gingival margin is termed 'clinical crown' and the tooth substance below the gingival margin is termed 'reserve crown'.

Premolars and molars have similar structure and form a functional grinding unit in each quadrant of the oral cavity. They are commonly named 'cheek teeth'. The cheek teeth in chinchillas and guinea pigs diverge from rostral to caudal (**Figure C11.3**). The occlusal surface consists of alternating enamel, dentin, and cementum with the presence of transversal enamel ridges or folds (lophodont).

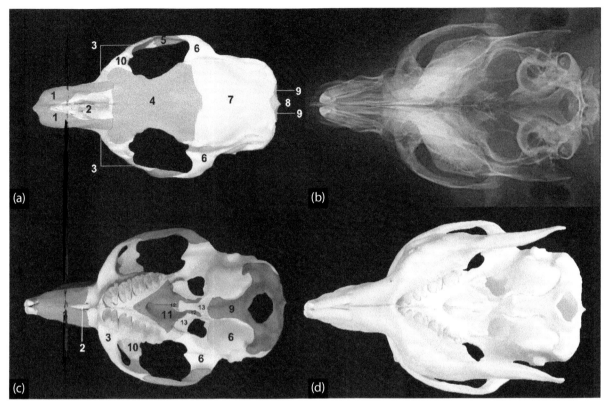

Fig. C11.6 **Normal skull and dentition of a guinea pig (a, c, d) and DV radiograph (b) of a normal adult guinea pig skull. DV (a) aspect of a skull with nasal bones removal and VD without (c) and with the mandible in position (d). 1, incisive bone; 2, nasal conchae; 3, maxilla; 4, frontal bone; 5, zygomatic bone; 6, temporal bone; 7, parietal bone; 8, interparietal bone; 9, occipital bone; 10, lacrimal bone; 11, palatine bone; 12, presphenoid bone; 13, basisphenoid.**

Deep longitudinal grooves are present on the buccal surface of the cheek teeth (**Figure C11.12**). The occlusal surface is nearly horizontal in chinchillas and degus, while in guinea pigs it is oblique (40 degrees). Each mandibular cheek tooth is in occlusion with the opposite maxillary tooth. In the resting jaw position, their occlusal planes are almost in contact. The occlusal surface of the premolars and molars in degus resembles a figure-of-eight (**Figure C11.13**).

In guinea pigs, the reserve crowns of the maxillary premolars and molars incline laterally within the alveoli, while those of the mandible incline medially.[12] The buccal surface of the maxillary premolars and molars and the lingual surface of the mandibular premolars/molars are covered with a continuous layer of cementum on the dentin. The remaining area of the tooth is covered by a layer of enamel with attached cementum pearls. Cementum pearls are seen all over the enamel surface except for in the two longitudinally folded grooves, which are filled with a special type of cementum called 'cartilage-like cementum'. Guinea pig premolars or molars are laminated teeth with two dental laminas composed of a pulp, dentin, and enamel covering. Interposed between the two dental laminas is the interdental septum, composed of a superior cartilaginous zone and a basal enamel organ. When viewed from the occlusal surface, two folds can be seen entering the tooth. These folds are made up of a thin enamel lining and are filled with cartilage-like cementum as described above. The periodontal ligament of the guinea pig molar is a complicated structure because it attaches alveolar bone to three types of tissue: enamel (via cemental pearls), dentin, and cartilage-like cementum.[13]

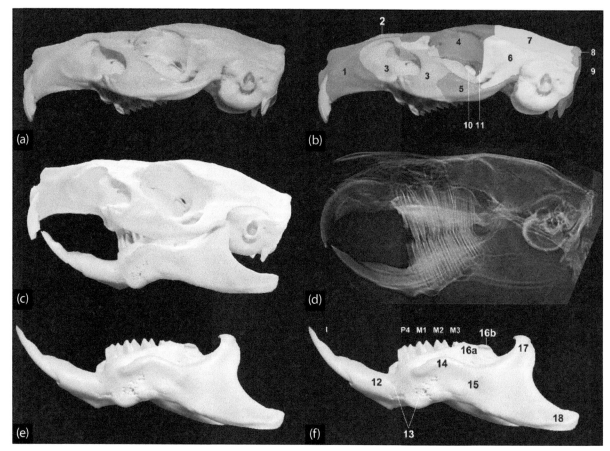

Fig. C11.7 Adult guinea pig skull. Unlabeled (a, e) and labeled (b, f) lateral aspects of a skull and mandible. A lateral view of a guinea pig skull with the mandible in position is shown in c. 1, incisive bone; 2, nasal bone; 3, maxilla; 4, frontal bone; 5, zygomatic bone; 6, temporal bone; 7, parietal bone; 8, interparietal bone; 9, occipital bone; 10, palatine bone; 11, presphenoid bone; 12, incisive part of the mandible; 13, mental foramina; 14, masseteric crest; 15, masseteric fossa; 16a,b, left and right coronoid process; 17, condylar process; 18, angular process.

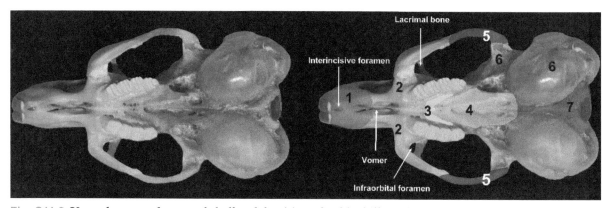

Fig. C11.8 Ventral aspect of a normal skull and dentition of a chinchilla with mandible removed. 1, incisive bone; 2, maxilla; 3, palatine bone; 4, sphenoidal bones; 5, zygomatic bone; 6, temporal bone, 7, occipital bone.

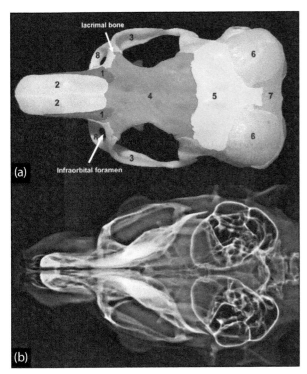

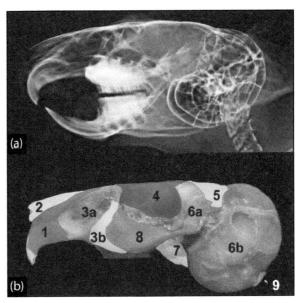

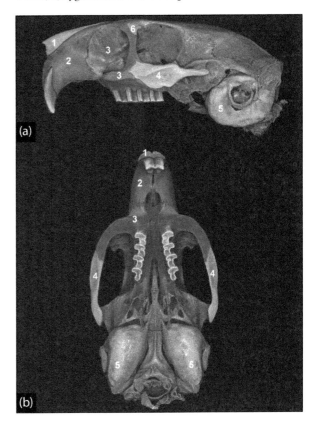

Fig. C11.9 Dorsal aspect of a normal skull (a) and DV radiograph (b) of a chinchilla. The distinctive features of the chinchilla skull include very large tympanic bullae, large infraorbital foraminae, reduced zygomatic arches, and an absence of a masseteric crest of the mandibles. 1, incisive bone; 2, nasal bone; 3, zygomatic arch; 4, frontal bone; 5, parietal bone; 6, frontal bone; 7, interparietal bone; 8, maxilla.

Fig. C11.10 Conventional right lateral radiograph of a normal adult chinchilla (a) and lateral aspect of a normal skull (b). 1, incisive bone; 2, nasal bone; 3, maxilla, 3a, infraorbital fossa; 3b, zygomatic process (maxilla); 4, frontal bone; 5, parietal bone; 6, temporal bone; 6a, zygomatic process; 6b, tympanic bulla; 7, sphenoidal bones; 8, zygomatic arch; 9, occipital bone.

Fig. C11.11 Micro-CT image of a degu skull (mandible removed) reconstructed as a 3D model: a, lateral view; b, ventrodorsal view. Reconstructed image is visualized using the volume rendering software Drishti. 1, nasal bone; 2, incisive bone; 3, maxilla; 4, zygomatic bone; 5, tympanic bulla; 6, lacrimal bone. (Courtesy Vladimír Jekl and Handschuh Stephan.)

Table C11.5 **Dentition of the Hystricognatha (porcupine/guinea pig-like rodents [e.g. guinea pigs, chinchillas and degus])**

	INCISORS	CANINES	PREMOLARS	MOLARS
Upper dental arch	1	0	1	3
Lower dental arch	1	0	1	3

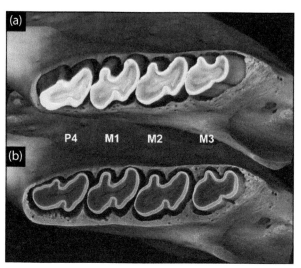

Fig. C11.13 **Micro-CT 3D reconstruction of a degus left mandible: occlusal view at a level of occlusal surface (a) and 3 mm below the alveolar ridge (b). Premolars and molars, which are largely composed of dentin, have similar structure and in each quadrant of the oral cavity they form a uniform functional grinding unit. The occlusal surface of degus premolars and molars resembles a figure-of-eight. Note the whitish enamel ridges and yellow to brown color of the dentinal grooves. (Courtesy Vladimír Jekl and Tomas Zikmund.)**

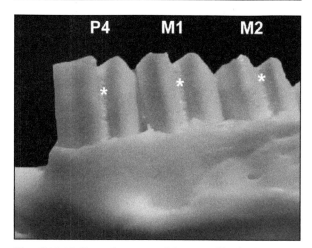

Fig. C11.12 **Buccal aspect of the mandibular left premolar and first two molars of a guinea pig. Guinea pig premolars or molars are laminated teeth with two dental laminas. Interposed between the two dental laminas is the interdental septum, which is seen as a deep fold from the buccal aspect of the teeth and is filled with acellular cementum (asterisks). With the mandibular premolars/molars, the enamel covering is present on the buccal surface; the lingual aspect is covered with a continuous layer of cementum on the dentin.**

POSITIONING AND RESTRAINT FOR RADIOGRAPHY OF THE SKULL

Radiography of the head must be performed in all cases of suspected dental or maxillofacial disease. As in rabbits, an understanding of the anatomy of the skull and teeth structure is crucial. Even though some authors[1] prefer manual restraint, other authors take radiographs under general anesthesia as even small amounts of angulation can cause severe distortion and misinterpretation. Procedure standardization is also more efficient with the animal under anesthesia. It is important that a radiographic method is established that is known to all who will interpret the radiographic images, especially in lateral oblique and intraoral views.

Conventional dorsoventral (DV), right lateral (RL), two lateral oblique, and rostrocaudal (RC) views are usually performed. Digital dental radiographs are particularly useful when evaluating tooth and skull pathology. A combination of intraoral and extraoral views is preferred as it provides the ability to interpret more subtle pathologic changes.

A ventrodorsal (VD) view with the patient in dorsal recumbency may impair respiration and therefore rodents should be repositioned into sternal recumbency as soon as possible. Patient oxygenation throughout the procedure is essential. If a facial mass is present, a cotton ball or wedge of foam can be used to aid proper positioning.

Assessment of tympanic bullae, temporomandibular joints, and teeth is possible using RC, lateral oblique (20–40°), and DV/VD views. Complete symmetry on the radiograph of DV or VD views confirms optimal positioning.

RADIOGRAPHIC VIEWS

Dorsoventral and ventrodorsal view

For the DV view (**Figures C11.5, C11.6, C11.9, C11.14, C11.15**), the patient is placed in sternal recumbency with its mandible resting on the cassette or sensor. The position of the head is maintained by using a bandage placed over the dorsal cervical region. Alternatively, a small box can be placed below the mandible to support the head. The forelimbs are taped cranially or left without any fixation. Exact positioning is achieved by gentle head manipulation, until the incisor interdental space, nasal philtrum, and the middle of the area between the eyes are in one straight line. The x-ray beam is centered on the middle of the line connecting the medial canthus of each eye. Complete symmetry on the radiograph confirms optimal positioning.

The VD view is performed with the patient in dorsal recumbency (**Figures C11.16, C11.17**). The head is extended and taped or held in place with a bandage so that the ventral margins of the mandibles are parallel with the cassette. Symmetry between the right and left sides should always be evaluated. The x-ray beam is centered on the middle of the line connecting the

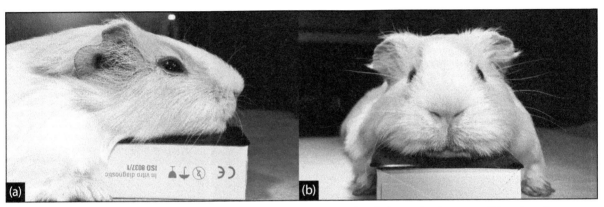

Fig. C11.14 **Positioning of a guinea pig for DV view (a, b) with its head elevated using a small box (e.g. for microscope slides as in this case). Exact positioning is achieved by gentle head manipulation until the incisor interdental space, nasal philtrum (b), and the middle of the area between the eyes are in one straight line. The x-ray beam is centered on the middle of the line connecting the medial canthus of each eye.**

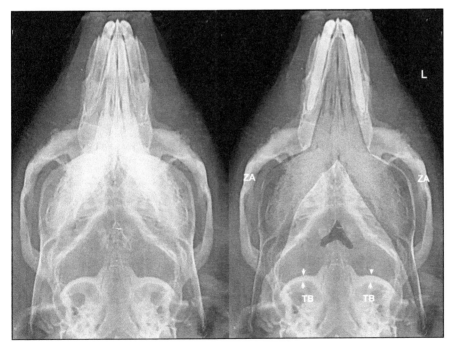

Fig. C11.15 **DV view of a guinea pig with subclinical otitis media confirmed by otoscopy. Note the massive mandible (blue) and zygomatic arches (ZA), maxillary incisors (yellow), and mild thickening (arrowheads) of both tympanic bulla bones (TB). The hyoid bone is marked red. (Courtesy Vladimír Jekl and Karel Hauptman.)**

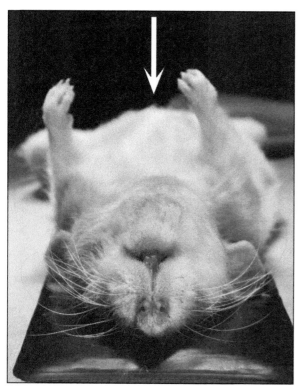

Fig. C11.16 **The VD view is helpful in cases of mandibular or neck masses, where proper DV positioning is very problematic to achieve. Arrow shows the direction of the x-ray beam.**

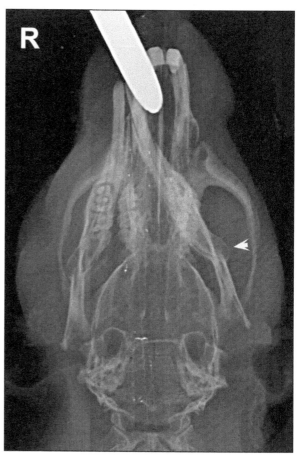

Fig. C11.17 **VD view of a rat. For better assessment of the incisor apex, a slight mandibular rotation is recommended to allow the apex (arrowhead) to be superimposed on the lucent orbital space.**

medial canthus of each eye. If the rostral part of the nasal cavity or maxillary incisors and premolars need to be evaluated, the mandible is gently displaced laterally to allow proper examination (**Figure C11.17**).

Rostrocaudal view

The patient is placed in dorsal recumbency with the nose pointing upwards and the long axis of the head perpendicular to the x-ray film (**Figures C11.5, C11.18–C11.21**). The head is supported with a wedge of foam or a bandage. The mouth is closed. An open mouth view does not provide additional information. The forelimbs are positioned parallel to the thorax. Larger rodents can be placed in a trough. The x-ray beam is centered between the eyes.

Lateral view

The lateral view of the head is performed with the patient in right or left lateral recumbency, depending on the locality of the lesion. If a rodent is undergoing screening for dental pathology, the right

lateral position is recommended as the standard view (**Figures C11.7, C11.10, C11.22–C11.24**). Cotton wool or a foam wedge can be used to support the nose and keep the head in the correct position. Proper positioning is where the nasal philtrum is parallel to the x-ray film and the incisors, bodies and rami of the mandibles, tympanic bullae, and all the bilateral anatomic structures are superimposed. The forelimbs must not be superimposed on the area of interest and are left parallel to the body or taped away from the skull. For assessment of the occlusal surfaces of the premolars and molars, the mouth can be kept slightly opened using a plastic syringe inserted between the incisors or using a bandage. The length of the syringe is cut to approximately 0.3–1 cm using scissors. The x-ray beam is centered on the medial canthus of the eye.

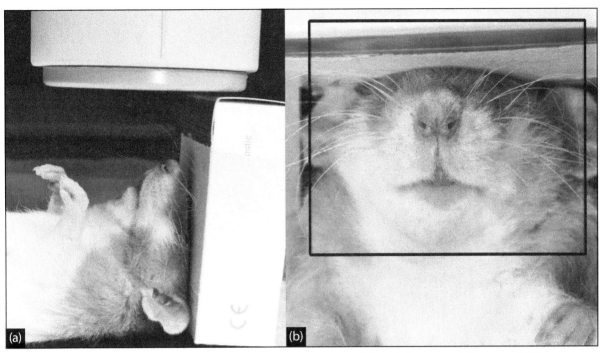

Fig. C11.18 Proper positioning of a rat for a RC view: lateral (a) and dorsal (b) views of the animal. The forelimbs are positioned parallel to the thorax. The x-ray beam is centered between the eyes (b).

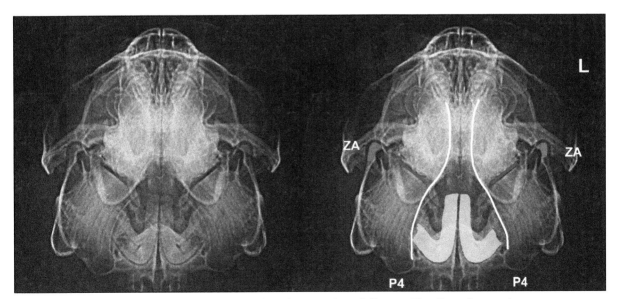

Fig. C11.19 RC view of an adult guinea pig with early stage dental disease. Blue lines denote the proper occlusal plane and alignment of the premolars and molars. Apices of the premolars and molars slightly elongate into the orbital area (red lines). Due to the normal bended curvature of the premolars and molars, the apices of the premolars (P4) seems to perforate the ventral mandibular cortex. Mandibular incisors (yellow), temporomandibular joints (green), and zygomatic arches (ZA) are radiographically normal in this patient. (Courtesy Vladimír Jekl and Karel Hauptman.)

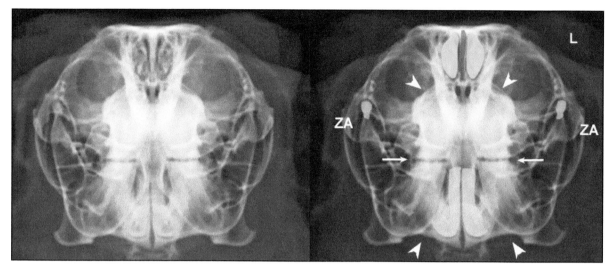

Fig. C11.20 **RC view of an adult chinchilla with normal dentition.** Arrows denote the proper occlusal plane and alignment of the premolars and molars. The apices of the premolars and molars do not elongate into the infraorbital/orbital area and do not penetrate the ventral mandibular cortex (arrowheads). The nasal cavity can also be evaluated on this view (vomer marked red, nasal cavity together with paranasal recess marked light blue, choanae marked dark blue). Mandibular incisors (yellow), temporomandibular joints (green), and zygomatic arches (ZA) are radiographically normal in this patient. (Courtesy Vladimír Jekl and Karel Hauptman.)

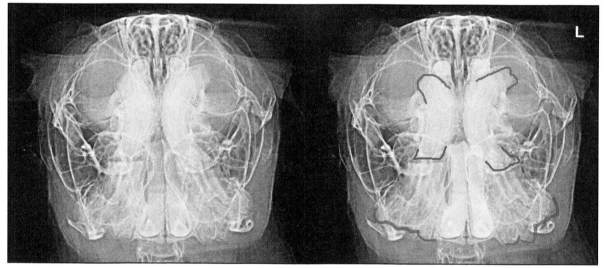

Fig. C11.21 **RC view of an adult chinchilla with severe dental disease.** Incisors are yellow colored and the clinical crowns of the mandibular incisors are elongated. The clinical crowns of the premolars and molars have increased angulation as well as maxillary buccal points (blue). The maxillary and mandibular reserve crowns of the premolars and molars have abnormal curvature and are apically elongated. The maxillary reserve crowns have penetrated the alveolar bone into the infraorbital fossa and orbit (red lines) and the mandibular reserve crowns have penetrated the ventral mandibular cortex (red lines). The temporomandibular joints (green circles) are radiographically normal in this patient. (Courtesy Vladimír Jekl and Karel Hauptman.)

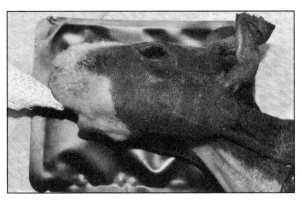

Fig. C11.22 Positioning of a guinea pig for lateral skull radiography. For optimal positioning, cotton wool or a foam wedge can be used to support the nose and keep the head in the correct position. Alternatively, gauze placed on the maxillary incisors can be used to keep the head in the correct position.

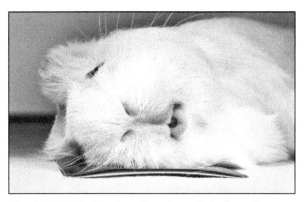

Fig. C11.23 Positioning of a guinea pig for lateral or lateral oblique skull radiography. Exact positioning is achieved by gentle head manipulation, until the nasal philtrum is parallel to the x-ray film and the incisors, bodies and rami of the mandibles, tympanic bullae, and all the bilateral anatomical structures are superimposed.

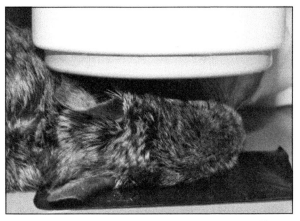

Fig. C11.24 Positioning of a degu for lateral skull radiography. In this case, the head was in the optimal position for lateral radiography.

In guinea pigs, because of the steep angle of the occlusal plane of the premolars and molars, it cannot be evaluated on the lateral view (**Figure C11.7**).[4]

Lateral oblique views

For lateral oblique views, the patient is placed in right or left lateral recumbency depending on the part of the head to be imaged. The mouth is closed or held open with a syringe inserted between the incisors or with the use of a bandage, based on practitioner preference. A foam wedge may be placed under the mandible to slightly elevate the nose; however, due to the size of the rodents being

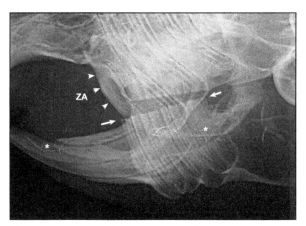

Fig. C11.25 Lateral oblique view of a guinea pig mandible using the conventional approach, where the head is rotated to an angle of 40° or the x-ray tube is adjusted to the desired angle. Note the superimposed premolar and molar teeth, normal straight occlusal plane (arrows), and zygomatic arch (ZA, arrowheads), which may imitate teeth structure. Thin opaque lines (asterisks) are artifacts associated with the presence of hair in the scanner or in the cassette/sensor. (Courtesy Vladimír Jekl and Karel Hauptman.)

examined, this is generally unnecessary. The head is rotated to an angle of 30–40° or the x-ray tube is adjusted to the desired angle (**Figure C11.25**). To minimize image distortion, the rotation should not be excessive. The x-ray beam is centered on the medial canthus of the eye.

Bohmer[1,11] described isolated views of the mandibles with the animal in ventral recumbency with the mouth held wide open using gauze bandages. The head is then raised steeply off the table (approximately 45°) and positioned such that the central beam is directed on to the middle intermandibular area cranially from the maxillary incisors and slightly caudally from the mandibular symphysis. In this way, both mandibles can be depicted largely in isolation without superimposition of the rostral part of the maxilla. For an isolated view of a maxilla, the patient is placed on the table in dorsal recumbency, and a relatively robust foam roller is placed under its neck so that the head is extended caudodorsally. If the apical parts of the posterior maxillary cheek teeth (M2/M3) are to be projected clearly, the patient's head is extended with a smaller angle (approximately 35°). Larger angles (approximately 45°) are chosen for isolated views of the apices of the two anterior cheek teeth (P4/M1). The entire intra- and extra-alveolar parts of the maxillary cheek teeth can be projected in isolation by slightly rotating the skull to the left (for the left half of the upper jaw) and to the right (for the right half of the upper jaw). This technique commonly requires hand-held positioning, which is against radiation safety regulation in some countries.

This author prefers the technique described by Minarikova et al.[14] where the guinea pig is placed in lateral recumbency with the mouth closed and the beam (tube head) directed into the proper position. This technique is the optimal radiographic view for assessment of the mandibular premolars and molars

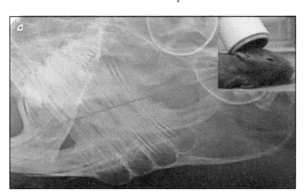

Fig. C11.26 Right lateral oblique view of a guinea pig mandible using the lateral oblique view (70°), but with the beam directed caudorostrally (the radiographic tube is at a 45° angle to the longitudinal head axis). (Courtesy Vladimír Jekl and Andrea Minarikova).

over their entire length and width without any superimposition. The beam is directed caudorostrally, with the radiographic tube at a 45° angle with the longitudinal head axis. Radiographs are then taken in different angles (45–70°) (**Figures C11.26, C11.27**). This technique is easily reproducible and does not need hand-held positioning.

Reference anatomic lines

One study[15] compared prepared skulls with the radiographs of identical animals, which provided species-specific anatomic reference lines that facilitate the objective assessment of the severity of dental disease in rabbits, guinea pigs, and chinchillas. This author uses these lines only as guidelines. Each radiograph should be thoroughly examined.

In a lateral view of a guinea pig head (**Figure C11.28A**), the first line connects the rostral end of the nasal bone with the dorsal notch of the tympanic bulla, about three-quarters of the height of the bulla. As the occlusal surfaces of guinea pig premolars and molars are strongly angled, the occlusal

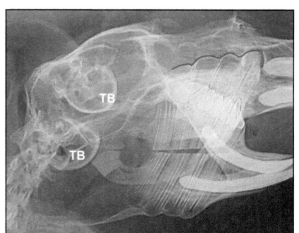

Fig. C11.27 Left lateral oblique view of a normal guinea pig skull using the lateral oblique view (70°), but with the beam directed caudorostrally (the radiographic tube is at a 45° angle to the longitudinal head axis). The occlusal plane can be easily evaluated. The apices of the left mandibular (blue) and the right maxillary (red) premolars and molars are easily seen on the radiograph. Incisor reserve crowns (yellow), tympanic bullae (TB), and the condylar process of the mandible (green) are normal. (Courtesy Vladimír Jekl and Andrea Minarikova.)

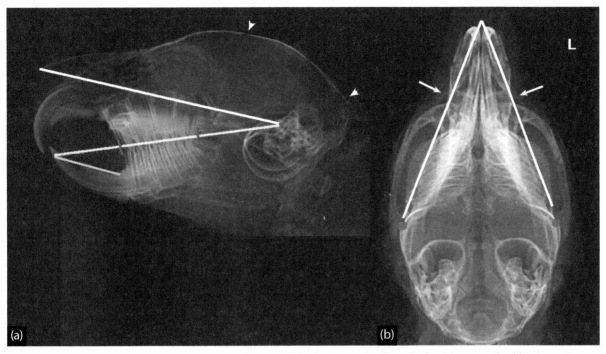

Fig. C11.28 Reference anatomic lines on lateral (a) and DV (b) views of a clinically healthy 4-week-old guinea pig skull. Note the nonfused bone sutures in this young animal (a, arrowheads). (b) The most informative reference line runs from the mesial border of the maxillary incisor to the most caudolateral part of the ipsilateral mandible, which lies at the level of the temporal zygomatic process (red circle). In healthy guinea pigs only the radiolucent apical bulla of the maxillary fourth premolar (the first cheek tooth) extends beyond this line (arrows).

plane does not present as a clear line on the lateral view (certain vagueness because of superimposition of the labial/palatal occlusal part of the maxillary and the buccal occlusal part of the mandibular premolars and molars), but it is mostly sufficiently visible to allow comparison with the next reference line. This is drawn from the point on the labial surface of the mandibular incisor where it is crossed by a line projected cranially from the mandibular bone plate (green line), to the notch of the tympanic bulla (yellow line).[15] This second reference line runs straight along the occlusal line of the mandibular premolar and molar teeth. If the teeth are healthy, it should also run through the wear surfaces of the maxillary and mandibular incisors when the mouth is closed, but this is rarely seen in practice as most guinea pigs have at least a minor degree of clinical crown elongation. The ventral mandibular cortex (blue line) should not be penetrated by any of the tooth apices, which should be distinctly radiolucent. The palatal and mandibular cortices converge rostrally when the mouth is closed (green lines). The greater the degree of intraoral tooth elongation

the less obvious this becomes in guinea pigs. The maxillary and mandibular tooth dental arches are each formed by four cheek teeth, the maxillary and mandibular arches being of matching lengths (red lines). A discrepancy between the length of the dental arches is an indicator of a dental disorder. In the DV view (**Figure C11.28B**) the most informative reference line runs from the mesial border of the maxillary incisor to the most caudolateral part of the ipsilateral mandible, which lies at the level of the temporal zygomatic process.[15] In healthy guinea pigs only the radiolucent apical bulla of the maxillary fourth premolar (the first cheek tooth) extends beyond this line.

In a lateral view of a chinchilla (**Figure C11.29**), the first reference line connects the dorsal margin of the maxillary incisor with the middle of the tympanic bulla. In healthy animals, the radiolucent germinative tissue at the apices of the maxillary cheek teeth should be on this line, with no calcified tooth structures extending dorsal to it. The second reference line begins at the tip of the maxillary incisors and extends caudally to pass through the tympanic

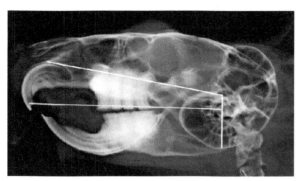

Fig. C11.29 **Reference anatomic lines on a lateral view of an adult chinchilla skull with advanced dental disease. Note the severe apical elongation of the maxillary premolars and molars.**

bulla at approximately three-quarters of its height. It runs almost parallel to the palatine bone and passes through the occlusal surfaces or tips of both incisors when they are of normal length and occlusion. This position will need to be estimated in incisor elongation. The reference line coincides with the normal occlusal plane. The ventral border of the mandible should be smooth and without any thinning or distortions associated with intruded apices.

Intraoral and extraoral views

Dental radiography has significant advantages over conventional radiography because of the greater resolution and detail provided. Small dental films or digital sensors can be used for intraoral radiography (20 × 30 mm; 20 × 40 mm; 27 × 54 mm). The use of special rabbit intraoral plates is recommended; however, they can be used only in larger rodents. Larger films are used for extraoral radiography to enable correct positioning and teeth examination (30 × 40 mm; 57 × 76 mm; 57 × 94 mm).

The parallel technique, which is typically performed with the patient in lateral recumbency, requires that the film and long axis of the tooth are parallel to each other and the x-ray beam directed perpendicularly to both the roots and x-ray sensor. This technique may be used for assessment of the occlusal surface of the premolars and molars. Furthermore, it is possible to evaluate the entire crown of mandibular molars with this method.

A bisecting angle technique can be performed with the patient in sternal or lateral recumbency (**Figures C11.30–C11.32**). Only the mandibular incisors can be examined with the patient in dorsal recumbency. The bisecting angle technique overcomes the difficulties of obtaining accurate images of teeth with different shapes and superimposing surrounding structures. In rodents, it is impossible to place a film parallel to maxillary incisors, premolars, and molars. Therefore, the x-ray beam is centered on the area of interest and positioned perpendicular to the bisecting angle. The bisecting angle is the line that bisects the angle created by the long axis of the sensor and the long axis of the tooth. Because of the relatively high curvature and very long reserve crowns of the maxillary incisors, the final image is typically foreshortened.

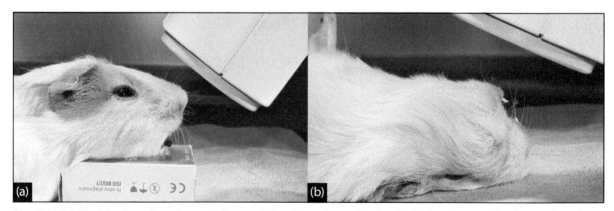

Fig. C11.30 **Positioning of a guinea pig for maxillary (a) and mandibular (b) incisor intraoral radiography using the bisecting angle technique. This technique can be performed with the patient in sternal (a, for maxillary teeth) or dorsal recumbency (b, for mandibular teeth). The animal is positioned with the palate parallel to the table and the film/sensor is carefully placed in the mouth, so that all target teeth will be on the film. The bisecting angle is calculated and the beam is directed onto the sensor (approximately 45°).**

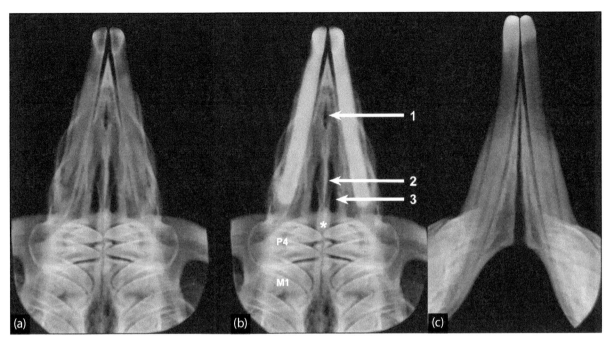

Fig. C11.31 Isolated view of the rostral part of the upper jaw (DV view, bisecting angle approximately 20°, a, b) and mandibular incisors (bisecting angle, approximately 40°, c). The cheek teeth in guinea pigs diverge from rostral to caudal, with the maxillary premolars located close to each other (asterisk). Guinea pig premolars or molars are laminated teeth with two dental laminas, and originating from two germinal centers. Maxillary incisors are marked yellow and apices of the maxillary molars are marked red. 1, interincisive foramen; 2, vomer; 3, incisive foramen.

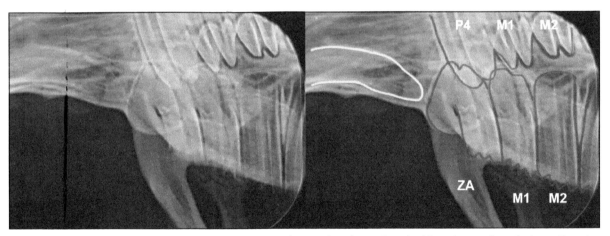

Fig. C11.32 Radiography of the right maxillary premolars and molars using the bisecting angle technique. Even in healthy dentition, the reserve crown of the premolars and molars can be seen partially distorted due to its normal curvature. The right maxillary second molar can be easily evaluated. Shape of the cheek teeth (periodontal space) is marked red; maxillary right incisor is marked yellow. (Courtesy Vladimír Jekl.)

Extraoral dental radiography can be used for examination of the maxillary premolars and molars. The patient is placed in lateral recumbency with the x-ray sensor placed just underneath the cheek teeth. For this technique, conventional left lateral, left lateral oblique, and DV views are suitable. With the use of small x-ray films and/or intraoral sensors, as well as the use of additional views, it is possible to evaluate all the incisors, premolars, and molars precisely, especially in larger rodents (**Figure C11.32**).

RADIOGRAPHIC INTERPRETATION

Proper interpretation of skull and dental radiographs is based on a sound knowledge of normal anatomy. When assessing the teeth on a radiograph, the following should be evaluated:

- Position.
- Size and shape.
- Contour.
- Internal structure.
- Density.
- Occlusal surface.
- Reserve crown.
- Periodontal ligament space.
- Alveolar bone.

DENTAL PATHOLOGY

Diseases of the oral cavity are common in small herbivorous mammals. In pet rabbits and rodents, many local and systemic conditions that affect the oral cavity have been described, including hereditary, infectious, metabolic (**Figure C11.33**), nutritional, and traumatic conditions as well as electrocution and neoplasms.

Clinical signs of dental disease are mostly non-specific and commonly include anorexia, progressive weight loss, change of feeding habits and feed preferences, deterioration of fur quality, and hypersalivation (**Figure C11.1**).[16–18] Fur chewing in chinchillas is in many cases associated with dental disease and is seen concurrently with excessive salivation. In some cases, dental disease can also be accompanied by moist dermatitis, epiphora, or exophthalmia. Any oral pathology may result in scant and smaller droppings, gastrointestinal hypomotility, and meteorism (excess gas in intestines).[10] In guinea pigs it can also be associated with soft droppings imitating diarrhea.

Incisor pathology

Hereditary pathologies, such as brachygnathia superior in rabbits, have been described in guinea pigs.[19] This author has seen a 3-month-old chinchilla with congenital brachygnatia superior, with subsequent incisor malocclusion as well as premolar and molar clinical crown elongation and malocclusion (**Figure C11.34**).

In Hystricomorpha (guinea pigs, chinchillas, and degus) incisor malocclusions generally occur secondary to coronal elongation of the cheek teeth or due to tooth fracture (**Figure C11.35**). In all rodents, dysplastic changes (uneven labial surface of incisors, horizontal ridges, **Figure C11.36**), or abnormal pigmentation are commonly seen in cases of chronic trauma, metabolic disturbances, or systemic diseases (e.g. secondary hyperparathyroidism, hypocalcemia).[11,20,21] Abnormal enamel pigmentation can also be seen in cases of accelerated incisor eruption after fractures.

Chronic incisor infection most commonly leads to a slight deviation of the tooth, structural changes of tooth substance in the form of transverse grooves, longitudinal fractures, and color changes, as well

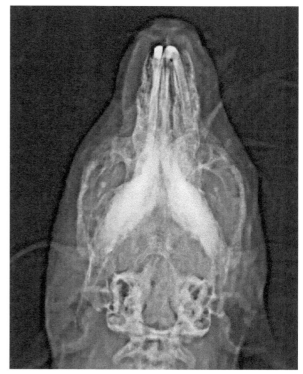

Fig. C11.33 **DV view of a guinea pig (Satin cross-bred) suffering from fibrous osteodystrophy. Total bone decalcification and loss of normal bone structure is obvious. Bone changes in Satin pure-bred or Satin cross-bred guinea pigs are associated with secondary renal hyperparathyroidism. (Courtesy Vladimír Jekl and Karel Hauptman.)**

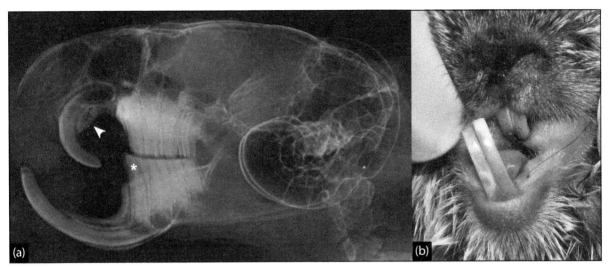

Fig. C11.34 Congenital brachygnathia superior in a 3-month-old chinchilla. Lateral skull radiograph (a) shows severe incisor malocclusion, shortened maxillary diastema (arrowhead), and elongated clinical crowns of all the premolars and molars. The tooth length of the mandibular cheek teeth gradually increase rostrally, with the highest crown of the premolar (asterisk). Note also incisor depigmentation (b).

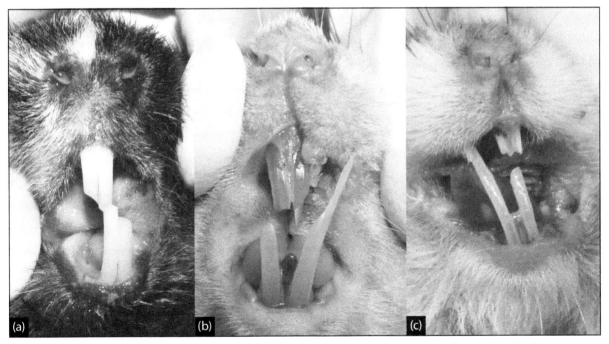

Fig. C11.35 Acquired incisor malocclusion in an adult guinea pig (a), a rat (b), and a hamster (c). Incisor malocclusion with lateral mandibular displacement (mandibular shift) in guinea pigs is mostly secondary to coronal elongation of the cheek teeth (a). Other etiologies include parodontopathies (b) or tooth fractures (c). (Courtesy Vladimír Jekl and Karel Hauptman.)

as enamel and dentin hypoplasia. Due to the pain, the tooth is no longer worn down correctly, which leads to secondary overgrowth and the formation of an abnormal occlusal plane.[11] The tooth becomes more mobile as the periodontal ligament enlarges, and purulent discharge from the alveolus is common. The changes described above, as well as tooth rotation around its long axis, increase

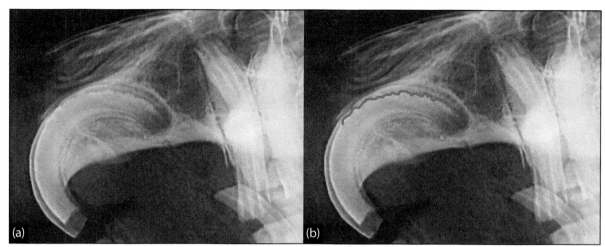

Fig. C11.36 Lateral extraoral view of a chinchilla suffering from severe dental disease (uneven size of maxillary incisors and apical (b, blue line) and coronal elongation of all the maxillary premolars and molars. Uneven labial/enamel incisor surface (b, red line) is associated with dysplastic changes of the germinal tooth tissue. (Courtesy Vladimír Jekl and Karel Hauptman.)

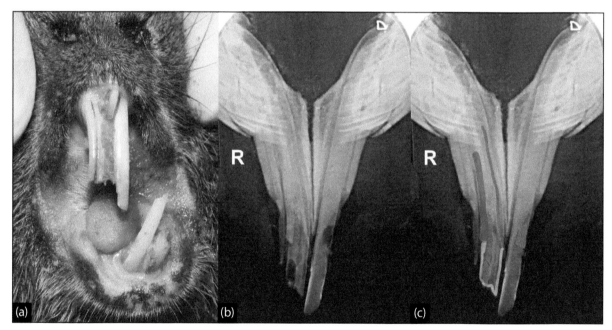

Fig. C11.37 Incisor malocclusion and teeth splitting in a 4-year-old guinea pig (a). Intraoral view of the mandibular incisors (b, c) showing tooth malformation and tooth splitting. In one alveolus, multiple isolated 'incisors' were present (blue, yellow, and red). This splitting of teeth is the result of an apical, pressure-related or infectious irritation. The tooth substance and periodontium progressively deteriorate with additional risk of periodontitis and caries lesions. Caries lesions are, in this patient, seen as radiolucent areas (green). Incisor splitting is an indication for extraction. (Courtesy Vladimír Jekl and Karel Hauptman.)

in transversal tooth diameter ('giant incisors') and longitudinal tooth splitting is commonly seen in guinea pigs (**Figure C11.37**). As a consequence of chronic inflammation and dysplastic/inflammatory change of the germinative tooth center, incisors can become depigmented, develop a rough surface, and become more fragile, which predisposes them to fractures and caries.

In this author's practice, periapical incisor inflammation and subsequent osteomyelitis is seen most commonly in rats (**Figure C11.38**), but can also be seen in other species (**Figures C11.39, C11.40**) or in animals after improper incisor trimming.

Fractures are mostly of traumatic origin (**Figure C11.35**). Other causes of total or partial incisor fractures are associated with iatrogenic damage due to improper incisor clinical crown adjustment.[3] A common consequence of these fractures is incisor malocclusion (**Figures C11.41, C11.42**).

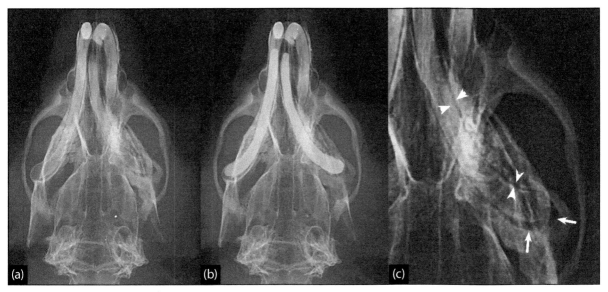

Fig. C11.38 **VD views of a rat head (a–c). Note the obvious periosteal reaction in the apical area of the left mandibular incisor with thickening of the alveolar bone (b, blue). Both mandibular incisors are marked in yellow. Note the normal thickness of the periodontal space (c, arrowheads) in comparison with the radiolucent area surrounding the teeth apex (c, arrows). Periapical inflammation and mandibular osteomyelitis was the final diagnosis. This incisor pathology is an indication for incisor extraction. The right tympanic bulla is more radiopaque than the left bulla, therefore another view (lateral oblique) and otoscopy is indicated to distinguish disease of the tympanic bulla (middle ear cavity). (Courtesy Vladimír Jekl and Karel Hauptman.)**

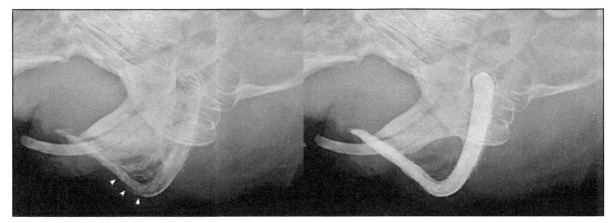

Fig. C11.39 **Lateral oblique view of a guinea pig mandible with a malformed left incisor with its aberrant growth (b, yellow) associated with mandibular osteomyelitis (b, blue). Arrowheads (a) indicate tooth resorptive lesions associated with inflammatory changes and caries. (Courtesy Vladimír Jekl and Karel Hauptman.)**

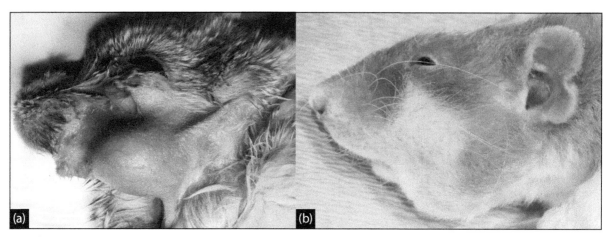

Fig. C11.40 Odontogenic abscesses in an adult chinchilla (a) and a rat (b). In chinchillas facial abscesses are usually associated with periapical inflammatory changes of the premolar or molar teeth, whereas in rats they are usually associated with incisor apical pathology. These abscesses are typically firm, cool, and with a wide base. (Courtesy Vladimír Jekl and Karel Hauptman.)

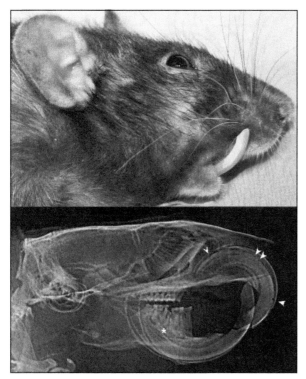

Fig. C11.41 Pronounced incisor malocclusion in a rat with severe mandibular as well as maxillary incisor overgrowth secondary to trauma (a). On the radiograph, the arrowheads indicate radiolucent areas in the enamel associated with aberrant enamel deposition. The clinical crown of the second molar is completely lytic and only the teeth roots are seen (asterisk). This pathology is associated with extensive caries. (Courtesy Vladimír Jekl and Karel Hauptman.)

Elodontoma (pseudo-odontoma, odontogenic dysplasia) is defined as a hamartoma (benign tumor-like lesions composed of an overgrowth of mature tissue that normally occurs in the affected part of the body but with disorganization and often one element predominating) of continuously developing odontogenic tissue and alveolar bone at the apical part of elodont teeth.[22] It seems that the formation of these tumor-like lesions is the result of crowding of the odontogenic tissue rather than excessive proliferation.[22] Early changes in squirrels and prairie dogs with these dysplastic tooth changes include abnormalities and irregularities with new dentin, clinically seen as superficial tooth folding and malformation.[17] Continued deposition of dysplastic tooth structure at the apices of the maxillary incisors is responsible for the formation of a space-occupying mass, which often obstructs the middle or caudal part of the nasal cavity, especially in squirrels and prairie dogs (**Figure C11.43**). True neoplastic masses (odontomas) associated with ectopic formation of tooth substances (especially in the nasal cavity) grow aggressively into the surrounding tissues and commonly obstruct the nasal cavities.[23] These pathologies are very common in degus,[24] but may also be seen in other small herbivorous mammals (**Figure C11.44**). In both these lesions, the most common presenting signs are reduced food intake, weight loss, general weakness, and/or dyspnea associates with narrowed nasal passages.[24]

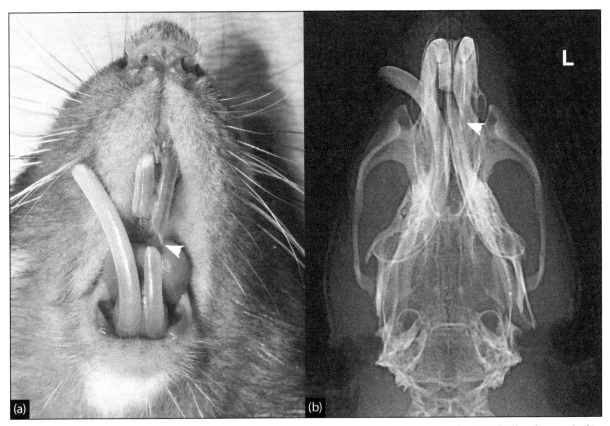

Fig. C11.42 Pronounced incisor malocclusion in the same rat as in Fig. C11.41 (a) and a DV skull radiograph (b). The mandibular incisors have generally decreased (lighter) enamel color with obvious elongation of the left tooth. The maxillary incisors have a rough labial surface and the left tooth has a sharp end (arrowheads). (Courtesy Vladimír Jekl and Karel Hauptman.)

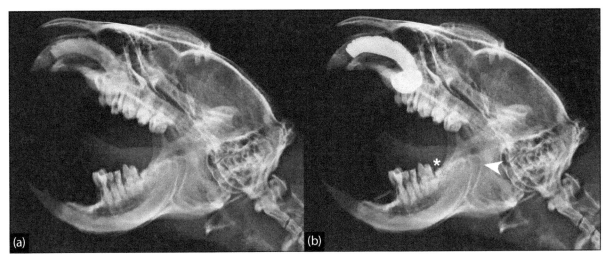

Fig. C11.43 Maxillary pseudo-odontoma in a prairie dog is seen as a bulging area at the incisor apex (yellow). Due to the dysplastic changes of the germinal tissue, enamel folds are recognized as the uneven labial surface of both incisors. The clinical crowns of the maxillary incisors are fractured. There is also horizontal bone loss at the rostral part of the mandible, with tooth loss associated with caries and periodontal disease. The missing clinical crown of the last mandibular molar is associated with dental caries (asterisk). (Courtesy Vladimír Jekl and Karel Hauptman.)

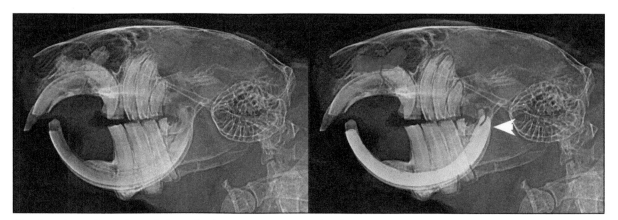

Fig. C11.44 Left 10° lateral view of a degu with incisor malocclusion (mandibular incisors marked yellow) and severe apical elongation of the mandibular incisors (arrowhead) and all the premolars and molars (red lines). Respiratory problems in this case were associated with odontoma (blue), which obstructed the nasal cavity. (Courtesy Vladimír Jekl and Karel Hauptman.)

Premolar and molar pathology

Acquired dental disease

In Hystricognatha (porcupine-like rodents), all the pre-molars and molars continue to erupt throughout life, so they are predisposed to the syndrome of acquired dental disease, which is a multifactorial disease/syndrome. The etiology of acquired dental disease seems to be related to a lack of proper tooth wear and/or calcium and phosphorus metabolic disorders, as is in found in other small herbivorous mammals.[2] All these factors lead to a reduction in cheek tooth wear rate, decreased length of the pulp, increased curvature of the tooth, clinical crown elongation (**Figure C11.2**), and apical elongation. As the dental disease develops and progresses, the cheek teeth will likely continue to grow at near the normal rate despite decreased or arrested eruption if the apical tissues can remodel rapidly and/or the apex penetrates through the periosteum.[6] Extensive apical cheek teeth elongation is commonly found in chinchillas and degus (**Figures C11.45, C11.46**).

In chinchillas, coronal cheek teeth elongation is most obvious in the maxillary dental arches, where premolars and molars curve buccally and form sharp spikes. In guinea pigs, mandibular premolars and first molars elongate coronally, causing a 'bridge'-like structure over the tongue (entrapment), which prevents feeding (**Figure C11.2**). In degus, the apices of the extensively elongated maxillary first premolars cause obstruction of the nasal passages and subsequent dyspnea (**Figure C11.47**).[25]

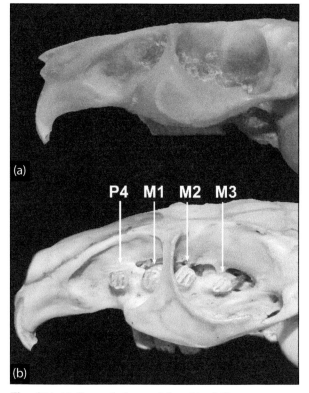

(a)

P4   M1   M2   M3

(b)

Fig. C11.45 Lateral views of the chinchilla skull. (a) Normal dentition of the maxillary left quadrant. (b) Advanced dental disease and severe apical elongation of maxillary cheek teeth. The premolar and first molar (first two cheek teeth) apices can be palpated in the infraorbital fossa. (Courtesy Vladimír Jekl.)

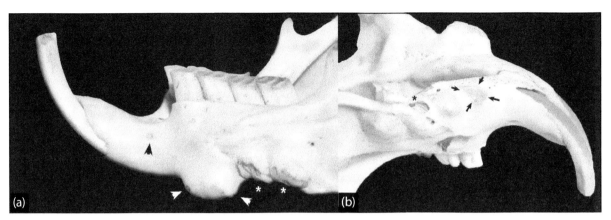

Fig. C11.46 Left lateral (a) and left ventrolateral (b) views of the mandible of the same chinchilla as in Fig. C11.45b. Apical cheek teeth elongation may be asymmetric and could imitate osteoproliferative lesions (a, white arrowheads). The apices of the mandibular premolars and molars have penetrated through the periosteum (a, b, asterisks). Note also the very thin bone 'overlying' the left mandibular premolar (b, black arrows). The mental foramen (a, black arrowhead) is located ventromesially to the fourth premolars (first cheek teeth). (Courtesy Vladimír Jekl.)

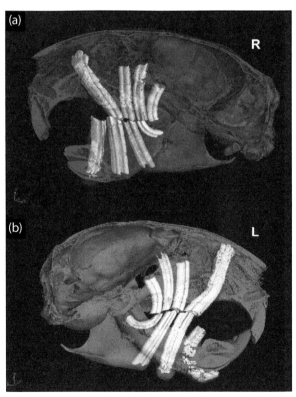

Fig. C11.47 Sagittal plane CT images of an adult degu reconstructed at two different image planes through the right (a) and left (b) maxillary dental arches, mediolateral view. Note the severe dental disease with significant apical elongation of the maxillary and mandibular premolars and molars. (The tomographic reconstruction was created using GE phoenix datos x 2.0 software; linear voxel size was 14 µm, 3D reconstruction visualized by Drishti software, Australian National University.) (Courtesy Vladimír Jekl and Tomas Zikmund.)

Apical elongation of mandibular cheek teeth can be palpated on the ventrolateral mandibular surface. In chinchillas, apical elongation of maxillary premolars and first molars may also be palpable rostrally to the orbit in the infraorbital fossa (Figures C11.45, C11.46, C11.48–C11.51). In chinchillas and degus, the main cause of partial or total obstruction of the lacrimal duct is bony remodeling around elongating maxillary premolar and first molar tooth apices.

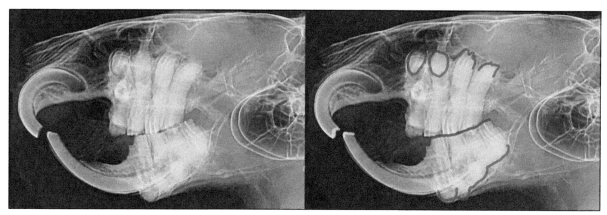

Fig. C11.48 Lateral view of a chinchilla with advanced dental disease. All the premolars and molars are apically elongated (red lines), have abnormal structure (loss of opaque enamel folds), and have uneven occlusal surface (blue line). The maxillary premolars and first molars are elongated laterally and perforate the lateral bone and periosteum. Radiographically, this is seen as the presence of a radiolucent zone around the whole apex (red circles). This abnormality is very common in chinchillas. The occlusal surface of the incisors is uneven (yellow lines) with apical elongation of mandibular incisors. (Courtesy Vladimír Jekl and Karel Hauptman.)

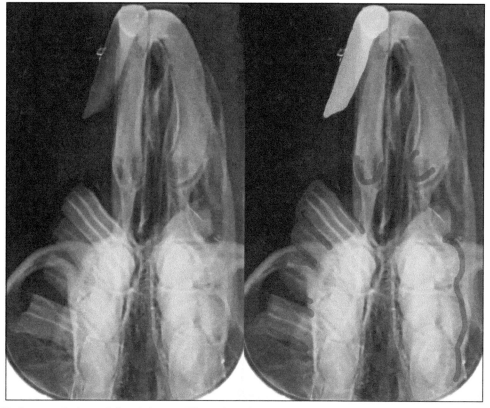

Fig. C11.49 Intraoral view of the right maxillary dental arch in a chinchilla. Note the obvious apical elongation (red lines) with perforation of the alveolar bone, and the presence of the apices and parts of the reserve crowns in the infraorbital fossa and retrobulbally. There is also severe incisor malocclusion and coronal elongation (yellow). The incisor apices are highlighted by blue lines. (Courtesy Vladimír Jekl and Karel Hauptman.)

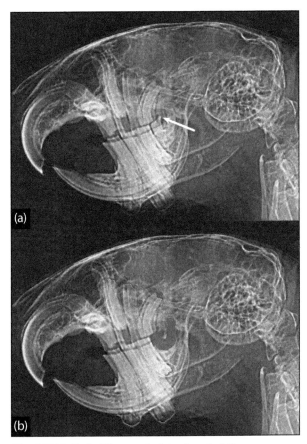

(a)

(b)

Fig. C11.50 Left 10° ventral–right dorsal oblique radiographic projection of the head of a degu showing apical and coronal elongation of all cheek teeth and uneven occlusal plane of cheek teeth. Bilateral assessment of the occlusal plane of cheek teeth is possible from this slightly oblique view. (a) Spur formation at the distal edge of the mandibular 3rd molar is visible (arrow). (b) The purple color emphasizes the diseased tooth. Red lines emphasize the location of abnormal apices. (Courtesy Vladimír Jekl and Karel Hauptman.)

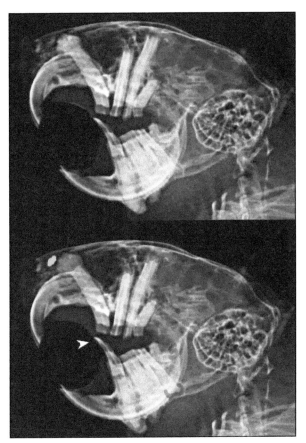

Fig. C11.51 Lateral view of the head of a degu that was presented with dyspnea. The radiograph shows severe coronal elongation and apical deformities of the cheek teeth with spike formation of the clinical crown of a mandibular premolar (arrow). Diseased apices of all the cheek teeth are clearly visible (red lines). The apical radiographic abnormality of a maxillary premolar (first cheek tooth) was indicative of a dysplastic change (pseudo-odontoma, blue color). The high radiopaque mass within the rostral part of the nasal cavity is indicative of chronic inflammatory changes with calcification or elodontoma (green). Histopathology confirmed the presence of pseudo-odontoma of the premolar and elodontoma within the nasal cavity. (Courtesy Vladimír Jekl and Karel Hauptman.)

Even a minor degree of cheek tooth clinical crown elongation has serious detrimental effects on incisor occlusion and jaw function (markedly reduced chewing efficiency), both of which further impede tooth wear. Gingival hyperplasia and alveolar bone growth frequently accompany elongation of the cheek teeth, resulting in little visible clinical crown elongation in many affected individuals and therefore radiography or CT is required to confirm the changes.[6,21]

The following pathologic changes of premolars and molars can be seen in radiographs of the cheek teeth: widening of the interproximal coronal surfaces, widening of the interdental spaces, coronal elongation, changes in the occlusal surfaces, presence of spikes, tooth torsion, tooth fracture, loss of normal tooth structure (enamel ridges loss, narrowing of the endodontic system), periapical/periodontal lysis, tooth resorptive lesions, and hypodontia. In guinea pigs, structurally abnormal teeth could be visible as 'giant teeth' with loss of enamel folds (**Figure C11.52**).

Periodontal disease

Periodontal disease (PD) is not as common in pet herbivorous rodents as it is in dogs and cats; however, one study described a 63% incidence of PD in chinchillas.[26] The presence of dental caries and PD in other exotic companion mammals has been reported or at least seen by this author (i.e. guinea pigs, degus, rats, prairie dogs), but information about the incidence of PD/caries is missing.[2,11,27] Healthy guinea pigs, chinchillas, and degus have complete elodont dentition with continuous eruption and attrition of all the teeth, so plaque accumulation and dental caries have no time to develop. In ill animals, it appears that the main cause of PD is acquired dental disease causing abnormal chewing patterns. This is due to the pathologic orthodontic tooth movements through jaw elongation, with widening of the interproximal spaces, subsequent accumulation of hair and debris, and abnormal periodontal tissue and tooth substance (i.e. enamel, dentin, and cementum) development.[3,10] Moreover, normal mastication and the natural cleaning mechanism of the oral cavity are disrupted in patients with acquired dental disease. Foreign materials and hair introduce bacteria and provide additional surface area for plaque accumulation, with possible secondary development of periodontitis, caries, osteoresorptive lesions, and abscess formation. If the diet is unsuitable, it may also provide higher levels of refined carbohydrates that enhance bacterial growth and accumulation, resulting in the periodontitis and caries formation.[28]

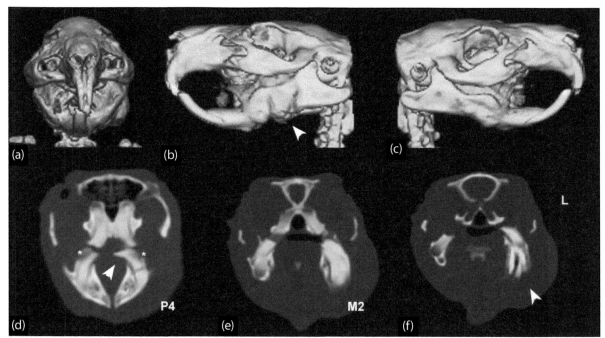

Fig. C11.52 **CT of an adult guinea pig with severe dental disease. 3D volume reconstruction of the skull (a–c) illustrates incisor malocclusion with right lateral mandibular displacement (a, rostrocaudal view) and the presence of osteoproliferative changes at the ventrolateral part of the mandible at the area of the mandibular last two molars (b, arrow). Axial views demonstrate abnormally curved and deformed reserve crowns of all the premolars, severe coronal elongation of the left mandibular premolar causing a 'bridge'-like structure over the tongue (entrapment), and abnormal occlusal plane. Areas of tooth lysis due to dental caries are also visible (asterisk). Axial views at the area of the mandibular M2 (e) and M2/M3 (f) show the presence of structurally abnormal 'giant' mandibular second molar (arrow). Apical lucency in the middle of the tooth (f) together with abnormal tooth structure is an indication for tooth extraction. (Courtesy Vladimír Jekl and Karel Hauptman.)**

Even though PD is an inflammatory and typically progressive disease process, in guinea pigs and chinchillas an edematous gingiva can result without signs of hyperemia or bleeding.[3] These findings were also demonstrated after experimental vitamin C deficiency or hypervitaminosis C. Final diagnosis of periodontitis is based on a thorough examination of the teeth as well as surrounding soft tissue and bone, periodontal probing, and dental imaging (**Figures C11.53–C11.55**).

The most common premolar and/or molar tooth pathology in Myomorpha (mice-like rodents) and Sciuromorpha (squirrel-like rodents) is PD and caries associated with a high carbohydrate diet (**Figures C11.42, C11.43**).

Odontogenic abscesses in rodents are not as common as in rabbits,[29] but a recent study in guinea pigs showed a 3.1% incidence (**Figure C11.40**).[3]

The radiographic and CT changes associated with PD include resorption of the alveolar margin, widening of the periodontal space, a defect in the path or loss of the opacity of the lamina dura, and destruction of alveolar bone.

Unlike in rabbits, most odontogenic abscesses of the mandible are retromasseteric in the guinea pig because of the anatomy of the cheek teeth and the masseter muscle. This makes the surgical approach even more challenging and is associated with a less favorable prognosis. The goal of surgery in these cases is to approach the abscess beneath the masseter muscle as far caudally as possible in order to preserve the cranial insertion of the muscle to the zygomatic arch.

Caries and osteoresorptive teeth lesions (Figures C11.53–C11.55)

Accumulation of dental plaque also predisposes to the development of caries. This initially depends on the presence of carbohydrates in the diet, particularly starch and sugars, which in acid production during bacterial digestion. The acid dissolves mineral from exposed tooth surfaces, which softens it and forms cavities in the enamel. In short-crowned teeth there is a significant risk of infection penetrating to the pulp and resulting in endodontic disease. This is less likely in continuously growing teeth as when eruption is arrested the pulp becomes shorter,

receding further from surfaces that may be affected by caries.[6]

Caries are common in chinchillas, with an incidence of more than 50% in chinchillas affected by acquired dental disease.[26] Cavities appear as

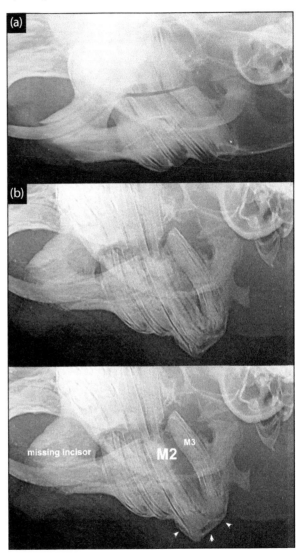

Fig. C11.53 **Lateral oblique radiographs of the right (a) and left (b) mandible of a guinea pig. The right mandibular dental arch is elongated apically and has an uneven occlusal surface. The left second and third molars are elongated apically and coronally, with periapical lucencies (arrowheads), apical deformity (red), and widened interdental space (blue) with loss of interdental alveolar bone. The typical tooth structure with enamel ridges is absent. (Courtesy Vladimír Jekl and Karel Hauptman.)**

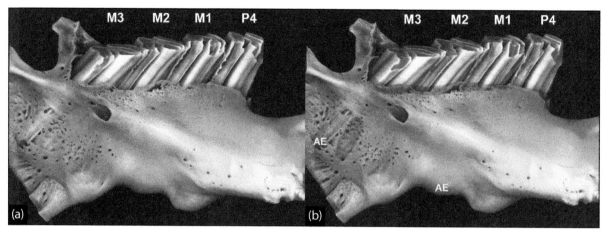

Fig. C11.54 **Micro-CT (a, b, medial views) of the left mandibular dental arch with horizontal and vertical bone loss (b, blue). Vertical bone loss is presented as a perforated bone area at the reserve crown and apical part of the last cheek tooth. Loss of tooth substance associated with caries resorptive lesions is visible at the occlusal and lingual surfaces of all teeth, especially P4 (b, red). Coronal and apical elongation (AE) of all the cheek teeth is also visible. (The tomographic reconstruction was created using GE phoenix datos x 2.0 software; linear voxel size was 14 μm, 3D reconstruction visualized by Drishti software, Australian National University.) (Courtesy Vladimír Jekl and Tomas Zikmund.)**

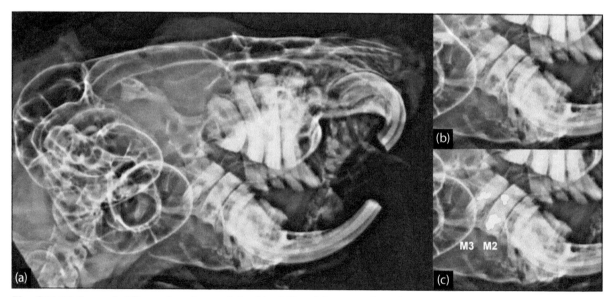

Fig. C11.55 **Lateral oblique views in an adult chinchilla with severe dental disease. Apart from the coronal and apical elongations, the presence of resorptive lesions should not be missed. On the detailed view (c), resorptive lesions can be seen at the gingival and apical levels of the second and third molar teeth (yellow). (Courtesy Vladimír Jekl and Karel Hauptman.)**

brown-to-black colored clinical crowns with associated loss of tooth substance. They can affect both the occlusal and the interproximal surface of cheek teeth.[21]

Osteoresorptive tooth lesions are very common in chinchillas.[26,30] The causes are likely either periodontitis, redirection of the resorption of alveolar bone towards the tooth itself, loss of blood supply (ischemic necrosis), hypomineralization, or decay. In chinchillas, tooth resorption leads to loss of the clinical crowns of the cheek teeth, followed by food impaction in the widened interproximal spaces and frequently the development of PD.[21] Periodontal inflammation and damage may be sufficient to induce odontoclastic resorption in affected animals. A further possibility is that the resorption of periapical bone occurring during remodeling to accommodate elongating tooth roots may become redirected towards the tooth itself.[11]

Neoplasia

Apart from odontomas, other tumors seen in the oral cavities of pet rodents include osteosarcoma, melanoma, and fibrosarcoma.[11,23] Several classifications have been proposed to describe odontogenic abnormalities in rodents and these are desribed in detail by Mancinelli and Capello.[31]

Other disorders

As premolars and molars of the Hystricomorph rodents are elodont, any systemic disease could affect enamel, dentin, and cementum formation.[32] In guinea pigs, dentition could be affected by hypovitaminosis C, hypervitaminosis C, and secondary renal hyperparathyroidism, which is seen relatively commonly in Satin pure-bred or Satin cross-bred individuals (see **Figure C11.33**).[33,34]

REFERENCES

1 Böhmer E (2001) Röntgendiagnostik bei Zahn- sowie Kiefererkrankungen der Hasenartigen und Nager. Teil 1: Tierartspezifische Zahn- und Kieferanatomie sowie Pathologie, Indikationen für die Rontgendiagnostik. *Tierärztl Prax* **29**:316–327.

2 Capello V, Lennox AM (2012) Small mammal dentistry In: *Ferrets, Rabbits and Rodents: Clinical Medicine and Surgery*, 3rd edn. (eds. KE Quesenberry, JW Carpenter) WB Saunders, St. Louis, pp. 452–471.

3 Minarikova A, Hauptman K, Jeklova E *et al*. (2015) Diseases in pet guinea pigs: a retrospective study in 1000 animals. *Vet Rec* **177**:200.

4 Gracis M (2008) Clinical technique: normal dental radiography of rabbits, guinea pigs, and chinchillas. *J Exot Pet Med* **17(2)**:78–86.

5 Berkovitz (1972) Ontogeny of tooth replacement in the guinea pig (*Cavia cobya*). *Arch Oral Biol* **17**:711–718.

6 Crossley DA (2005) Pathophysiology of continuously growing teeth. In: *Proceedings of 2nd Slovenian – Croatian Congress on Exotic Pets and Wild Animals*, Ljubljana, pp. 21–28.

7 Martin T (1999) Phylogenetic implications of glires (Eurymylidae, Mimotonidae, Rodentia, Lagomorpha) incisor enamel microstructure. *Zoosyst Evol* **75(2)**:257–273.

8 Ohshima H, Nakasone N, Hashimoto E *et al*. (2005) The eternal tooth germ is formed at the apical end of continuously growing teeth. *Arch Oral Biol* **50**:153–157.

9 Müller J, Clauss M, Codron D *et al*. (2014) Tooth length and incisal wear and growth in guinea pigs (*Cavia porcellus*) fed diets of different abrasiveness. *J Anim Physiol Anim Nutr* **99(3)**:591–604.

10 Jekl V (2009) Dentistry. In: *BSAVA Manual of Rodents and Ferrets*, 2nd edn. (eds. M Keeble, A Meredith) British Small Animal Veterinary Association, Gloucester, pp. 86–95.

11 Böhmer E (2015) *Dentistry in Rabbits and Rodents*. John Wiley and Sons, Chichester.

12 Breazile JE, Brown EM (1976) Anatomy. In: *The Biology of the Guinea Pig*. (eds. JE Wagner, PJ Manning) Academic Press, New York, pp. 53–62.

13 Jayawardena CK, Takano Y (2006) Nerve-epithelium association in the periodontal ligament of guinea pig teeth. *Arch Oral Biol* **51**:587–595.

14 Minarikova A, Hauptman K, Knotek Z *et al*. (2015) Optimal positioning of the guinea pig head for the radiographic examination. *International Conference on Avian and Herpetological and Exotic Mammal Medicine*, ICARE, p. 384.

15 Böhmer E, Crossley D (2009) Objective interpretation of dental disease in rabbits, guinea pigs and chinchillas. Use of anatomical reference lines. *Tieraerztl Prax* **37(K)(4)**:250–260.

16 Crossley DA (2001) Dental diseases in chinchillas in the UK. *J Small Anim Pract* **42**:12–19.

17 Capello V, Gracis M, Lennox AM (2005) *Rabbit and Rodent Dentistry Handbook*. Zoological Education Network Inc., Lake Worth.

18 Jekl V, Hauptman K, Knotek Z (2008) Quantitative and qualitative assessments of intraoral lesions in 180 small herbivorous mammals. *Vet Rec* **162**:442–449.

19 Rest JR, Richards T, Ball SE (1982) Malocclusion in inbred strain-2 weanling guinea pigs. *Lab Anim* **16**:84–87.

20 Jekl V, Hauptman K, Knotek Z (2011) Diseases in pet degus: a retrospective study in 300 animals. *J Small Anim Pract* **52(2)**:107–112.

21 Mans C, Jekl V (2016) Anatomy and disorders of the oral cavity of chinchillas and degus. *Vet Clin North Am Exot Anim Pract* **19(3)**:843–869.

22 Boy SC, Steenkamp G (2006) Odontoma-like tumours of squirrel elodont incisors: elodontomas. *J Comp Pathol* **135:**56–61.

23 Jekl V, Hauptman K, Skoric M *et al.* (2008) Elodontoma in a degu (*Octodon degus*). *J Exot Pet Med* **17:**216–220.

24 Jekl V, Hautpman K, Minarikova A *et al.* (2011) Actinomycosis in a chinchilla. *Proceedings of the 20th European Congress of Veterinary Dentistry*, Chalkidiky, pp. 133–135.

25 Jekl V, Zikmund T, Hauptman K (2016) Dyspnea in a degu (*Octodon degu*) associated with maxillary cheek teeth elongation. *J Exot Pet Med* **25(2):**128–132.

26 Crossley DA, Dubielzig RR, Benson KG (1997) Caries and odontoclastic resorptive lesions in a chinchilla (*Chinchilla laniger*). *Vet Rec* **141:**337–339.

27 Mans Ch, Donnelly TM (2013) Update on diseases of chinchillas. *Vet Clin North Am Exot Anim Pract* **16:**383–406.

28 Pavlica Z (2007) Parodontopathies in exotic pets. *Proceedings of the Czech Association of Zoo and Wildlife Veterinarians - Veterinary Dentistry Conference - Exotic Pets*, Brno, pp. 21–28.

29 Schweda MC, Hassan J, Böhler A *et al.* (2014) The role of computed tomography in the assessment of dental disease in 66 guinea pigs. *Vet Rec* **175:**538.

30 Crossley DA, Jackson A, Yates J *et al.* (1998) Use of computed tomography to investigate cheek tooth abnormalities in chinchillas (*Chinchilla laniger*). *J Small Anim Pract* **39(8):**385–389.

31 Mancinelli E, Capello V. (2016) Anatomy and disorders of the oral cavity of rat-like and squirrel-like rodents. *Vet Clin North Am Exot Anim Pract* **19(3):**871–900.

32 Jekl V, Krejcirova L, Buchtova M *et al.* (2011) Impact of pelleted diets with different mineral compositions on the crown size of mandibular cheek teeth and mandibular relative density in degus (*Octodon degus*). *Vet Rec* **168(24):**641.

33 Stoffels-Adamowicz E (2014) *The Satin Syndrome in Guinea Pigs. Master's Dissertation.* Faculty of Veterinary Medicine, Ghent University, p. 109.

34 Legendre LFJ (2016) Anatomy and disorders of the oral cavity of guinea pigs. *Vet Clin North Am Exot Anim Pract* **19(3):**825–842.

CHAPTER 12

ADVANCED AND FUTURE OPTIONS FOR ORAL AND MAXILLOFACIAL IMAGING

Brook A. Niemiec

INTRODUCTION

There are numerous imaging options currently available to the veterinarian for diagnosis and treatment planning of oral and maxillofacial conditions. These include: skull radiographs, dental radiographs, magnetic resonance imaging (MRI), computed tomography (CT), and cone-beam CT (CBCT). All options have advantages and disadvantages. It is important to note that successful therapy often depends on the information obtained from appropriate imaging. This chapter will cover the various modalities (other than dental radiographs) and their strengths and weaknesses with regard to this area of veterinary medicine.

SKULL RADIOGRAPHS

This is the most universally available imaging modality. Most veterinary clinics have x-ray capability and skull images offer a good overall view of the maxillofacial structures. However, the benefits of these images are generally compromised by the difficulty in separating the different sides of the mandible and maxilla, making evaluation of the individual oral

hard tissues challenging (**Figure 12.1**). In addition, skull films typically lack the required radiographic detail to effectively evaluate dental conditions such as root fractures or periodontal and endodontic disease (**Figure 12.2**). Finally, a major limitation of skull radiographs is their relative lack of resolution when compared with dental radiographs or other imaging modalities. Because 30–60% of bone mineralization must be lost before it is recognized radiographically, radiology will always *underestimate* the amount of bone loss.

The temporomandibular joint (TMJ) can be imaged with skull radiographs. If well positioned, skull radiographs can be useful in the diagnosis of condylar fractures and TMJ luxation (**Figure 12.3**). However, these images lack the fine detail necessary for proper treatment of other TMJ issues such as subluxation, dysplasia, or minor areas of ankylosis.

One of the biggest disadvantages of skull films is the relative inability to effectively diagnose periodontally and endodontically infected teeth and pathologic fractures resulting from weakened bone associated with chronic periodontal or

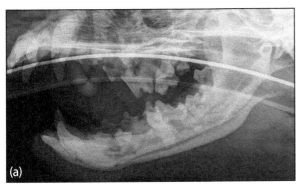
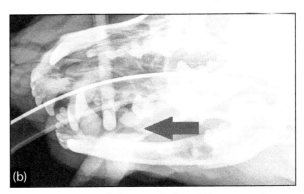

Fig. 12.1 Lateral skull radiograph of the mandible of a dog (a). There is no obvious pathology. However, when the image is obliqued and the fracture distracted, it becomes visible (arrow) (b). Note that good evaluation is still not possible.

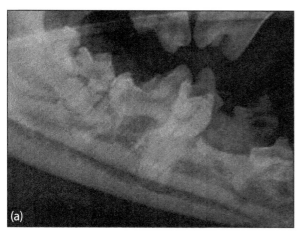
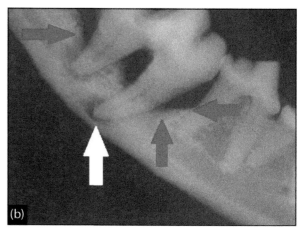

Fig. 12.2 **Well collimated lateral skull film of a dog (a) with a distal ventral swelling, suspected to be dental in origin. No significant findings are observed. (b) Intraoral dental radiograph of the right mandibular first molar (409) of the dog in (a) reveals significant alveolar bone loss (red arrows) and a secondary class II perio-endo lesion (white arrow).**

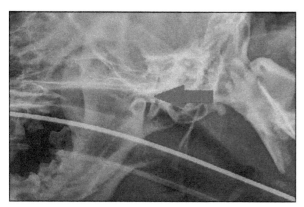

Fig. 12.3 **Well positioned skull film of the temporomandibular joint of a dog. This image allows for fairly good evaluation of the joint (arrow), but not as good as would be expected with MRI or CT.**

endodontic disease. In fact, it is quite common for patients to present to dental specialists for a non-union jaw fracture that was treated elsewhere without dental radiographs. Dental radiographs will reveal the bone loss associated with periodontal infection and guide the practitioner to proper treatment, reduction, and fixation (**Figure 12.4**).

An additional limitation of skull films (as well as dental radiographs) is the fact that it is a 2D image of a 3D space. This does not provide ideal information for treatment planning of fractures or neoplasia. Finally, it is difficult to evaluate fracture reduction in three dimensions (i.e. the ventrodorsal and rostrocaudal reduction may be good, but the lateral

alignment may be way off). Orthogonal images are possible (albeit difficult) with dental radiographs, but not with skull images.

MAGNETIC RESONANCE IMAGING

MRI technology does not utilize radiation and instead uses a very strong magnetic field and a radio signal.[1] As with CT images, MRI examines very small 'slices' of the patient and puts them together via computer processing. MRI technology provides the best soft tissue detail (**Figure 12.5a**) and has an additional advantage for oral imaging due to its ability to separate cortical from cancellous bone.[2,3] MRI can also be very effective for imaging the TMJ (**Figure 12.5b**).[4] In addition, it is very good at determining the extent of dental caries, as well as the presence of endodontic involvement.[5,6] However, the lack of good bone resolution with MRI significantly limits its application in oral surgery.[7] Other imaging modalities are far superior for oral and maxillofacial surgery.

COMPUTED TOMOGRAPHY

CT images are produced by making multiple radiographs of the area, which are then digitized. A computer can then be used to processes the digitized information to reconstruct the object in 3D.[8] CT is thought to be the best

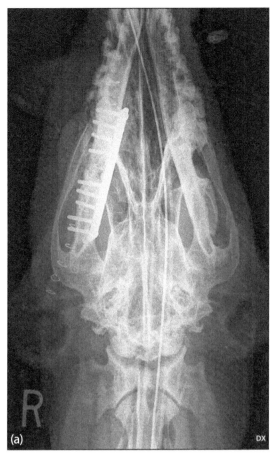

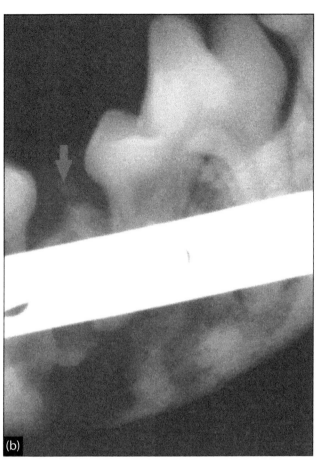

Fig. 12.4 (a) Skull film of a nonhealing distal right mandibular fracture in a dog apparently properly reduced and fixed with a bone plate. (b) Dental radiographs confirmed the infected distal root of the first molar (arrow), which was creating the nonunion fracture. Extraction of this root and subsequent stabilization by a veterinary dentist resulted in healing.

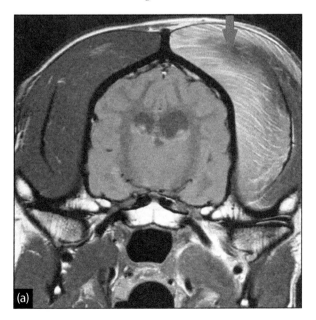

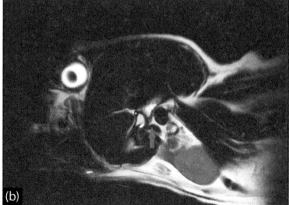

Fig. 12.5 (a) MR image of a dog with significant swelling on the right (arrow), which was subsequently diagnosed as neoplasia. (b) Lateral MR image of a dog demonstrating the temporomandibular joint (arrow).

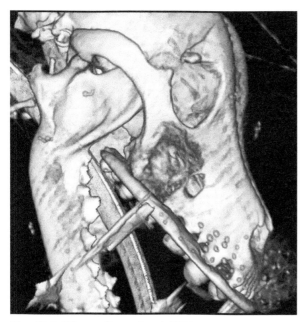

Fig. 12.6 **Three-dimensional CT image.**

modality for surgical treatment planning in maxillofacial surgery cases.[9–13] CT images provide 3D reconstruction and good detail, which allows for excellent surgical planning and improved results (**Figure 12.6**).[14] This appears to be true for all facets of major oral surgery including:

- Fracture repair.
- Neoplastic resection and reconstruction.
- Nasal imaging for treatment planning (**Figure 12.7a**).[15,16]
- TMJ surgery (**Figure 12.7b**).

CT technology represents a quantum leap forward in maxillofacial diagnosis, with improved surgical outcomes. All practices providing advanced oral surgery should have access to a fairly recent unit. This author has treated several cases where CT provided crucial information that was not appreciated

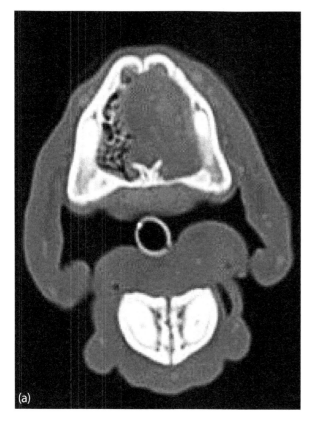

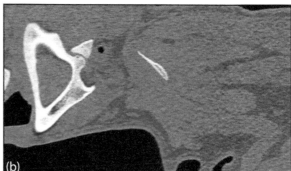

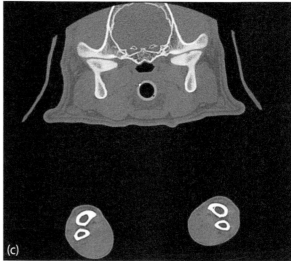

Fig. 12.7 (a) CT image of a nasal tumor in a dog. Lateral (b) and VD (c) CT images of a dog with temporomandibular joint dysplasia.

with skull films or dental radiographs. CT imaging is further enhanced by the use of 3D printers, which can produce a full scale model of the patient's jaw/skull. This is incredibly valuable for treatment planning and educational (client and student) purposes (**Figure 12.8**).

CT may also be superior to dental radiographs at determining alveolar bone height.[17,18] In addition, high-res CT appears to be more effective than dental radiology at finding and mapping furcational defects from periodontal disease.[19]

Despite the obvious advantages, there are several limitations to this diagnostic modality when it comes

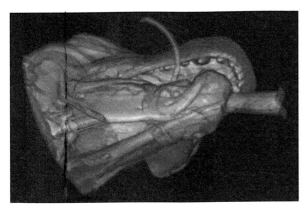

Fig. 12.8 **Three-dimensional printing for treatment planning.**

to general dental practice. Chief of these is decreased resolution compared with dental radiographs and CBCT, which is necessary for endodontic and restorative diagnosis/therapy.[20] Other limitations include: cost and inconvenience (intra- and postoperative imaging is difficult to impossible). In many instances, a CT scan must be performed at a place distant to the surgery site, and thus often requires an additional anesthesia.

CONE-BEAM COMPUTED TOMOGRAPHY:

CBCT[21] is a diagnostic imaging modality that is gaining favor due to its numerous positive attributes. CBCT has been proven to be superior to dental radiographs in the detection of small areas of bone loss and endodontically involved teeth (**Figure 12.9**).[22–25] In addition, it is superior in detecting failed endodontic therapy (**Figure 12.10**).[26] Most (but not all)[27,28] studies report that it is superior to other imaging techniques for detecting vertical root fractures.[29–33] CBCT also appears to be the best imaging technique for mapping root canal morphology and finding extra roots/canals.[34–36]

CBCT provides better evaluation of alveolar bone loss created by periodontal disease,[37–40] and is

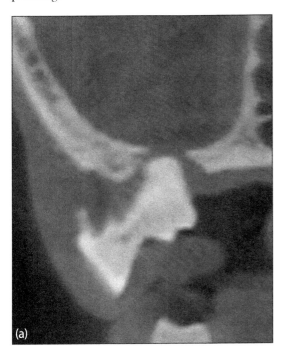

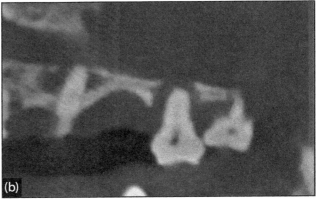

Fig. 12.9 **(a) Palatal root of a tooth showing a communication with the orbital floor. (b) A mesiodistal cut through the same root shows the extent of the periodontal lesion.**

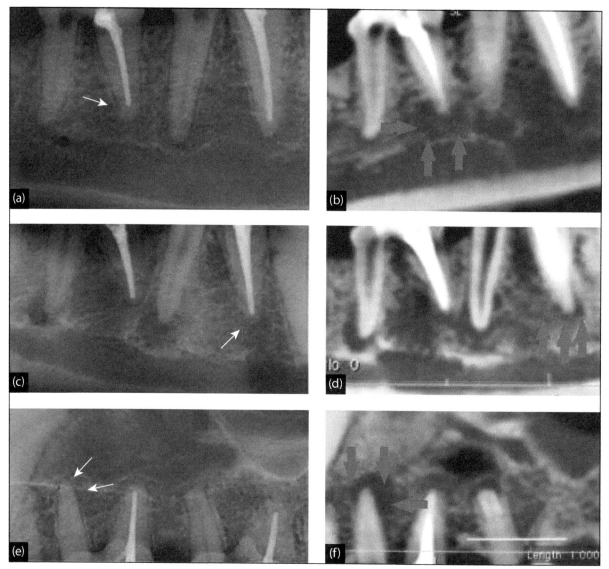

Fig. 12.10 **Comparison of canine endodontic success using digital dental radiographs (a, b, e) and CBCT (b, d, f). In all three images, there are roots that appear successful on dental radiographs (a, c, e; white arrows), but have significant periapical pathology (b, d, f; red arrows).**

also valuable for orthodontic therapy planning and follow-up.[41,42] In addition, CBCT has proven superior in the diagnosis of most pathologic conditions.[43] CBCT provides 3D imaging capabilities and offers real life representations of oral structures, which can be invaluable for surgical treatment planning (**Figure 12.11**).[44–47] These images also provide fairly accurate measurements,[48] have exceedingly high resolution, and are less affected by metal artifacts. This imaging modality offers easy accessibility and

handling, a small footprint, and can be used within the dental suite. These advantages may allow for intra- and postoperative images.

CBCT is also much faster than standard dental radiographs and provides the advantage of not having to reposition the patient for various images.[49] CBCT also provides a panoramic view of the area, as opposed to 2D images.[49] The 3D view allows for easy separation of the mesial roots of the maxillary P4, as opposed to the multiple images typically required

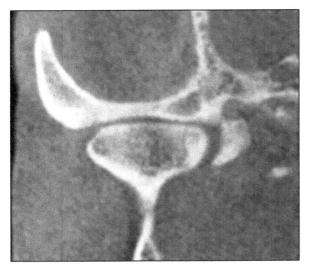

Fig. 12.11 **Normal temporomandibular joint anatomy.**

with standard intraoral dental radiographs.[49,50] In addition, it allows easy imaging of the maxillary cheek teeth in cats without the zygomatic arch interference seen in standard dental radiographs.[51] Finally, CBCT has been shown to create significantly less radiation than standard CT, but there is significant variability in exposure with different systems depending on scan size.[52,53]

In addition to the great detail and 3D image capability of CBCT, recent digital enhancements have made it even more precise. In fact, it appears that the software may be very important in determining image quality. These enhancements can reveal even smaller details than standard CB units. However, at this time, these advanced CBCT systems are generally only used in research applications.

While these positive attributes are significant (especially for evaluation of small areas of diseased bone and infected teeth), there are limitations to this technology. The most significant limitation is the small detector size, which creates a limited field of view and low scan volume. This means that the entire traumatized/diseased area may not be imaged, which can make treatment planning challenging. Furthermore, truncation artifacts are created because the acquired projections do not necessarily contain the entire object. There may be a low contrast range with limited soft tissue information, and increased scatter and 'noise' may

further reduce contrast. CBCT is very susceptible to movement artifacts and requires a higher radiation dose than digital dental radiographs.[27] Finally, one veterinary study revealed that CBCT did not appear to provide consistent resolution in veterinary patients.[54] However, a further veterinary study showed CBCT to be superior to standard CT.[55]

In summary, CBCT appears to be excellent for the diagnosis and treatment of endodontic disease, but it may be more valuable in human endodontics due to the greater variation of human root canal systems. In addition, it has distinct advantages in the diagnosis of periodontal disease and cysts. Without the high-end software, resolution is sacrificed. Also, the increased dose of radiation and other limitations has led to less than enthusiastic recommendations for its use in general.[56,57] Finally, due the small focal area of CBCT, standard CT is considered superior in most cases of maxillofacial trauma or neoplasia. At the time of writing, digital dental radiology in combination with standard CT is the recommended imaging combination. However, as costs decrease and resolution increases, CBCT may overtake dental radiographs in the near future.

PANORAMIC RADIOGRAPHS

Panoramic radiographs (**Figure 12.12**) are quite common and useful in human dentistry. It is particularly valuable in orthodontic and implant dentistry. Panoramic radiographs provide a view of the entire dental arch on one image, allowing for effective evaluation of tooth relationships. However, this technology is not currently available for veterinary patients. The main reason for this is the great variability in head size and shape in veterinary patients. To be useful, numerous machines with various sized and/or shaped tube heads would be required in each practice, and the computer program significantly upgraded to account for this variability. Further, the requirement for general anesthesia and intubation would limit the ability to effectively determine occlusal relationships unless alternate intubation (e.g. pharyngotomy) is performed.

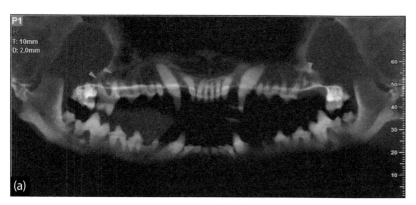

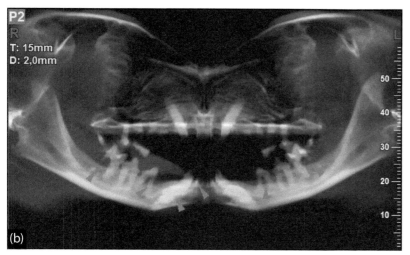

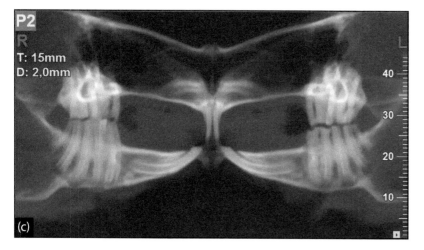

Fig. 12.12 Panoramic images. (a) Panoramic image of a dog revealing significant alveolar bone loss associated with the right maxillary P4 and a retained root of the maxillary left maxillary fourth premolar (arrowheads). (b) A feline case demonstrating significant alveolar bone loss and tooth resorption lesions (arrowheads). (c) Panoramic image of a rabbit.

CONCLUSIONS

There are several options for imaging oral and maxillofacial structures for diagnosis, treatment planning, postoperative evaluation, and follow-up examinations.

Dental radiographs are the current minimum standard of practice for dental treatment and oral surgery and should be available for intra- and postoperative imaging.[49] Dental radiographs provide excellent resolution and the ability to be used within the dental suite. CBCT has similar positives to dental radiographs, with better resolution and potential for 3D rendering. If financially feasible, this modality should be considered as an additional imaging system, especially in specialty practices.

At present, standard CT is the modality of choice for oral and maxillofacial trauma and oncologic surgery. CT provides an overall view of the entire surgical area, good resolution, and 3D reconstruction of the area. The major limitations to this technology are its cost, poor evaluation of the periapical structures, and that they are typically distant from the dental suite.

Panoramic radiology is very valuable in human dentistry, but due to variation in skull size and shape of animal patients, it is not currently available in veterinary medicine. Similarly, MRI, while excellent for soft tissue diagnosis, is not generally indicated for bony oral conditions. Finally, skull films are generally considered insufficient for proper diagnosis and therapy of dental and oral conditions, with the exception of TMJ conditions (in the absence of CT).

REFERENCES

1 Dennis R (1993) Magnetic resonance imaging and its application to veterinary medicine. *Vet Int* **6(2)**:3–10.

2 Gray CF, Redpath TW, Smith FW (1996) Pre-surgical dental implant assessment by magnetic resonance imaging. *J Oral Implantol* **22(2)**:147–153.

3 Revenaugh AF (2000) Computed tomography and magnetic resonance imaging in veterinary dentistry and oral surgery diagnostics. In: *An Atlas of Veterinary Dental Radiology*. (eds. DH Deforge, BH Colmery) Iowa State University Press, Ames, pp. 261–263.

4 Harms SE, Wilk RM (1987) Magnetic resonance imaging of the temporomandibular joint. *Radiographics* **7(3)**:521–542.

5 Vidmar J, Cankar K, Nemeth L *et al.* (2012) Assessment of the dentin-pulp complex response to caries by ADC mapping. *NMR Biomed* **25(9)**:1056–1062.

6 Tymofiyeva O, Boldt J, Rottner K *et al.* (2009) High-resolution 3D magnetic resonance imaging and quantification of carious lesions and dental pulp in vivo. *MAGMA* **22(6)**:365–374.

7 Adams WH, Daniel GB, Pardo AD *et al.* (1995) Magnetic resonance imaging of the caudal lumbar and lumbosacral spine in 13 dogs (1990–1993). *Vet Radiol Ultrasound* **36(1)**:3–13.

8 Feeney DA, Fletcher TF, Hardy RM (1991) *Atlas of Correlative Imaging Anatomy of the Normal Dog*. WB Saunders, Philadelphia.

9 Yu H, Shen SG, Wang X *et al.* (2013) The indication and application of computer-assisted navigation in oral and maxillofacial surgery: Shanghai's experience based on 104 cases. *J Craniomaxillofac Surg* **41(8)**:770–774.

10 Yu HB, Shen GF, Zhang SL *et al.* (2008) [Application of computer assisted navigation in the treatment of temporomandibular joint ankylosis]. *Shanghai Kou Qiang Yi Xue* **17(5)**:452–456.

11 Foley BD, Thayer WP, Honeybrook A *et al.* (2013) Mandibular reconstruction using computer-aided design and computer-aided manufacturing: an analysis of surgical results. *J Oral Maxillofac Surg* **71(2)**:e111–119.

12 Markiewicz MR, Bell RB (2011) Modern concepts in computer-assisted craniomaxillofacial reconstruction. *Curr Opin Otolaryngol Head Neck Surg* **19(4)**:295–301.

13 Hirsch DL, Garfein ES, Christensen AM *et al.* (2009) Use of computer-aided design and computer-aided manufacturing to produce orthognathically ideal surgical outcomes: a paradigm shift in head and neck reconstruction. *J Oral Maxillofac Surg* **67(10)**:2115–2122.

14 Abboud M, Guirado JL, Orentlicher G *et al.* (2013) Comparison of the accuracy of cone beam computed tomography and medical computed tomography: implications for clinical diagnostics with guided surgery. *Int J Oral Maxillofac Implants* **28(2)**:536–542.

15 Park RD, Beck ER, LeCouteur RA (1992) Comparison of computed tomography and radiography for detecting changes induced by malignant nasal neoplasia in dogs. *J Am Vet Med Assoc* **201(11)**:1720–1724.

16 Lefebvre J, Kuehn NF, Wortinger A (2005) Computed tomography as an aid in the diagnosis of chronic nasal disease in dogs. *J Small Anim Pract* **46(6)**:280–285.

17 Fuhrmann RA, Bücker A, Diedrich PR (1995) Assessment of alveolar bone loss with high resolution computed tomography. *J Periodontal Res* **30(4)**:258–263.

18 Langen HJ, Fuhrmann R, Diedrich P *et al.* (1995) Diagnosis of infra-alveolar bony lesions in the dentate alveolar process with high-resolution computed tomography. Experimental results. *Invest Radiol* **30(7)**:421–426.

19 Fuhrmann RA, Bücker A, Diedrich PR (1997) Furcation involvement: comparison of dental radiographs and HR-CT-slices in human specimens. *J Periodontal Res* **32(5)**:409–418.

20 Loubele M, Guerrero ME, Jacobs R *et al.* (2007)
    A comparison of jaw dimensional and quality
    assessments of bone characteristics with cone-beam
    CT, spiral tomography, and multi-slice spiral CT.
    Int J Oral Maxillofac Implants **22(3):**446–454.

21 Ahmad M, Jenny J, Downie M (2012) Application
    of cone beam computed tomography in oral and
    maxillofacial surgery. *Aust Dent J* **57(Suppl 1):**82–94.

22 Wu MK, Shemesh H, Wesselink PR (2009)
    Limitations of previously published systematic reviews
    evaluating the outcome of endodontic treatment.
    Int Endod J **42(8):**656–666.

23 de Paula-Silva FW, Wu MK, Leonardo MR *et al.*
    (2009) Accuracy of periapical radiography and cone–
    beam computed tomography scans in diagnosing
    apical periodontitis using histopathological findings as
    a gold standard. *J Endod* **35(7):**1009–1012.

24 Estrela C, Bueno MR, Leles CR *et al.* (2008) Accuracy
    of cone beam computed tomography and panoramic
    and periapical radiography for detection of apical
    periodontitis. *J Endod* **34(3):**273–279.

25 Patel S, Wilson R, Dawood A *et al.* (2012) The
    detection of periapical pathosis using digital periapical
    radiography and cone beam computed tomography -
    part 2: a 1-year post-treatment follow-up. *Int Endod J*
    45(8):711–723.

26 de Paulo-Silva FWG, Santamaria M, Leonardo MR
    et al. (2009) Cone-beam computerized tomographic,
    radiographic, and histologic evaluation of periapical
    repair in dogs' post-endodontic treatment.
    Oral Surg Oral Med Oral Path Oral Radiol Endod
    108(5):786–805.

27 Bechara B, McMahan CA, Noujeim M *et al.* (2013)
    Comparison of cone beam CT scans with enhanced
    photostimulated phosphor plateimages in the
    detection of root fracture of endodontically treated
    teeth. *Dentomaxillofac Radiol* **42(7):**201–214.

28 da Silveira PF, Vizzotto MB, Liedke GS *et al.* (2013)
    Detection of vertical root fractures by conventional
    radiographic examination and cone beam computed
    tomography: an in vitro analysis. *Dent Traumatol*
    29(1):41–46.

29 Khedmat S, Rouhi N, Drage N *et al.* (2012) Evaluation
    of three imaging techniques for the detection of vertical
    root fractures in the absence and presence of gutta–
    percha root fillings. *Int Endod J* **45(11):**1004–1009.

30 Hassan B, Metska ME, Ozok AR *et al.* (2009)
    Detection of vertical root fractures in endodontically
    treated teeth by a cone beam computed tomography
    scan. *J Endod* **35(5):**719–722.

31 Ozer SY (2010) Detection of vertical root fractures of
    different thicknesses in endodontically enlarged teeth
    by cone beam computed tomography versus digital
    radiography. *J Endod* **36(7):**1245–1249.

32 Khasnis SA, Kidiyoor KH, Patil AB *et al.* (2014)
    Vertical root fractures and their management.
    J Conserv Dent **17(2):**103–110.

33 Edlund M, Nair MK, Nair UP (2011) Detection of
    vertical root fractures by using cone-beam computed
    tomography: a clinical study. *J Endod* **37(6):**768–772.

34 Baziar H, Daneshvar F, Mohammadi A *et al.* (2014)
    Endodontic management of a mandibular first molar
    with four canals in a distal root by using cone-beam
    computed tomography: a case report. *J Oral Maxillofac
    Res* **5(1):**e5.

35 Zhang R, Wang H, Tian YY *et al.* (2011) Use of cone-
    beam computed tomography to evaluate root and
    canal morphology of mandibular molars in Chinese
    individuals. *Int Endod J* **44(11):**990–999.

36 Silva EJ, Nejaim Y, Silva AV (2013) Evaluation of root
    canal configuration of mandibular molars in a Brazilian
    population by using cone-beam computed tomography:
    an in vivo study. *J Endod* **39(7):**849–852.

37 Grimard BA, Hoidal MJ, Mills MP (2009)
    Comparison of clinical, periapical radiograph, and
    cone-beam volume tomography measurement
    techniques for assessing bone level changes following
    regenerative periodontal therapy. *J Periodontol*
    80(1):48–55.

38 Vandenberghe B, Jacobs R, Yang J (2008) Detection
    of periodontal bone loss using digital intraoral and
    cone beam computed tomography images: an in
    vitro assessment of bony and/or infrabony defects.
    Dentomaxillofac Radiol **37(5):**252–260.

39 Misch KA, Yi ES, Sarment DP (2006) Accuracy of
    cone beam computed tomography for periodontal
    defect measurements. *J Periodontol* **77(7):**1261–1266.

40 Mol A, Balasundaram A (2008) In vitro cone beam
    computed tomography imaging of periodontal bone.
    Dentomaxillofac Radiol **37(6):**319–324.

41 Merrett SJ, Drage NA, Durning P (2009) Cone beam
    computed tomography: a useful tool in orthodontic
    diagnosis and treatment planning. *J Orthod*
    36(3):202–210.

42 Dudic A, Giannopoulou C, Martinez M *et al.*
    (2008) Diagnostic accuracy of digitized periapical
    radiographs validated against micro-computed
    tomography scanning in evaluating orthodontically
    induced apical root resorption. *Eur J Oral Sci*
    116(5):467–472.

43 Ahmad M, Freymiller E (2010) Cone beam computed tomography: evaluation of maxillofacial pathology. *J Calif Dent Assoc* **38(1):**41–47.

44 de Oliveira-Santos C, Souza PH, de Azambuja Berti-Couto S *et al.* (2012) Assessment of variations of the mandibular canal through cone beam computed tomography. *Clin Oral Investig* **16(2):**387–393.

45 Ghaeminia H, Meijer GJ, Soehardi A *et al.* (2009) Position of the impacted third molar in relation to the mandibular canal. Diagnostic accuracy of cone beam computed tomography compared with panoramic radiography. *Int J Oral Maxillofac Surg* **38(9):**964–971.

46 Ghaeminia H, Meijer GJ, Soehardi A *et al.* (2011) The use of cone beam CT for the removal of wisdom teeth changes the surgical approach compared with panoramic radiography: a pilot study. *Int J Oral Maxillofac Surg* **40(8):**834–839.

47 Umar G, Obisesan O, Bryant C *et al.* (2013) Elimination of permanent injuries to the inferior alveolar nerve following surgical intervention of the "high risk" third molar. *Br J Oral Maxillofac Surg* **51(4):**353–357.

48 Halperin-Sternfeld M, Machtei EE, Horwitz J (2014) Diagnostic accuracy of cone beam computed tomography for dimensional linear measurements in the mandible. *Int J Oral Maxillofac Implants* **29(3):**593–599.

49 Roza MR, Silva LAF, Barriviera M *et al.* (2011) Cone beam computed tomography and intraoral radiography for diagnosis of dental abnormalities in dogs and cats. *J Vet Sci* **12(4):**387–392.

50 Niemiec BA, Furman R (2004) Canine dental radiography. *J Vet Dent* **21:**186–190.

51 Niemiec BA, Furman R (2004) Feline dental radiography. *J Vet Dent* **21:**252–257.

52 Cohenca N, Simon JH, Roges R *et al.* (2007) Clinical indications for digital imaging in dento-alveolar trauma. Part 1: traumatic injuries. *Dent Traumatol* **23:**95–104.

53 Mah JK, Danforth RA, Bumann A *et al.* (2003) Radiation absorbed in maxillofacial imaging with a new dental computed tomography device. *Oral Surg Oral Med Oral Pathol Oral Radiol Endod* **96:**508–513.

54 Van Thielen B, Siguenza F, Hassan B (2012) Cone beam computed tomography in veterinary dentistry. *J Vet Dent* **29(1):**27–34.

55 Soukup JW, Drees R, Koenig LJ *et al.* (2015) Comparison of the diagnostic image quality of the canine maxillary dentoalveolar structures obtained by cone beam computed tomography and 64-multidetector row computed tomography. *J Vet Dent* **32(2):**80–86.

56 Patel S, Durack C, Abella F *et al.* (2014) European Society of Endodontology position statement: the use of CBCT in endodontics. *Int Endod J* **47(6):**502–504.

57 American Academy of Oral and Maxillofacial Radiology (2013) Clinical recommendations regarding use of cone beam computed tomography in orthodontics. Position statement by the American Academy of Oral and Maxillofacial Radiology. *Oral Surg Oral Med Oral Pathol Oral Radiol* **116(2):**238–257.

Brook Niemiec (San Diego)	www.vetdentaltraining.com
Patrick Vail and Tony Woodward (Colorado Springs)	www.wellpets.com
Ira Luskin (Baltimore)	www.animaldentalcenter.com
Brett Beckman (Florida)	www.veterinarydentistry.net
Cindy Charlier (Chicago)	www.vdent.org
Veterinary Dental Forum	www.avdf.org
European Veterinary Dental Congress	www.evds.org
Accesia (Sweden)	http://academy.accesia.se//?lang=en&action=@ HemStatic.html

Note: Page numbers in *italic* refer to tables.

T - #0983 - 101024 - C384 - 261/194/21 [23] - CB - 9781482225433 - Gloss Lamination